FIRST AID FOR THE®
Obstetrics & Gynecology Clerkship
Fourth Edition

LATHA GANTI, MD, MS, MBA, FACEP
Professor of Emergency Medicine and Neurology
University of Central Florida College of Medicine
Vice Chair for Research and Academic Affairs
HCA UCF Emergency Medicine Residency of Greater Orando
Orlando, Florida

MATTHEW KAUFMAN, MD
Associate Director
Department of Emergency Medicine
Richmond University Medical Center
Staten Island, New York

SHIREEN MADANI SIMS, MD
Associate Professor and Clerkship Director
Department of Obstetrics and Gynecology
University of Florida College of Medicine
Gainesville, Florida

Mc
Graw
Hill
Education

New York   Chicago   San Francisco   Athens   London   Madrid   Mexico City
Milan   New Delhi   Singapore   Sydney   Toronto

First Aid for the®: Obstetrics & Gynecology Clerkship, Fourth Edition

2 3 4 5 6 7 8 9   DSS   22 21 20 19 18

ISBN 978-1-259-64406-1
MHID 1-259-64406-5

NOTICE

Medicine is an ever-changing science. As new research and clinical experience broaden our knowledge, changes in treatment and drug therapy are required. The authors and the publisher of this work have checked with sources believed to be reliable in their efforts to provide information that is complete and generally in accord with the standards accepted at the time of publication. However, in view of the possibility of human error or changes in medical sciences, neither the authors nor the publisher nor any other party who has been involved in the preparation or publication of this work warrants that the information contained herein is in every respect accurate or complete, and they disclaim all responsibility for any errors or omissions or for the results obtained from use of the information contained in this work. Readers are encouraged to confirm the information contained herein with other sources. For example and in particular, readers are advised to check the product information sheet included in the package of each drug they plan to administer to be certain that the information contained in this work is accurate and that changes have not been made in the recommended dose or in the contraindications for administration. This recommendation is of particular importance in connection with new or infrequently used drugs.

This book was set in Electra LT Std by MPS Limited.
The editors were Bob Boehringer and Cindy Yoo.
The production supervisor was Catherine Saggese.
Project management was provided by Gaurav Prabhu.

This book is printed on acid-free paper.

Cataloging-in-Publication data for this title is on file with the Library of Congress.

McGraw-Hill Education books are available at special quantity discounts to use as premiums and sales promotions or for use in corporate training programs. To contact a representative, please visit the Contact Us pages at www.mhprofessional.com.

Contents

Contents

Introduction

This clinical study aid was designed in the tradition of the *First Aid* series of books, formatted in the same way as the other titles in this series. Topics are listed by bold headings to the left, while the "meat" of the topic comprises the middle column. The outside margins contain mnemonics, diagrams, summary or warning statements, "pearls," and other memory aids. These are further classified as "exam tip" noted by the ♟ symbol, "ward tip" noted by the ✋ symbol, and "typical scenario" noted by the ⚲ symbol.

The content of this book is based on the American Professors of Gynecology and Obstetrics (APGO) and the American College of Obstetricians and Gynecologists (ACOG) recommendations for the OB/GYN curriculum for third-year medical students. Each of the chapters contain the major topics central to the practice of obstetrics and gynecology and closely parallel APGO's medical student learning objectives. This book also targets the obstetrics and gynecology content on the USMLE Step 2 examination.

The OB/GYN clerkship can be an exciting hands-on experience. You will get to deliver babies, assist in surgeries, and see patients in the clinic setting. You will find that rather than simply preparing you for the success on the clerkship exam, this book will also help guide you in the clinical diagnosis and treatment of the many interesting problems you will see during your obstetrics and gynecology rotation.

Acknowledgments

We would like to thank the following faculty for their help in the preparation of the fourth edition of this book:

Eugene C. Toy, MD
Assistant Dean for Educational Programs
Director, Doctoring Courses
Professor and Vice Chair of Medical Education
Department of Obstetrics and Gynecology
McGovern Medical School at University of Texas Health Science Center (UTHealth) at Houston
Houston, Texas

Patti Jayne Ross, MD
Clerkship Director
Department of Obstetrics and Gynecology
The University of Texas–Houston Medical School
Houston, Texas

How to Contribute

To continue to produce a high-yield review source for the obstetrics and gynecology clerkship, you are invited to submit any suggestions or correction. Please send us your suggestions for:

- New facts, mnemonics, diagrams, and illustrations
- Low-yield facts to remove

For each entry incorporated into the next edition, you will receive personal acknowledgment. Diagrams, tables, partial entries, updates, corrections, and study hints are also appreciated, and significant contributions will be compensated at the discretion of the authors. Also let us know about material in this edition that you feel is low yield and should be deleted. You are also welcome to send general comments and feedback, although due to the volume of e-mails, we may not be able to respond to each of these.

The preferred way to submit entries, suggestions, or corrections is via electronic mail. Please include name, address, school affiliation, phone number, and e-mail address (if different from the address of origin). If there are multiple entries, please consolidate into a single e-mail or file attachment. Please send submissions to:

firstaidclerkships@gmail.com

Otherwise, please send entries, neatly written or typed or on disk (Microsoft Word) to:

Bob Boehringer
Executive Editor
McGraw-Hill Education
Two Penn Plaza, 9th Floor
New York, NY 10121

All entries become property of the authors and are subject to editing and reviewing. Please verify all data and spellings carefully. In the event that similar or duplicate entries are received, only the first entry received will be used. Include a reference to a standard textbook to facilitate verification of the fact. Please follow the style, punctuation, and format of this edition if possible.

How to Succeed in the Obstetrics & Gynecology Clerkship

How to Behave on the Wards

BE ON TIME

Most OB/GYN teams begin rounding between 5 and 7 AM. If you are expected to "pre-round," you should give yourself at least 10 minutes per patient to see the patient and learn about the events that occurred overnight. Like all working professionals, you will face occasional obstacles to punctuality, but make sure this is infrequent. When you first start a rotation, try to show up at least 15 minutes early until you get the routine figured out.

DRESS IN A PROFESSIONAL MANNER

Even if the resident wears scrubs and the attending wears stiletto heels, you must dress in a professional, conservative manner. Wear a white coat over your clothes unless discouraged (i.e., when you are on labor and delivery or in the operating room). Recommended attire (professional versus scrubs) can vary based on rotation and clinical site, so it is a question that should be addressed to the team on the first day of the rotation.

> **Men** should wear long pants covering the ankle, dress shoes, a long-sleeved collared shirt, and a tie. No jeans, no sneakers, no short-sleeved shirts. Facial hair should be well groomed.
> **Women** should wear long pants or knee-length skirt or dress, and a top with a modest neckline. No jeans, no sneakers, no bare midriffs, no open-toed shoes.
> **Both men and women** may wear scrubs occasionally, during overnight call, in the operating room, or in the labor and delivery unit. You never know what to expect on labor and delivery, so as a general guideline, always keep a spare pair of scrubs available on your hospital-issued scrub card. Operating room attire such as masks, hats, and shoe covers should only be worn in the operating or delivery room, and should be discarded as soon as those areas are exited. Scrubs should not be worn outside the hospital (i.e., between home and the hospital).

ACT IN A PLEASANT MANNER

The rotation is often difficult, stressful, and tiring. You will have a smoother experience if you are nice to be around. Be friendly and try to learn everyone's name. If you do not understand or disagree with a treatment plan or diagnosis, do not "challenge." Instead, say, "I'm sorry, I don't quite understand, could you please explain? . . ." Be very aware of your tone.

Be aware of your demeanor and reactions. It is always good to approach each rotation with an open mind, but there will be times when you are bored or just not in the mood. Try to appear interested and engaged to attendings and residents. When someone is trying to teach you something, be respectful and look grateful, not tortured. If you seem uninterested, that attending or resident is unlikely to try to take the time to teach you again.

A crucial aspect of being a good doctor is to always treat patients professionally and with respect. It is a good idea to start exhibiting this behavior at the student level. Your relationship with patients is one factor that is used to assess your performance in all clerkships. Thus, having a good rapport with your patients is usually noted by attendings and residents, and this is likely to be reflected in your final evaluations. However, if a resident or attending spots you behaving in an impolite or unprofessional manner, it will damage your evaluation quicker than any dumb answer on rounds ever could. Also, be nice to the nurses—really nice! If they like you, they can make your life a lot easier and make you look good in front of the residents and attendings.

BE AWARE OF THE HIERARCHY

The way in which this will affect you will vary from hospital to hospital and team to team, but it is always present to some degree. In general, address your questions regarding ward functioning to interns or residents when the attending isn't present. Address your medical questions to residents or attendings; make an effort to be somewhat informed on your subject prior to asking. But please don't ask a question just to show off what you know. It's annoying to everyone and is always very obvious. You are more likely to make a favorable impression by seeming interested and asking real questions when they come up.

Don't be afraid to ask questions, but be conscious of the time and number of questions asked during rounds, so that everyone can finish their work and go home at a reasonable time. Do not ever answer a question from an attending that was clearly directed at one of the residents or another student.

ADDRESS PATIENTS AND STAFF IN A RESPECTFUL WAY

Address patients as Sir or Ma'am, or Mr., Mrs., or Miss. Don't address patients as "honey," "sweetie," etc. Although you may feel that these names are friendly, patients may think you have forgotten their name, that you are being inappropriately familiar, or both. Address all physicians as "doctor," unless told otherwise. While your resident may tell you to call them by their first name, remember to call them "doctor" in front of patients.

BE HELPFUL TO YOUR RESIDENTS

Take responsibility for the patient you have been assigned. You should aim to know everything there is to know about her including her history, test results, details about her medical problems, prognosis, and general plan of care. Keep your interns or residents informed of new developments that they might not be aware of, and ask them for any updates as well. Communicate with the nurses to make sure you are aware of overnight or other new developments. Work independently and try to anticipate the needs of your team and your patients.

If you have the opportunity to make a resident look good, take it. If a new complication develops with a patient, make sure to tell the resident about it so they can be best prepared to take care of the patient and answer questions from the attending. Look up recent literature, if appropriate, and share it with your team (ideally before discussing with the attending). Don't hesitate to give credit to a resident for some great teaching in front of an attending. These things make the resident's life easier; he or she will be grateful, and the rewards will come your way.

After rounds, assess what needs to be done for your patients, and take ownership of their care. Pay attention to what was discussed on rounds so you can know what information to obtain or what follow-up phone calls to make. Volunteer to do things that will help out. Observe and anticipate. If a resident is always hunting around for some tape to perform a dressing change during rounds, get some tape ahead of time and be prepared to help.

RESPECT PATIENTS' RIGHTS

1. All patients have the right to have their personal medical information kept private. This means do not discuss the patient's information with family members without that patient's consent, and do not discuss any patient in hallways, elevators, or cafeterias.
2. All patients have the right to refuse treatment. This means they can refuse treatment by a specific individual (you, the medical student) or of a specific type (Pap smear). Patients can even refuse lifesaving treatment. The only exceptions to this rule are a patient who is deemed to not have the capacity to make decisions or understand situations—in which case a health care proxy should be sought—or a patient who is suicidal or homicidal.
3. All patients should be informed of the right to seek advance directives on admission. This is often done by the admissions staff, in a booklet. If your patient is chronically ill or has a life-threatening illness, address the subject of advance directives with the assistance of your attending.

VOLUNTEER MORE

Be self-motivated. Volunteer to help with procedures or difficult tasks. Volunteer to give a short talk on a topic of your choice. Volunteer to take additional patients. Volunteer to stay late. The more unpleasant the task, the better. Give more of yourself unsolicited.

BE A TEAM PLAYER

Help other medical students with their tasks; teach them information you have learned. Make your fellow medical students look good if you have the opportunity. Support your supervising intern or resident whenever possible. Never steal the spotlight, steal a procedure, or make a fellow medical student look bad. Don't complain—no matter how hard you have worked or how many hours you have been at the hospital, your residents have done more.

BE HONEST

If you don't understand, don't know, or didn't do it, make sure you are honest about it. Never say or document information that is false (i.e., don't say "bowel sounds normal" when you did not listen).

KEEP PATIENT INFORMATION HANDY

Use a clipboard, notebook, or index cards to keep patient information, including a miniature history and physical, labs, and test results at hand.

PRESENT PATIENT INFORMATION IN AN ORGANIZED MANNER

Here is a template for the "bullet" presentation:

This is a [age]-year-old [ethnicity] female with a history of [major history such as abdominal surgery, pertinent OB/GYN history] who presented on [date] with [major symptoms, such as pelvic pain, fever], and was found to have [working diagnosis]. [Tests done] showed [results]. Yesterday the patient [state important changes, new plan,

new tests, new medications]. This morning the patient feels [**state the patient's words**], and the physical exam is significant for [**state major findings**]. Plan is [**state plan**].

The newly admitted patient generally deserves a longer presentation following the complete history and physical format (see below).

Some patients have extensive histories. The whole history can and probably should be present in the admission note, but in a ward presentation it is often too much to absorb. In these cases learn how to generate a good summary that maintains an accurate picture of the patient. This usually takes some thought, but it's worth it.

DOCUMENT INFORMATION IN AN ORGANIZED MANNER

A complete medical student initial history and physical is thorough and organized. Make sure you are not just checking boxes in a template in the electronic medical record. You should be thinking about every section of the history you take and documenting appropriately (see page 7).

How to Organize Your Learning

One of the best things about the OB/GYN clerkship is that you get to see a lot of patients. The patient is the key to learning, and is the source of most satisfaction and frustration on the wards. Starting OB/GYN can make you feel like you're in a foreign land. A lot of your studying from the first 2 years doesn't help much. Your experiences on other clerkships do not necessarily help much, either. There is a new language and new way of thinking to absorb. You have to start from scratch in some ways, and it will help enormously if you can skim through this book before you start. Get some of the terminology straight, get some of the major points down, and it won't seem so strange.

SELECT YOUR STUDY MATERIAL

We recommend:

- This review book, *First Aid for the® Obstetrics & Gynecology Clerkship*, 4th edition.
- A full-text online journal database, such as *www.mdconsult.com*.
- An online peer-reviewed resource, such as Up-To-Date®, which is now available in most hospitals and academic centers.
- A small book to look up drugs, such as *Pocket Pharmacopoeia* (Tarascon Publishers, $8), or you can use the app.

AS YOU SEE PATIENTS, NOTE THEIR MAJOR SYMPTOMS AND DIAGNOSIS FOR REVIEW

Your reading on the symptom-based topics above should be done with a specific patient in mind. For example, if a postmenopausal patient comes to the office with increasing abdominal girth and is thought to have ovarian cancer, read about ovarian cancer that night. It helps to have a real patient in mind to "hang" a diagnosis on for improved recall.

PREPARE A TALK ON A TOPIC

You may be asked to give a small talk once or twice during your rotation. If not, you should volunteer! The ideal topic is slightly uncommon but not rare, and pertains to a patient on the service. To prepare a talk on a topic, read about it in a major textbook and a review article not more than 2 years old, and then search online for recent developments or changes in treatment.

How to Prepare for the Clinical Clerkship and USMLE Step 2 Exam

If you have read about your core illnesses and core symptoms, you will know a great deal about medicine. To study for the clerkship exam, we recommend:

2–3 weeks before exam: Read this entire review book, taking notes.
10 days before exam: Read the notes you took during the rotation on your core content list and the corresponding review book sections. Begin doing practice test questions through whatever resource you prefer (i.e., the U Wise test questions at the APGO website).
5 days before exam: Read this entire review book, concentrating on lists and mnemonics. Continue working through practice test questions.
2 days before exam: Exercise, eat well, skim the book, and go to bed early.
1 day before exam: Exercise, eat well, review your notes and the mnemonics, and go to bed on time. Do not have any caffeine after 2 PM.

Other helpful studying strategies are detailed below.

STUDY WITH FRIENDS

Group studying can be very helpful. Other people may point out areas that you have not studied enough and may help you focus on the goal. If you tend to get distracted by other people in the room, limit this to less than half of your study time.

STUDY IN A BRIGHT ROOM

Find the room in your house or in your library that has the best, brightest light. This will help prevent you from falling asleep. If you don't have a bright light, get a halogen desk lamp.

EAT LIGHT, BALANCED MEALS

Make sure your meals are balanced, with lean protein, fruits and vegetables, and fiber. A high-sugar, high-carbohydrate meal will give you an initial burst of energy for 1–2 hours, but then you'll drop.

TAKE PRACTICE EXAMS

The point of practice exams is not so much the content that is contained in the questions but the training of sitting still for 3 hours and trying to pick the best answer for each and every question. You can also use practice questions to assess where the gaps in your knowledge are in order to guide your future studying.

TIPS FOR ANSWERING QUESTIONS

All questions are intended to have one best answer. When answering questions, follow these guidelines:

Read the answers first. For all questions longer than two sentences, reading the answers first can help you sift through the question for the key information.

Look for the words "EXCEPT," "MOST," "LEAST," "NOT," "BEST," "WORST," "TRUE," "FALSE," "CORRECT," "INCORRECT," "ALWAYS," and "NEVER." If you find one of these words, circle or underline it for later comparison with the answer.

Evaluate each answer as being either true or false. Example:
Which of the following is *least* likely to be associated with pelvic pain?
A.   endometriosis **T**
B.   ectopic pregnancy **T**
C.   ovarian cancer **F**
D.   ovarian torsion **T**

By comparing the question, noting LEAST, to the answers, "C" is the best answer.

Terminology

G (gravidity) 3 = total number of pregnancies, including normal and abnormal intrauterine pregnancies, abortions, ectopic pregnancies, and hydatidiform moles. (*Remember, if patient was pregnant with twins, **G** = 1.*)
P (parity) 3 = number of deliveries >500 g or >20 weeks' gestation, stillborn (dead) or alive. (*Remember, if patient was pregnant with twins, **P** = 1.*)
Ab (abortus) 0 = number of pregnancies that were lost before the 20th gestational week or in which the fetus weighs <500 g.
LC (living children) 3 = number of successful pregnancy outcomes. (*Remember, if patient was pregnant with twins, **LC** = 2.*)

Or use the "FPAL" (Florida Power And Light) system if it is used at your medical school:

F = number of Full **Term** deliveries (3)
P = number of **Preterm** deliveries (0)
A = number of **Abortions** (0)
L = number of **Living children** (3)

Sample Obstetric Admission History and Physical

MS3 H&P
Date
Time
Estimated gestational age (EGA): 38^5/$_7$ weeks
Last menstrual period (LMP): First day of LMP
Estimated date of confinement: Due date (*specify how it was determined*) by LMP or by _____ wk US
Chief complaint (CC): Uterine contractions (UCs) q 7 min since 0100

History of present illness (HPI): 25 yo Hispanic female, G3P2002, 38⁵/₇ weeks' GA, dated by LMP (10/13/09) and consistent with US at 10 weeks' GA, who presented to L&D with CC of uterine contractions q 7 min. She reports that fetal movement is present, denies leakage of fluid, vaginal bleeding, headaches, visual changes, or right upper quadrant pain. Prenatal care (PNC) at Montefiore Hospital (12 visits, first visit at 7 weeks' GA), uterine size = to dates, prenatal BP range 100–126/64–83. Problem list includes h/o + group B *Streptococcus* (GBS) and a +PPD with subsequent negative chest x-ray. Patient admitted in early active labor with a vaginal exam (VE) 4/90/–2.

Past Obstetric History

1. '12 SVD @ 40+2 weeks, girl, wt 3700 g, St. Joseph's Hospital
No complications during pregnancy, delivery, and puerperium
No developmental problems in childhood
2. '14 SVD @39+4 weeks , boy, wt 3900 g, St. Joseph's Hospital
Postpartum hemorrhage, atonic uterus, methergine given and hemorrhage resolved
No developmental problems in childhood

Past Gynecological History

13 yo/28 days/regular (age at first menstrual cycle/how often/regular or irregular)
No significant history of PID, intermenstrual bleeding, dyspareunia, postcoital bleed
Last pap smear: 3/4/15—normal, no h/o abnormal Pap smear
Last mammogram: 3/15/16—normal
Contraception: None
Blood group: O–, anti D prophylaxis given at 30 weeks' GA
Allergies: NKDA
Medications: PNV, Fe
Past Medical Hx: H/o asthma (asymptomatic × 7 yrs), UTI × 1 @ 30 wks' s/p Macrobid 100 mg × 3d, neg PPD with subsequent neg CXR
Surgical Hx: Negative
Social Hx: Denies h/o alcohol, smoking, drug abuse. Feels safe at home
Family Hx: Mother—DM II, father—HTN
ROS: Bilateral low back pain. Denies chest pain, shortness of breath, nausea, vomiting, fever, chills

PE

General appearance: Alert and oriented (A&O), no acute distress (NAD)
Vital signs: T, BP, P, R
HEENT: No scleral icterus, pale conjunctiva
Neck: Thyroid midline, no masses, no lymphadenopathy (LAD)
Lungs: CTA bilaterally
Back: No CVA tenderness
Heart: II/VI SEM
Breasts: No masses, symmetric
Abdomen: Gravid, nontender
Fundal height: 36 cm
Estimated fetal weight (EFW): 3500 g by Leopold's
Presentation: Vertex
Extremities: Mild lower extremity edema, nonpitting, 2+ DTRs
Pelvis: Adequate
Sterile speculum exam (SSE): (Nitrazine?, Ferning?, Pooling?); membranes intact
Sterile Vaginal Exam (SVE): 4 cm/90%/–2 (dilatation/effacement/station)
US (L&D): Vertex presentation confirmed, anterior placenta, AFI = 13.2
Fetal monitor: Baseline FHR = 150, accelerations present, no decelerations, moderate variability. Toco = q 5 min

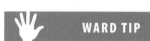
WARD TIP

A good way to elicit information about complications in previous pregnancies is to ask if the baby went home from the hospital with mom.

Assessment

25 yo G3P2002 @ 38^{5}/$_{7}$ weeks' GA presented with regular painful contractions.

1. Early active labor.
2. Group B strep +
3. H/o + PPD with subsequent – CXR
4. H/o UTI @ 30 wks' GA, s/p Rx—resolved
5. H/o asthma—stable × 7 yrs, no meds

Plan

1. Admit to L&D
2. NPO except ice chips
3. CBC, T&S, STD panel (if not done third trimester)
4. D5 LR @ 125 cc/hr
5. Penicillin 5 million units IV load, then 2.5 million units IV q 4 hr (*for GBS*)
6. External fetal monitors (EFMs)
7. Epidural when patient desires

Sample Delivery Note

Always date, time, and sign your notes.

25 yo P3003 s/p spontaneous vaginal delivery (SVD) of viable male infant over a second-degree perineal laceration @ 12:35 PM. Infant was bulb suctioned on the perineum. Nuchal cord × 1 was reduced. The infant was delivered with gentle downward traction. The cord was doubly clamped and cut; the infant was handed to the awaiting nurse. Cord blood and arterial pH was obtained. The placenta was delivered spontaneously, intact, with 3-vessel cord. No vaginal or cervical lacerations were noted. The second-degree laceration was repaired with 3-0 vicryl in layers using local anesthesia. Rectal exam was within normal limits. EBL = 450 cc. Apgars 8 & 9, wt 3654 g. Mom and baby stable.

Sample Postpartum Note

See what your residents do; low-risk patients might not need heart and lung exam.

S: Pt ambulating, voiding, tolerating a regular diet. Lochia = menses. Denies preeclampsia symptoms.

O: *T_{max}: 99.1 $T_{current}$: 98.6 BP:128/70 (117–130/58–76) HR: 86 (76–100) RR: 18*
Heart: RRR
Lungs: CTA bilaterally
Fundus: Firm, mildly tender to palpation, 1 fingerbreadth below umbilicus
Perineum: Intact, no edema
Extremities: No edema, nontender
Postpartum Hgb: 9.7
VDRL: NR, HIV neg, HBsAG neg

A: S/p SVD, PP day #1—progressing well, afebrile, stable

P: Continue postpartum care

Sample Post-SVD Discharge Orders

1. D/c pt home
2. Pelvic rest × 6 weeks
3. Postpartum check in 4–6 weeks
4. D/c meds:
   a. $FeSO_4$ 325 mg, 1 tab PO TID, #90 (For Hgb < 10; opinions vary on when to give Iron supplementation postpartum)
   b. Colace 100 mg, 1 tab PO BID PRN no bowel movement, #60 (A side effect of iron supplementation is constipation)
   c. Ibuprofen 600 mg, 1 tab PO q 4 hours, PRN pain, #60

Sample Post–Cesarean Delivery Note

S: Pt reports pain well controlled, passing flatus, minimal ambulation, tolerating oral intake. Lochia < menses. Foley in place.
O: T_{max}: 99.1 $T_{current}$: 98.6 BP: 128/70 (117–130/58–76) HR: 86 (76–100) RR: 18
I&O *(urinary intake and output):* Last 8 hr = 750/695
Heart: RRR without murmurs
Lungs: CTA bilaterally
Fundus: Firm, tender to palpation, 1 fingerbreadth above umbilicus; normal abdominal bowel sounds (NABS)
Incision: Without erythema/edema; C/D/I (clean/dry/intact)
Extremities: 1 + pitting edema bilateral LEs, nontender
Postpartum Hgb: 11
VDRL: NR, HIV neg, HBsAG neg
A: S/p primary low-transverse c/s for arrest of descent, POD # 1– afebrile, + flatus, stable
P: 1. D/c Foley
   2. Strict I&O—Call HO if UO < 120 cc/4 hr
   3. Advance diet as tolerated
   4. Heplock IV (once patient tolerates clears)
   5. Ambulate qid
   6. Incentive spirometry 10 × hr
   7. Percocet 5/325 mg, 1–2 tabs PO q 4–6 hr PRN (as needed) for pain

WARD TIP

Reporting about flatus and bowel movements is important after a C-section. These are less relevant after an SVD.

Sample Discharge Orders Post–Cesarean Delivery

1. D/c patient home
2. Pelvic rest × 4 wks
3. Incision check in 1 wk
4. Discharge meds:
   a. Percocet 5/325mg, 1–2 tabs PO q 4–6 hr PRN pain, #30
   b. Ibuprofen 600 mg, 1 tab PO q 6 hr, PRN pain, #60
   c. Colace 100 mg, 1 tab PO bid, #60

High-Yield Facts in Obstetrics

Reproductive Anatomy

An adequate knowledge of the normal female anatomy is essential in obstetrics and gynecology. Each time a physician delivers a baby or performs a gynecologic surgery, he or she must be well versed in the anatomy of the region. This chapter will discuss the major structures of the pelvis. The major blood supply to the pelvis is from the **internal iliac artery (hypogastric artery)** and its branches. The lymphatics drain to the inguinal, pelvic, or para-aortic lymph nodes. The major parasympathetic innervation is via **S2, S3, S4**, which forms the pudendal nerve. The major sympathetic innervation is via the aortic plexus, which gives rise to the **internal iliac plexus.**

(hypogastric)

Sympathetics follow blood vessels.

Vulva

A 30-year-old female presents to the emergency room with a lump in the vulva and acute onset of pain for 2 days. The pain has gradually ↑ and she is unable to sit. She reports no fever, chills, nausea, or vomiting. She has no medical conditions and takes no medications. On exam, the right labium majorum is noted to be swollen. A 4 × 4-cm fluctuant tender mass is palpated at the 8 o'clock position; no drainage is noted. What is the most likely diagnosis? What is the best treatment?

Answer: Bartholin's gland abscess. The best treatment is incision and drainage followed by marsupialization, packing, or placement of Word catheter. Can consider broad-spectrum antibiotics. If an older patient with recurrent Bartholin's abscess or cysts, consider adenocarcinoma and take a biopsy.

The vulva consists of all structures visible externally from the pubis to perineum. It includes the labia majora, labia minora, mons pubis, clitoris, vestibule of the vagina, vestibular bulb, and the greater vestibular glands (see Figure 1-1). The vestibule itself contains the urethral opening, vaginal opening, bilateral Bartholin gland ducts, and bilateral Skene's (paraurethral) glands.

- **Clitoris:** Homologue of the male penis. Composed of a glans, a corpora, and two crura. Rarely exceeds 2 cm in length, and normal diameter is 1.5 cm.
- **Bartholin glands:** Located at 4 o'clock and 8 o'clock of the vaginal orifice, and are typically nonpalpable. They function in secreting mucous to provide vaginal lubrication and are homologous to the bulbourethral glands in males.
- **Skene's glands:** Ducts of these glands open on either side of the urethral orifice.

BLOOD SUPPLY

From branches of the external and internal pudendal arteries, which are subdivisions of the hypogastric artery (internal iliac).

LYMPH

Medial group of superficial inguinal nodes.

NERVE SUPPLY

Pudendal branches:
- **Anterior parts of vulva:** Ilioinguinal nerves and the genital branch of the genitofemoral nerves.
- **Posterior parts:** Perineal nerves and posterior cutaneous nerves of the thigh.

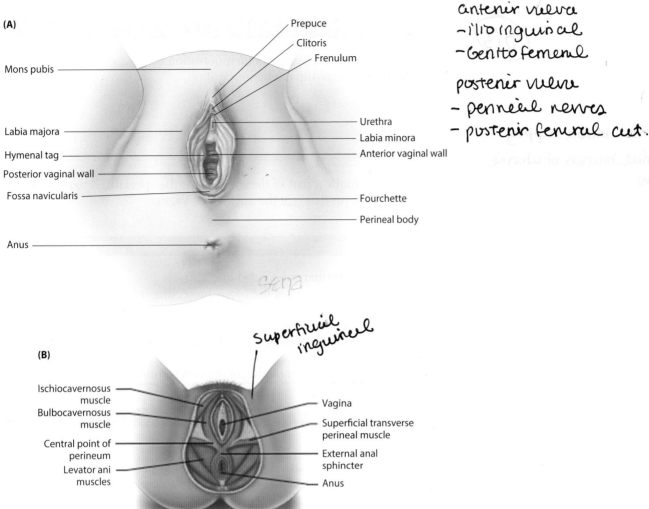

FIGURE 1-1. **(A) External female genitalia.** (Reproduced, with permission, from Cunningham FG, Leveno KJ, Bloom SL, et al. *Williams Obstetrics*, 23rd ed. New York: McGraw-Hill Education, 2010: Fig. 2-2.). **(B) Perineal anatomy.** (Reproduced, with permission, from Ganti L. *Atlas of Emergency Medicine Procedures*. New York: Springer Nature; 2016.)

Vagina

The vagina is a tubular, muscular structure that extends from the vulva to the cervix. Exteriorly, the vaginal orifice is located anterior to the perineum and posterior the urethra.

BLOOD SUPPLY

- Hypogastric artery (anastomotic network):
  - **Vaginal branch of the uterine artery** is the primary supply to the vagina.
  - **Middle rectal and inferior vaginal branches of the hypogastric artery** (internal iliac artery) are secondary blood supplies.
- Anastomoses with cervical arteries.

[handwritten margin notes:]

anterior vulva
- ilio inguinal
- Genito femeral

posterior vulva
- perineal nerves
- posterior femural cut.

superficial inguineal

vaginal arterial supply:
- vaginal branches of uterine artery
- vaginal branches of hypogastric artery.
- middle rectal artery (branch of the hypogastric artery).

vaginal blood supply
-vaginal branch of uterine
artery

NERVE SUPPLY

- **Hypogastric plexus:** Sympathetic innervation.
- **Pelvic nerve:** Parasympathetic innervation.

Cervix

The cervix is actually a part of the uterus. It is the specialized narrow inferior portion of the uterus that is at the apex of the vagina.

COMPONENTS

The cervix can be further subdivided into:
- **Portio vaginalis:** Portion of the cervix projecting into the vagina.
- **External os:** Lowermost opening of the cervix into the vagina.
- **Ectocervix:** Portion of the cervix exterior to the external os.
- **Endocervical canal:** Passageway between the external os and the uterine cavity.
- **Internal os:** Uppermost opening of the cervix into the uterine cavity.

CERVICAL EPITHELIUM

A 36-year-old G3P3 woman has an abnormal Pap smear, showing a low-grade squamous intraepithelial lesion (LSIL). The colposcopic biopsy shows cervical intraepithelial neoplasia II. She undergoes a loop electroexcision procedure (LEEP). What portion of the cervix must be completely excised to ensure proper treatment?

Answer: The transformation zone should be completely excised because that is where the majority of cervical cancers arise.

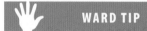

WARD TIP

Colposcopy: Magnified view of the cervix, vagina, and vulva.

Both **columnar** and **stratified nonkeratinized squamous** epithelia cover the cervix.
- The stratified nonkeratinized squamous epithelium covers the ectocervix.
- The columnar epithelium lines the endocervical canal.
- The **squamocolumnar junction** is where the two types of epithelium meet.
- The **transformation zone** is the area of metaplasia where columnar epithelium changes to squamous epithelium. It is the most important cytologic and colposcopic landmark, as this is where over 90% of lower genital tract neoplasias arise.

BLOOD SUPPLY

Cervical and vaginal branch of the uterine artery, which arises from the internal iliac artery.

(hypogastric artery)

NERVE SUPPLY

Hypogastric plexus.

Uterus

The uterus is a muscular organ that lies posterior to the bladder and anterior to the rectum in the pelvis of a nonpregnant woman. In pregnancy, the uterus enlarges with the growth of the fetus and progressively becomes an abdominal as well as a pelvic organ.

COMPONENTS

- **Fundus:** Uppermost region of uterus.
- **Corpus:** Body of the uterus.
- **Cornu:** Part of uterus that connects to the fallopian tubes bilaterally.
- **Cervix:** Inferior part of the uterus that protrudes into the vagina.

HISTOLOGY

- **Myometrium:** The smooth muscle layer of uterus. It is subdivided into three layers:
  1. Outer longitudinal
  2. Middle oblique
  3. Inner longitudinal
- **Endometrium:** The mucosal layer of the uterus, made up of columnar epithelium.

BLOOD SUPPLY

- **Uterine arteries:** Arise from hypogastric artery (internal iliac artery).
- **Ovarian arteries:** Arise from the aorta, and anastamose with uterine vasculature.

NERVE SUPPLY

- **Superior hypogastric plexus**
- **Inferior hypogastric plexus**
- **Common iliac nerves**

Fallopian (Uterine) Tubes

The fallopian tubes extend from the superior lateral aspects of the uterus through the superior fold of the broad ligament laterally to the ovaries.

ANATOMIC SECTIONS, FROM LATERAL TO MEDIAL

- **Infundibulum:** The most distal part of the uterine tube. Gives rise to the fimbriae. Helps to sweep the egg that is released from the ovary into the tube.
- **Ampulla:** Widest section. This is where fertilization takes place.
- **Isthmus:** Narrowest part. This is where tubal sterilizations are performed.
- **Intramural part:** Pierces uterine wall and connects to the endometrial cavity.

Infundibulum — sweep egg
ampulla — fertilization
isthmus — occlusion

Total hysterectomy = Uterus and cervix are removed (ovarian status unknown). Supracervical hysterectomy = Uterus removed, cervix retained (ovarian status unknown).
Although you may hear patients refer to a "partial hysterectomy," this is not a term used to describe a hysterectomy. When patients say this, they usually mean that the ovaries were retained. To describe removal of the ovaries and Fallopian tubes, you would say, "bilateral salpingo-oohporectomy."

WARD TIP

The ureter travels under the uterine artery. Think "water under the bridge."

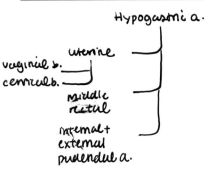

Hypogastric a.
vaginal b. *uterine*
cervical b.
middle rectal
internal + external pudendal a.

WARD TIP

The tubes are occluded at the isthmus for permanent sterilization via laparoscopy, via mini infra-umbilical incision immediately postpartum, or at the time of cesarean delivery.

WARD TIP

Most common location for ectopic pregnancy = Ampulla of fallopian tube.

[handwritten notes in left margin:]
1st tri: 0-12 wks
2nd tri: 13-27 wks
3rd tri: 28-40 wks.

BLOOD SUPPLY

From uterine and ovarian arteries.

NERVE SUPPLY

Pelvic plexus (autonomic) and ovarian plexus.

Ovaries

The ovaries lie on the posterior aspect of the broad ligament and fallopian tubes. They are attached to the broad ligament by the mesovarium and are not covered by peritoneum. Each ovary functions in ova development and hormone production.

BLOOD SUPPLY

Both ovarian arteries arise from the aorta at the level of L1. Ovarian veins drain into the inferior vena cava on the right side and the renal vein on the left.

NERVE SUPPLY

Derived from the aortic plexus.

HISTOLOGY

The ovaries are covered by tunica albuginea, a fibrous capsule. The tunica albuginea is covered by germinal epithelium.

Ligaments of the Pelvic Viscera

impnres

A 22-year-old G2P1001 at 32 weeks' gestation complains of sharp lower abdominal pain. The pain worsens with walking and with rest. She has no loss of fluid, vaginal bleeding, fever, trauma, sick contacts, or recent travel. Her last intercourse was 3 weeks ago. Fetal movement is present. Non-stress test (NST) is reassuring and no contractions are noted. Her cervix is closed on exam. Urinalysis (UA) is negative. What is this patient's most likely diagnosis?

Answer: Round ligament pain. Round ligament pain is a diagnosis of exclusion. The round ligaments begin near the uterine cornua, pass through the inguinal canal, and end up in the labia majora. The key finding is worsening pain with movement and improvement with rest. It can be treated with acetaminophen and rest.

Some ligaments of the pelvis act only as support structures, but others also carry the blood supply for essential organs.

- **Broad ligament:** Peritoneal fold extends from the lateral pelvic wall to the uterus and adnexa. Contains the fallopian (uterine) tube, round ligament, uterine and ovarian blood vessels, lymph, ureterovaginal nerves, and ureter (see Figure 1-2).

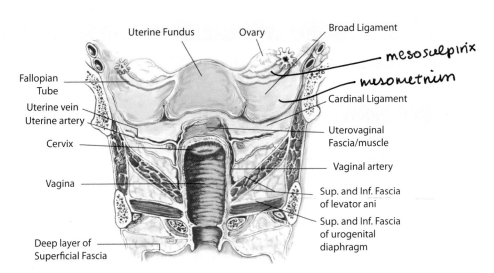

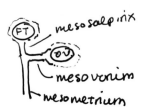

FIGURE 1-2.   Supporting structures of the pelvic viscera. (Reproduced, with permission, from Lindarkis NM, Lott S. *Digging Up the Bones: Obstetrics and Gynecology.* New York: McGraw-Hill, 1998: 2.)

- **Infundibulopelvic (IP) ligament (aka suspensory ligament of the ovary):** Contains the ovarian artery and vein and connects the ovary to the pelvic wall.
- **Round ligament:** The remains of the gubernaculum; extends from the corpus of the uterus down and laterally through the inguinal canal and terminates in the labia majora.
- **Cardinal ligament (Mackenrodt ligament):** Extends from the cervix (near the level of the internal cervical os) and lateral vagina to the pelvic side wall; most **important support** structure of the uterus. It contains the uterine artery and vein.
- **Uterosacral ligaments:** Each ligament extends from an attachment posterolaterally to the supravaginal portion of the cervix and inserts into the fascia over the sacrum. Provides some support to the uterus.

· pubocenical ligament.

WARD TIP

Most hysterectomies start by ligation and transection of the round ligament.

— "transverse ligament"

EXAM TIP

Most common site for ureteral injury during hysterectomy = level of cardinal ligament (ureter passes under the uterine artery).

Muscles

Various muscles of the pelvis make up the perineum. Most of the support is provided by the pelvic and urogenital diaphragms.
- **Pelvic diaphragm** forms a broad sling in the pelvis to support the internal organs. It is composed of the levator ani complex (iliococcygeus, puborectalis, pubococcygeus muscles) and the coccygeus muscles.
- **Urogenital diaphragm** is external to the pelvic diaphragm and is composed of the deep transverse perineal muscles, the constrictor of the urethra, and the internal and external fascial coverings. It helps maintain urinary continence.
- **Perineal body** is the central tendon of the perineum, which provides much of the support. The median raphe of the levator ani, between the anus and vagina. Bulbocavernosus, superficial transverse perineal, and external anal sphincter muscles converge at the central tendon.

WARD TIP

Pelvic organ prolapse is caused by a defect in the pelvic diaphragm.

WARD TIP

The perineal body is cut when episiotomy is performed.

BLOOD SUPPLY

Internal pudendal artery and its branches, inferior rectal artery, and posterior labial artery.

NERVE SUPPLY

Pudendal nerve, which originates from S2, S3, S4 levels of the spinal cord.

Pelvis

The adult pelvis is composed of four bones: the sacrum, the coccyx, and two innominate bones. The innominate bones are formed from the fusion of the ilium, ischium, and pubis (see Figure 1-3).

■ **Sacrum:** Consists of five vertebrae fused together to form a single wedge-shaped bone. It articulates laterally with two iliac bones to form the sacro-iliac joints. The **sacral promontory** is the first sacral vertebrae, and it can be palpated during a vaginal exam. It is important landmark for clinical pelvimetry.

■ **Coccyx:** Composed of four vertebrae fused together to form a small triangular bone that articulates with the base of the sacrum.

■ **Ischial spines:** Extend from the middle of the posterior margin of each ischium.

PELVIC SHAPES

There are four major shapes: **gynecoid, android, platypelloid,** and **anthropoid.** These shapes are differentiated based on the measurements of the pelvis. Gynecoid is the ideal shape for vaginal delivery, having a round to slightly oval pelvic inlet. (See Intrapartum chapter, Table 5-5.)

WARD TIP

Pelvimetry assesses the shape and capacity of the pelvis in relation to the ability of a baby to pass through it.

WARD TIP

The ischial spines serve as landmarks in determining the station of the fetus. Leading edge of the fetus head at the ischial spine = 0 station.

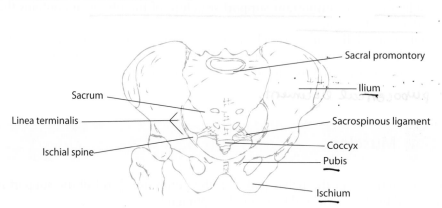

FIGURE 1-3.   Bony pelvis.

artenies:

[vulva - external/internal pud a. (hypogast.)
 vagina - vaginal b. of uterine a.   "
 cervix - cervical b. of uterine a.   "
 uterus - uterine a.   "
 fallopian tube - uterine + ovarian a.   "
 ovary - ovarian a (aorta)

CHAPTER 2

Diagnosis of Pregnancy

gynecoid

android

anthropoid

platypelloid

It is essential to make an accurate diagnosis of pregnancy and establish the estimated date of delivery, because this determines the patient's future pre-natal care. This chapter will discuss how to diagnose pregnancy, including symptoms of pregnancy, use of human chorionic gonadotropin (hCG), fetal heart rate (FHR), and ultrasound.

Naegele's Rule

 A 25-year-old G0P0 presents with complaints of absent menses for 2 months. Prior to this, she had regular menses every 28 days, lasting for 4 days each month. She is sexually active and reports using condoms regularly. What is the best test to evaluate her condition?

Answer: Urine pregnancy test (UPT). Pregnancy must be considered in any woman of reproductive age with complaints of amenorrhea or irregular menses, even if she is using contraception. Including or excluding pregnancy will significantly narrow the list of differential diagnoses.

280 days = 40 whs.

WARD TIP

Naegele's rule assumes two things:
1. A normal gestation is 280 days.
2. All patients have a 28-day menstrual cycle.

Naegele's rule is used to calculate the estimated date of confinement (EDC; i.e., due date, or estimated date of delivery (EDD)) ±2 weeks.
- First day of patient's last normal menstrual period (LMP), minus 3 months, plus 7 days, plus 1 year.
- Example: If LMP = July 20, 2017, then EDC = April 27, 2018.

WARD TIP

When determining the estimated date of confinement (EDC), use the first day of bleeding of the last menstrual period (LMP).

Signs and Symptoms

A woman's body goes through drastic physiologic changes from the day she conceives to weeks after the delivery of her baby. It is important to differentiate the normal physiologic changes of pregnancy from other pathological conditions. This section will discuss signs and symptoms that are indicative of pregnancy.
- **Cessation of menses:** Pregnancy is highly likely if 10 or more days have passed from the time of expected menses in a woman who previously had regular cycles.
- **Breast changes:**
  - ↑ breast tenderness.
  - ↑ in breast size.
  - Nipples become larger, more pigmented, and more erectile.
  - Areolae become broader and more pigmented.
  - Colostrum may be expressed from the nipples.
  - Striations on the skin.
- **Skin changes:**
  - Striae gravidarum (aka stretch marks): Reddish, slightly depressed streaks on the abdomen, breast, and thighs.
  - Linea nigra: Midline of the abdominal wall becomes darkly pigmented.
  - Chloasma or melasma gravidarum (aka mask of pregnancy): Irregular brown patches of varying size on the face and neck.

WARD TIP

Use Naegele's rule to calculate the estimated due date from the LMP.
EDC = (LMP + 1 year + 7 days) − 3 months

pregnancy :
- cessation of menses
- breast tenderness/enlargement
- nausea/vomiting
- soften/nippened cervix + chadwicks sign

- Angiomas: Red elevation at a central point with branching vasculature present on the face, neck, chest, and arms due to estrogens.
  - Palmar erythema.
- **Uterine changes:**
  - On bimanual exam, the uterus feels soft and elastic.
  - The uterus ↑ in size throughout the pregnancy (its size correlates to gestational age). By week 12, it is about the size of a grapefruit and the fundus of the uterus becomes palpable above the pubic symphysis (see Table 2-1).
- **Cervical changes:** Cervix becomes softer.
- **Changes in cervical mucus:** Cervical mucus can be dried on a slide and evaluated via microscope.
  - **Fernlike pattern:** Not pregnant—estrogen effect.
  - **Beaded or cellular pattern:** Pregnant—progesterone effect.
- **Vaginal mucosa discoloration:** With pregnancy and ↑ blood flow, the vagina appears dark bluish or purplish-red.
- **Perception of fetal movement:** A primigravida may report fetal movement at approximately 20 weeks' gestation, and a multipara at 18 weeks' gestation.
- **Nausea and/or vomiting** (aka morning sickness): Nausea and/or vomiting occurs in approximately 70–85% of pregnancies, most notably at 2–12 weeks gestation. It frequently occurs in the morning, but it can occur throughout the day. **Hyperemesis gravidarum** is persistent vomiting that typically occurs early in pregnancy. When severe, it can result in weight loss, dehydration, acidosis (from starvation), alkalosis (from loss of HCl in vomitus), and hypokalemia. *↳ ketosis*
- **Hair growth changes:** Prolonged anagen (the growing hair phase).
- **Fetal heart rate (FHR) detection** (discussed later in this chapter).
- **Urologic changes:** ↑ pressure from the enlarging uterus results in ↑ urinary frequency, nocturia, and bladder irritability.

WARD TIP

A nonpregnant cervix feels like the cartilage of the nose. A pregnant cervix feels like the lips of the mouth. Hegar's sign = softening of the cervix.

WARD TIP

Estrogen → increased sodium chloride in mucus → crystallization → ferning pattern.
Progesterone → decreased sodium chloride in mucus → no crystallization → beading.

WARD TIP

Chadwick's sign: Bluish discoloration of the vaginal and cervical mucosa due to vascular congestion in pregnancy.

WARD TIP

Quickening: First fetal movements felt by the mother.

TABLE 2-1.   Fundal Height During Pregnancy

WEEKS PREGNANT	FUNDAL HEIGHT
12	Barely palpable above pubic symphysis
15	Midpoint between pubic symphysis and umbilicus
20	At the umbilicus
28	8 cm above the umbilicus
32	6 cm below the xyphoid process
36	2 cm below xyphoid process
40	4 cm below xiphoid process[a]

[a]Due to engagement and descent of the fetal head, the fundal height at 40 weeks is typically less than the fundal height at 36 weeks.

Handwritten notes (right margin):
- Breast
- menstrual
- skin/hair (anagen)
- uterine, cervical, vaginal Δ's
- nausea/vomiting
- urologic Δ's

Human Chorionic Gonadotropin (hCG)

A 25-year-old female presents with vaginal spotting and right lower quadrant pain. Her abdomen is slightly tender to palpation in the right lower quadrant. There is minimal dark blood in the vaginal vault, and her cervix is closed. Quantitative serum hCG is 4000 mIU/mL. A transvaginal ultrasound (TVUS) shows no evidence of pregnancy inside the uterus. What is the most likely diagnosis?

Answer: Ectopic pregnancy. A gestational sac should be seen inside the uterus on a transvaginal ultrasound with an hCG level of 1500 mIU/mL. If the pregnancy is not in the uterus, then an investigation must be carried out for an ectopic pregnancy.

Detection of hCG in the mother's serum and urine is used to diagnose pregnancy. This section discusses the various aspects of the hormone, as well as how it is used in the diagnosis of abnormal pregnancies.

OVERVIEW

- hCG can be detected in maternal serum and urine.
- It is a glycoprotein made by trophoblasts.
- Composed of two subunits—α and β:
  - α subunit is similar in luteinizing hormone (LH), follicle-stimulating hormone (FSH), thyroid-stimulating hormone (TSH).
  - β subunits are unique: Urine and serum tests are based on antibody specificity to β subunit of hCG.
- **Function:** Helps sustain the corpus luteum during the **first 7 weeks.** After the first 7 weeks, the placenta makes its own hormones to sustain the pregnancy.
- Can be detected in the maternal serum or urine 6–12 days after fertilization (3–3.5 weeks after the LMP).
- ↑ by 66–100% every 48 hours prior to 10 weeks. In general, hCG should double every two days.
- Peaks at 10 weeks' gestation. (100k) - rule of 10s.
- Nadirs at 14–16 weeks.
- Keep in mind that pregnancy tests detect not only hCG produced by the syncytiotrophoblast cells in the placenta, but also:
  - Hydatidiform mole.
  - Choriocarcinoma.
  - Germ cell tumors.
  - hCG produced by breast cancers and large cell carcinoma of the lung.
- A gestational sac can be visualized with transvaginal ultrasound (TVUS) when hCG levels are >1500. If hCG is >1500 and no evidence of intrauterine pregnancy, think *ectopic pregnancy*.

PREGNANCY TEST USING hCG

hCG can be detected in plasma and urine. Each test has specific uses, which are discussed below.

Urine hCG

- Preferred method to diagnose normal pregnancy.
- Total urine hCG closely parallels plasma concentration.
- First morning specimens are more accurate. hCG concentration is higher in the morning.

- Assays detect 25 mU/mL of hCG, and diagnose pregnancy with 95% sensitivity by 1 week after the first missed menstrual period.
- **False negatives** may occur if:
  - The test is performed too early (i.e., before the first missed period).
  - The urine is very dilute.
- **False positives** may occur with:
  - Proteinuria (confirm with plasma hCG).
  - Urinary tract infection (UTI).

Plasma hCG

Used when quantitative information is needed:
- To aid in the diagnosis of ectopic pregnancy.
- Monitoring trophoblastic tumors.
- Screening for fetal abnormalities.
- Serial levels to monitor complications of pregnancy.
- Does not provide cost-effective additional information in diagnosing routine pregnancy since it is positive <1 week before urine hCG.

Fetal Heart Rate (FHR)

Hearing the fetal heartbeat confirms the presence of a viable pregnancy. **Electronic Doppler device** can detect fetal heart tones as early as 10 weeks' gestation.

Ultrasound (US)

US is a noninvasive tool that serves multiple purposes in the setting of a pregnancy.

INDICATIONS

- Confirm an intrauterine pregnancy (especially important if an ectopic is suspected).
- Document the viability of embryo. Fetal cardiac activity can be seen when the embryo measures ≥5 mm.
- Diagnose multiple gestations.
- Estimate gestational age.
- Screen for fetal structural anomalies.

LIMITATIONS

- Ultrasound dating becomes progressively less accurate after 20 weeks' gestation.
- US measures the size of the fetus, not the gestational age.
- Biologic variation in size ↑ as gestation advances.

WARD TIP

Normal fetal heart rate ranges from 110 to 160 bpm.

WARD TIP

If fetal heart tones are not auscultated by 10 weeks' gestation, an US evaluation should be performed to document a viable intrauterine pregnancy.

EXAM TIP

Up to 12 weeks, the crown-rump length is predictive of gestational age within 4 days.

WARD TIP

Early pregnancy US is more precise in establishing the EDC:
US done in T1 can vary by ± 4 days.
US done in T2 can vary by ± 14 days.
US done in T3 can vary by ± 21 days.

WARD TIP

US dating is used for all pregnancies and is considered more reliable than menstrual data.

- US:
  - intrauterine
  - viable
  - multiple gestations
  - gestational age
  - structural abnormalities.

NOTES

Physiology of Pregnancy

Pregnancy causes changes in the female body from the time of conception. The body prepares not only for the development and growth of a fetus, but also for delivery. These alterations can potentially cause serious complications during pregnancy.

Conception

OVULATION

Ovulation is necessary for normal fertilization to occur:

- The ovum must leave the ovary and be carried into the fallopian tube.
- The unfertilized ovum is surrounded by its zona pellucida.
- This oocyte has completed its first meiotic division and carries its first polar body.

FERTILIZATION

Fertilization typically occurs within 24 hours after ovulation in the ampulla of the fallopian tube:

- The sperm penetrates the zona pellucida of the ovum. The male and female nuclear material combine to form a single cell called a zygote.
- Fertilization signals the ovum to complete meiosis II and to discharge an additional polar body.

PREIMPLANTATION

- The zygote starts to undergo cleavage (divide). At the 16 cells' stage, it is called a **morula**.
- The morula divides to form a multicellular **blastomere**.
- The blastomere passes from the fallopian tube into the uterine cavity.
- The embryo develops into a **blastocyst** as it freely floats in endometrial cavity after conception (see Table 3-1).
- Each cell of the preimplantation embryo is **totipotent**; each cell can form all different types of cells in the embryo.

IMPLANTATION

- On day 5–6 after ovulation, the blastocyst adheres to the endometrium with the help of adhesion molecules on the secretory endometrial surface.
- After attachment, the endometrium proliferates around the blastocyst.

PLACENTATION

- During week 2, cells in the outer cell mass differentiate into **trophoblasts.**
- A trophoblastic shell forms the initial boundary between the embryo and the endometrium.
- The trophoblasts nearest the myometrium form the placental disk; the other trophoblasts form the chorionic membranes.

Handwritten margin notes:

- before ovulation, all eggs are arrested in prophase I of meiosis I
- after ovulation, cells arrest in metaphase of meiosis II.

oogonium (2n)
↓ (divisions-mitosis)
1° oocyte (2n)
↓
2° oocyte
↓
ovum.

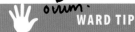

WARD TIP

Fertilization occurs in the ampulla of the fallopian tube.

EXAM TIP

Human chorionic gonadotropin (hCG) is detectable in maternal serum after implantation has taken place, approximately 8–11 days after conception.

EXAM TIP

The decidua produces steroids and proteins that are related to the maintenance and protection of the pregnancy from immunologic rejection.

TABLE 3-1. **Embryology**

Week	Preembryonic Period
1	Fertilization and start of implantation.
2	Formation of yolk sac and embryonic disk.
3	First missed menstrual period; formation of primitive streak and neural groove.
Embryonic Period	
4	Primitive heartbeat; crown-rump length (CRL) approximately 4.0 mm.
5	Hand and foot plates develop.
6	Hand plates develop digital rays; upper lip, nose, and external ear formed.
7	Umbilical herniation (intestines begin growth outside abdominal cavity).
8	Human appearance; tail has disappeared; CRL approximately 30 mm.
Previable Fetal Period	
9	Eyes closing or closed.
10	Intestines in abdomen; thyroid, pancreas, and gallbladder development.
11	Fetal kidneys begin excreting urine into amniotic fluid; fetal liver begins to function; baby teeth formed in sockets.
12	Sex distinguishable externally; fetal breathing movements begin; colonic rotation; fetus active; first-trimester ends.
14	Head and neck take an erect, straight-line alignment.
16	↑ fetal activity; ultrasound can determine sex; myelination of nerves and ossification of bones begin.
18	Egg cells, ovaries, and uterus develop in females.
20	Head and body (lanugo) visible; testes begin descent in males.
22	Fetus can hear, will reflexively move in response to loud noise.
Viable Fetal Period	
24	Fetal lungs develop alveoli and secrete surfactant, fetus generally capable of breathing air by week 27.
28	Third trimester begins; eyelids unfuse; muscle tone ↑.
30	Cerebral gyri and sulci, which began to form in week 26, are now prominent and begin accelerated formation.
32	Fetal immune system functioning and capable of responding to mild infections.
34	Vernix thickens.
36	Fetus capable of sucking; meconium present in fetal intestines.
40	Due date.

EXAM TIP

First trimester (T1): 1–12 weeks
Second trimester (T2): 13–27 weeks
Third trimester (T3): 28–40 weeks or term
Term: 37–42 weeks

 WARD TIP

The most common cause for abnormal maternal serum screen for aneuploidy is incorrect gestational age.

estriol
progesterone.

POSTIMPLANTATION

- The endometrium, or lining of the uterus, during pregnancy is termed *decidua*.
- Maternal RBCs may be seen in the trophoblastic lacunae in the second week postconception.

THE PLACENTA

The placenta continues to adapt over T2 and T3. It is the primary producer of steroid hormones after 7 weeks' gestation. The human placenta is **hemochorionic;** transfer of materials between mother and fetus is via maternal blood coming in contact with placental villi. There is no direct mixing of maternal and fetal blood.

Reproductive Tract

UTERUS

- The uterus is a thin-walled, muscular structure that is capable of expanding to hold the fetus, placenta, and amniotic fluid.
- Enlargement of the uterus is due to hypertrophy and hyperplasia of the myometrial smooth muscle.
- Early in pregnancy, this process is primarily stimulated by estrogen. As pregnancy progresses, ↑ in uterine size is due to mechanical distention.
- Throughout the pregnancy, these muscle cells will spontaneously contract.
  - These contractions, also known as Braxton Hicks contractions, are spontaneous and irregular with an intensity ranging from 5 to 25 mm Hg.
  - They may ↑ in frequency during the last month of pregnancy.
- Perfusion of the placenta depends on uterine blood flow, which comes from uterine and ovarian arteries.
- Blood flow ↑ as a result of vasodilation from the effects of estradiol and progesterone.
- Blood vessels lie between the various layers of uterine muscle. These muscle cells contract after delivery thereby constricting the blood vessels.

WARD TIP

Braxton Hicks contractions do not cause cervical change.

CERVIX

- The cervix is composed of smooth muscle and connective tissue. ↓ amount of collagen and accumulation of water cause the cervix to soften and become cyanotic.
- Other changes include ↑ vascularity of the entire cervix and hypertrophy and hyperplasia of the glands.
- ↑ in gland activity leads to the formation of a mucous plug.
  - The mucous plug is composed of immunoglobulins and cytokines, which act as a barrier to bacteria.
  - Cervical effacement causes expulsion of the mucous plug as the cervical canal shortens in labor.

"thinning"

VAGINA

The vagina also undergoes changes during pregnancy in preparation for labor/delivery.

- The tissue becomes more vascular leading to a purplish tinge—Chadwick's sign.
- The vaginal walls prepare for distention by increasing the thickness of the mucosa, loosening of the connective tissue, and hypertrophy of smooth muscle cells.
- The vaginal secretions become thicker with a white color due to influence of progesterone. Additionally, the secretions are more acidic in nature as a result of ↑ *Lactobacillus acidophilus*. This inhibits growth of most pathogens and favors growth of yeasts.

SKIN

The skin undergoes changes in pigmentation and vascularity as a result of pregnancy.
- The ↑ in pigmentation is due to melanocyte-stimulating hormone, estrogen, and progesterone.
  - Linea nigra: Dark line/discoloration of the abdomen that runs from umbilicus to pubis.
  - Darkening of the nipple and areola.
  - Facial chloasma/melasma: Light to dark brown hyperpigmentation in exposed areas (face or neck).
- High levels of estrogen cause vascular spiders and palmar erythema.
- Certain dermatologic conditions are unique to pregnancy. See Table 3-2.

BREASTS

- Breasts may ↑ in size and become painful.
- After a few months of pregnancy, the breast may express a thick, yellow fluid called colostrum.

Handwritten margin notes:

MSH/prog:
- melasma
- linea nigra
- hyperpig of nipples/areola

Estrogen
- spider angiomata
- palmar erythema
- striae gravidarum
- hair - anagen.

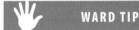

TABLE 3-2. Pruritic Dermatologic Disorders Unique to Pregnancy

DISEASE	ONSET	PRURITUS	LESIONS	DISTRIBUTION	INCIDENCE	↑ INCIDENCE FETAL MORBIDITY/ MORTALITY	INTERVENTION
Pruritic urticarial papules and plaques of pregnancy (PUPPP) (polymorphic eruption of pregnancy)	T2–T3	Severe	Erythematous urticarial papules and plaques	Abdomen, thighs, buttocks, occasionally arms and legs	Common (1:160–1:300)	No	Topical steroids, antipruritic drugs (hydroxyzine, diphenhydramine, calamine lotion
Intrahepatic cholestasis of pregnancy (bile not properly excreted from the liver)	T3	Severe	Excoriations common	Generalized, palms, soles	Common (1–2%)	Stillbirth	Check serum bile acids, liver function tests, antipruritics, ursodeoxycholic acid, fetal testing

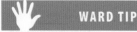
Metabolic Changes

- Ideal weight gain:
    T1: 1.5–3 lb gained
    T2 and T3: 0.8 lb/wk
- As both baby and placenta grow, the mother's body ↑ its energy needs. By the last trimester, requirements ↑ by 300 kcal/day.

WATER METABOLISM

- Water retention is a normal part of pregnancy. Often, pitting edema of the ankles and legs is seen in pregnant women, especially at the end of the day. This is due to several factors, including:
    - ↑ venous pressure in the lower extremities due to compression of the vena cava and pelvic veins by the gravid uterus.
    - ↓ in interstitial colloid osmotic pressure.
    - ↑ hydration of connective tissue leading to laxity and swelling of connective tissue and joints that mainly occur in T3.

CARBOHYDRATE METABOLISM

- First 20 weeks:
    - Insulin sensitivity ↑ in first half of pregnancy.
    - Lower fasting glucose levels allow for glycogen synthesis and fat deposition.
- After 20 weeks:
    - Insulin resistance develops and plasma insulin levels rise.
    - Higher levels of both insulin and glucose stimulate utilization of glucose and lipids for energy.
    - As a result, pregnant women will have mild fasting hypoglycemia, postprandial hyperglycemia, and hyperinsulinemia.

Hematologic Changes

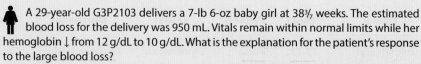

A 29-year-old G3P2103 delivers a 7-lb 6-oz baby girl at 38³/₇ weeks. The estimated blood loss for the delivery was 950 mL. Vitals remain within normal limits while her hemoglobin ↓ from 12 g/dL to 10 g/dL. What is the explanation for the patient's response to the large blood loss?

Answer: The patient remained hemodynamically stable despite a large blood loss due to the normal ↑ in blood volume that takes place in the second trimester. The ↑ in blood volume buffers the anticipated blood loss at the time of delivery.

BLOOD VOLUME

- Maternal blood volume ↑ during pregnancy by 50%. ↑ blood volume is needed to:
    - Meet the demands of the enlarged uterus.
    - Protect the mother and the fetus against impaired venous return.
    - Protect the mother from blood loss at the time of delivery.
- Expanded volume is composed of plasma and erythrocytes but proportionately more plasma. ↑ erythrocyte production is reflected by ↑ reticulocyte count.

- Both hemoglobin and the hematocrit ↓ slightly.
  - Hemoglobin averages 12.5 g/dL.
  - Levels below 11.0 g/dL, especially late in pregnancy, should be considered abnormal.

IRON

- Iron requirements ↑ in pregnancy to about 1000 mg/day.
- Most of the iron is used for hematopoiesis, especially in the last half of pregnancy.
- The amount of iron from the diet is insufficient to meet the needs of the pregnancy, so patients must take supplemental iron. The most common side effect of this supplementation is constipation.

IMMUNOLOGY

- During pregnancy, humoral and cell-mediated immunological functions are suppressed. During T3:
  - ↑ granulocytes, ↑ CD8 T lymphocytes.
  - ↓ in CD4 T lymphocytes, ↓ monocytes.
- The leukocyte count varies during normal pregnancy. Usually, it ranges from 5000/µL to 12,000/µL. During labor, counts can rise to 25,000/µL; however, it averages 14,000–16,000/µL.
- Markers of inflammatory states such as leukocyte alkaline phosphatase, C-reactive protein, and erythrocyte sedimentation rate (ESR) also rise.

COAGULATION

> A 36-year-old G3P2002 at 32 weeks' gestation presents with a sudden onset of shortness of breath, dyspnea, and palpitations that has been ongoing for 1 hour and is now worsening. She reports no sick contacts, cough, fever, or leg swelling. She has no medical conditions and has a negative family history. On exam, she is afebrile, pulse is 120, respirations 25, and BP 120/80. She appears to be in distress. There are absent breath sounds on the right side. Her legs show 1+ pitting edema bilaterally. Fetal heart rate is reassuring. Pulse oximetry is 75% on room air. What is the most likely diagnosis?
>
> **Answer:** Pulmonary embolus (PE). Estrogen causes an ↑ in clotting factors, resulting in a hypercoagulable state in pregnancy. Pregnant patients are at ↑ risk for pulmonary embolus and deep venous thrombosis (DVT) during the pregnancy and immediately after delivery.

- Pregnancy is a hypercoagulable state (risk factor for stroke, pulmonary emboli, DVT).
  - ↑ concentrations of all clotting factors, except factors XI and XIII.
  - ↑ fibrinogen.
  - ↑ resistance to activated protein C.
  - ↓ protein S.
- The average platelet count is ↓ slightly.

Cardiovascular System

- Changes in cardiac function begin in the first 8 weeks of pregnancy.
- Cardiac output is ↑ as early as the fifth week of pregnancy due to:
  - ↓ systemic vascular resistance.
  - ↑ heart rate.

Al ⎱
Fe ⎰ – constipation
Mg – diarrhea.

weight gain during preg:
1.) BMI <18.5: 28–30 lbs
2.) BMI 18.5–24.9: 25–35 lbs
3.) BMI 25–29.9: 15–25 lbs
4.) BMI >30: 11–20 lbs.

– ↑ clotting except 11/13
– ↑ fibrinogen
– ↓ Protein c/s.

EXAM TIP

$\uparrow CO = \downarrow SVR + \uparrow HR$.

$\downarrow ERV, RV \rightarrow \downarrow FRC$

$\uparrow TV, IRV \rightarrow \uparrow IC$

$\Delta VC = 0$

$\downarrow TLC$

WARD TIP

Patients with hypertensive heart disease may develop progressive or sudden deterioration in pregnancy.

WARD TIP

Normal acid-base status in pregnancy = compensated respiratory alkalosis (more CO_2 blown off).

WARD TIP

In pregnancy, the higher rate of renal clearance leads to reduced effective dose of antibiotics and other medications.

- As the diaphragm rises, the heart is displaced to the left and upward and rotates slightly.
- Systolic ejection murmurs along left sternal border occur in 96% of pregnant women due to ↑ flow across aortic and pulmonic valves.
- Diastolic murmurs are never normal and should be evaluated by a cardiologist.
- Blood pressure ↓ in midpregnancy and rises during the last trimester. Diastolic pressure ↓ more than systolic.

Respiratory System

- As a result of the expanding uterus, diaphragm rises about 4 cm, the subcostal angle widens, and thoracic circumference ↑ about 6 cm.
- Respiratory rate unchanged.
- ↑ tidal volume, minute ventilatory volume, and minute oxygen uptake.
- ↓ functional residual capacity and residual volume due to the elevated diaphragm.
- Normal acid-base status in pregnancy is **respiratory alkalosis** due to more CO_2 being blown off. pH = 7.45

Urinary System

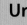 A 31-year-old G1P0 at 24 weeks presents for her routine prenatal visit. She has no complaints. However, urinalysis showed large nitrites, large leukocytes, and small blood. What is the next step?

Answer: The patient should be empirically treated for a urinary tract infection (UTI). The antibiotics can be modified once the urine culture results are available. Due to the changes caused by progesterone, pregnant women are at ↑ risk for developing asymptomatic bacteriuria, and UTIs can progress to pyelonephritis if left untreated. Pyelonephritis in pregnant women can lead to sepsis and respiratory failure; it is the most common non-obstetric cause for hospitalization in pregnancy, so prevention is key.

KIDNEYS

- ↑ glomerular filtration rate, creatinine clearance, renal plasma flow.
- ↓ serum creatinine, blood urea nitrogen.
- Renal tubules lose some of their resorptive capacity: Amino acids, uric acid, and glucose are not completely absorbed. Sodium is retained in higher levels in the pregnant female.

trace proteinuria; glycosuria are normal.

URETERS

- Dilate due to compression from uterus at the pelvic brim and the effect of progesterone.
- Dilation R > L due to the dextroversion of the uterus.
- Dilated ureters cause ↑ glomerular size and ↑ fluid flow → enlarged kidneys.
- Decreased ureteral peristalsis and increased ureteral compression cause urinary stasis which can lead to asymptomatic bacteriuria and pyelonephritis.

BLADDER

- ↓ tone, ↑ capacity progressively during pregnancy.
- ↑ urinary frequency is due to bladder compression by an enlarged uterus.
- Stress incontinence develops as a result of relaxation of bladder supports.

WARD TIP

Right hydronephrosis is a normal finding in pregnancy.

Gastrointestinal Tract

- The stomach, appendix, and intestines are displaced upward by the enlarging uterus.
- Effects of progesterone:
  - ↓ lower esophageal sphincter tone → heartburn.
  - ↓ bowel peristalsis → constipation.
- **Hemorrhoids,** common in pregnancy, are caused by constipation and elevated pressure in veins below the level of the uterus.

WARD TIP

Pain from appendicitis may occur much higher in the abdomen because the gravid uterus pushes the appendix up.

- heartburn / GERD
- constipation
- hemorrhoids
- cholestasis + gallstones.

LIVER

- **Alkaline phosphatase** activity in serum almost doubles during pregnancy. Serum aspartate transaminase, alanine transaminase, γ-glutamyl transferase, and bilirubin levels are slightly lower.
- Serum albumin ↓, but total albumin ↑ because of a greater volume of distribution.

GALLBLADDER

Contractility of the gallbladder is reduced, leading to an increased residual volume and cholestasis.

- Progesterone impairs gallbladder contraction by inhibiting cholecystokinin-mediated smooth muscle stimulation.
- Estrogen inhibits intraductal transport of bile acids, also contributing to cholestasis.

EXAM TIP

Cholestasis with increased lipids and cholesterol leads to higher incidence of gallstones, cholecystitis, and biliary obstruction.

Endocrine System

PITUITARY GLAND

The pituitary gland ↑ in size and weight during pregnancy.

Prolactin
- Main function is to ensure milk **production**.
- Levels ↑ throughout pregnancy due to estradiol.

Oxytocin
- Responsible for lactation, especially milk **letdown**.
- ↑ throughout the pregnancy.
- Released by nipple stimulation and infant crying.
- Causes uterine contractions.

WARD TIP

Pitocin is synthetic oxytocin. It is used to start or enhance labor.

EXAM TIP

Thyroxine-stimulating hormone (TSH) is unchanged during pregnancy.

WARD TIP

Pregnant women have elevated thyroxine-binding globulin (TBG) and therefore will have elevated total thyroxine and T_3, normal free T_4, and normal thyroid-stimulating hormone.

THYROID GLAND

- Total thyroxine levels and thyroxine-binding globulin ↑ in response to high estrogen levels. However, *free* thyroxine remains normal and the mother remains euthyroid.
- Thyroxine-stimulating hormone is a sensitive marker for thyroid disease.
- The gland does not ↑ in size; therefore, all goiters need to be investigated.

PARATHYROID GLAND

- In the mother, parathyroid hormone ↓ in first trimester but then rises progressively during the remainder of the pregnancy. Estrogens block the action of parathyroid hormone on bone resorption, resulting in ↑ hormone levels, which allow the fetus to have adequate calcium supply.
- The fetus has ↑ calcitonin levels allowing for bone deposition.

CHAPTER 4

Antepartum

This chapter focuses on the care provided for the pregnant patient prior to delivery. The prenatal (or antepartum) course often influences the outcome of the pregnancy. During this time, patients are encouraged to maintain healthy practices and abstain from practices that are harmful for the pregnancy. Regular visits at specific intervals are used to screen patients and fetus for abnormal medical conditions that may develop.

Prenatal Care

The goal of prenatal care is as follows:
1. Determine the health status of mother and fetus.
2. Determine gestational age.
3. Initiate plan for obstetrical care (routine versus high risk).
4. Lower maternal/perinatal morbidity/mortality.
5. Enhance pregnancy, childbirth experience for patient/family.

DEFINITIONS

- **Gestational age (GA):** The time of pregnancy counting from the first day of the last menstrual period (LMP).
- **Developmental age:** The time of pregnancy counting from fertilization.
- **First trimester:** 0–12 weeks.
- **Second trimester:** 13–27 weeks.
- **Third trimester:** 28 weeks–birth.
- **Embryo:** Fertilization–8 weeks.
- **Fetus:** 9 weeks–birth.
- **Previable:** <24 weeks.
- **Preterm:** 20–36 weeks.
- **Term:** 37–42 weeks.

TERMINOLOGY OF REPRODUCTIVE HISTORY

The mother's pregnancy history is described in terms of gravidity (G) and parity (P).
- **Gravidity** is the total number of pregnancies, regardless of the outcome.
- **Parity** is the number of pregnancies that have reached a gestational age of ≥20 weeks. It can be further subdivided into term births, preterm births, abortions, and living children.
- A woman that is gravida 3, para 1201 (G3P1201) has been pregnant three times, has had one term birth, two preterm births, no abortions, and has one live child.

FREQUENCY OF OBSTETRIC VISITS

- <28 weeks: Every month.
- 28–36 weeks: Every 2–3 weeks.
- 36–41 weeks: Once per week.
- 41–42 weeks: Twice per week for fetal testing.
- 42 weeks or more: Plan for delivery.
- See Table 4-1.

WARD TIP

Gravidity: The number of times a woman has been pregnant.

Parity: The number of times a woman has had a pregnancy that led to a birth after 20 weeks' gestation or an infant >500 g.

EXAM TIP

Parity: **FPAL** (Remember "Florida Power and Light")
Full term
Preterm
Abortuses
Living Children

TABLE 4-1. **Prenatal Visits**

FIRST VISIT	11–13 WEEKS	16–20 WEEKS	26–28 WEEKS
1. History and physical (H&P)	1. H&P	1. H&P	1. H&P
2. Labs:	2. Fetal exam:	2. Fetal exam:	2. Fetal exam:
■ Hct/Hgb	■ Fetal heart tones	■ Fetal heart	■ Fetal heart
■ Rh factor	3. Urine dip: Protein, glucose, leukocytes	■ Fundal height	■ Fundal height
■ Blood type	4. First-trimester screen or cfDNA	3. Urine dip: Protein, glucose, leukocytes	3. Labs: *"Recheck"*
■ Antibody screen		4. Fetal ultrasound: Anatomy, dating	■ Complete blood count
■ Pap smear		5. Quad screen (if FTS or cfDNA not selected)	■ Ab screen (if Rh neg)
■ *Gonorrhea* and *Chlamydia* cultures		6. Genetic amniocentesis (if indicated)	■ Diabetes screen
■ Urine analysis (protein, glucose, ketones)			■ Urine dip: Protein, glucose, leukocytes
■ Urine culture			4. Give anti D immunoglobulin if indicated (28 weeks)
■ Infection screen: Rubella, syphilis, hepatitis B, human immunodeficiency virus (HIV), tuberculosis (TB)			
■ Cystic fibrosis screen			
■ Hemoglobin electrophoresis (as needed)			
3. Discuss plan for genetic testing.			

every visit
–H&P
–Fetal exam–heart tones, fundal height. (>36–present)
–urine dip: glucose, protein, leukocytes
>36

WEEK 32	WEEK 36	WEEK 38	WEEK 39	WEEK 40
1. H&P	1. H&P	1. H&P	1. H&P	1. H&P
2. Fetal exam:	2. Fetal exam:	2. Fetal exam:	2. Fetal exam:	2. Fetal exam:
■ Fetal heart	■ Fetal heart	■ Fetal heart	■ Fetal heart	■ Fetal heart
■ Fundal height	■ Fundal height	■ Fundal height	■ Fundal height	■ Fundal height
3. Urine dip: protein, glucose, leukocytes	■ Fetal presentation	■ Fetal presentation	■ Fetal presentation	■ Fetal presentation
	3. Urine dip: Protein, glucose, leukocytes	3. Urine dip: Protein, glucose, leukocytes	3. Urine dip: Protein, glucose, leukocytes	3. Urine dip: Protein, glucose, leukocytes
	4. Group B strep culture	4. Cervical exam (frequency is controversial)		
	5. STD panel including HIV— required in some states			

11–13: 1ST T screen or cfDNA
16–20: Quad/amnio's; Fetal US.
26–28: Diabetes screen, anti-D immunoglobin
36: GBS culture; STD panel.

FIRST VISIT

History

■ Biographical: Age, race, occupation, marital status.

■ Obstetrical: Gravidity, parity, prior labor/deliveries (vaginal, cesareans), complications, infant status, birth weight.

■ Menstrual: Last menstrual period (LMP), menstrual irregularities.

■ Contraceptive use: What type and when was it last used?

■ Medical: Asthma, diabetes, hypertension, thyroid disease, cardiac disease, seizures, rubella, previous surgeries, sexually transmitted infections, allergies, medications, smoking, alcohol, recreational drugs.

■ Family history: Multiple gestations, diabetes, hypertension, bleeding disorders, hereditary disorders, mental retardation, anesthetic problems.

EXAM TIP

Remember that alcohol use has the highest correlation with congenital abnormalities.

Physical Exam

- Vitals: Blood pressure (BP), weight, height, temperature, heart rate.
- Head, neck, heart, lungs, back.
- Pelvic:
    - External genitalia: Bartholin's gland, condyloma, herpes, other lesions.
    - Vagina: Discharge, inflammation.
    - Cervix: Polyps, growths.
    - Uterus: Masses, irregularities, size compared to gestational age.
    - Adnexa: Masses.
    - Clinical pelvimetry: Following are dimensions of a gynecoid pelvis shape:
        - Pelvic inlet: Diagonal conjugate >12.5 cm. Distance between the inferior border of symphysis pubis to sacral promontory.
        - Midpelvis: Ischial spines blunt, >10 cm.
        - Pelvic outlet: Intertuberous diameter >8 cm, pubic arch >90 degrees.

WARD TIP

Patient's history and physical determine whether the patient receives routine or high-risk care.

SUBSEQUENT VISITS

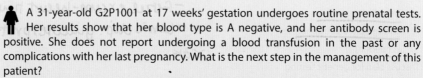

A 31-year-old G2P1001 at 17 weeks' gestation undergoes routine prenatal tests. Her results show that her blood type is A negative, and her antibody screen is positive. She does not report undergoing a blood transfusion in the past or any complications with her last pregnancy. What is the next step in the management of this patient?

Answer: The next step is to identify the antibody. There are many types of antibodies, and in a patient that is Rh negative, it should not be assumed that she has Rh antibodies.

History

Ask each patient the following at each subsequent visit:

- Presence of fetal movement.
- Vaginal bleeding.
- Leakage of fluid.
- Contractions/abdominal pain.
- Preeclampsia symptoms:
    - Headache.
    - Visual disturbances.
    - Right upper quadrant pain.

Physical Exam

After thorough initial exam, each subsequent exam must record four findings:

- BP.
- Urine dip for protein, glucose, leukocytes.
- Fundal height.
- Fetal heart rate.

Routine Initial Tests

- Complete blood count (CBC).
- Blood type.
- Rh status.
- Antibody screen.
- Urinalysis (UA).
- Urine culture.
- Rapid plasma reagin (RPR).

- Human immunodeficiency virus (HIV).
- Hepatitis B surface antigen (HBsAg).
- Rubella.
- Tuberculin skin test (if patient meets criteria).
- Gonorrhea.
- Chlamydia.
- Pap smear (if not up to date, and only if over age 21).
- Cystic fibrosis screen.
- Hemoglobin electrophoresis (if in high risk group).

Routine Timed Tests

Certain prenatal tests should occur at specific times during pregnancy (see Table 4-1):

- >10 weeks:
  - Cell-free fetal DNA (cfDNA); screens for Down syndrome, Trisomy 13, Trisomy 18, Turner syndrome, and sex chromosomes.
  - Sequencing of cell-free fetal DNA in the maternal circulation.
- 11–13 weeks:
  - First trimester screen; screens for Down syndrome and (depending on lab) Trisomy 18.
  - Nuchal translucency (NT) measured via ultrasound.
  - Maternal serum pregnancy-associated plasma protein A (PAPP-A) and free β-human chorionic gonadotropin (β-hCG).
  - In Down syndrome, the NT is ↑, PAPP-A ↓, free β-hCG ↑.
- 16–18 weeks: Quad screen (range 15–21 weeks).
  - Unconjugated estriol.
  - α-fetoprotein.
  - β-hCG.
  - Inhibin A.
- 18–20 weeks:
  - Ultrasound for anatomy/dating.
- 24–28 weeks:
  - One hour 50-g glucose tolerance test (GTT) to screen for gestational diabetes. └→ challenge.
- 28 weeks:
  - Recheck antibody screen, administer RhoGAM if indicated.
- 35–37 weeks:
  - Group B streptococcus (GBS) culture. (rectovaginal)
  - Third-trimester HIV testing (and/or full STD panel) is mandated by law in some states.

Handwritten margin note:

Down syndrome
↑ NT
↑ hCG
↓ PAPPA

Quad
MSAFP
β hCG
estriol
Inhibin A

FUNDAL HEIGHT

As the fetus grows, the leading edge of the uterus or the fundus grows superiorly in the abdomen, toward the maternal head. Fundal height (in centimeters) roughly corresponds to gestational age (in weeks).

- Uterus at level of pubic symphysis: 12 weeks.
- Uterus between pubic symphysis and umbilicus: 16 weeks.
- Uterus at the level of umbilicus: 20 weeks.
- Uterine height correlates to weeks' gestation: 20–36 weeks.

Fundal height (cm) should correlate to gestational age (weeks) ±3. If not, consider inaccurate dating (most common), multiple gestations, or molar pregnancy. Past approximately 36 weeks' gestation, the fundal height may not correspond to the gestational age due to the fetal descent into the pelvis.

WARD TIP

Most common cause of size not equal to date—incorrect gestational age. Order an US to establish the correct dates.

Fetal Surveillance

When the mother is diagnosed with a medical condition that can affect the fetus, or when the fetus is diagnosed with a condition that may result in a poor outcome, several tests can be used to monitor the health of the fetus. They include fetal movement counts, non-stress test (NST), contraction stress test (CST), biophysical profile (BPP), the modified BPP (mBPP), and Doppler ultrasonography. In general, they are performed in T3, but may be done earlier. These tests assess for chronic uteroplacental insufficiency and cannot predict acute events. The choice and frequency of testing depend on indication, gestational age, medical condition, and experience of the practitioner.

FETAL MOVEMENT COUNTS

Fetal movement counts, or kick counts, may be performed at home by the patient in order to monitor the baby's health. The patient should select a time at which the fetus usually is active, usually after a meal or at night before bed. The level of activity differs for each baby, and most have sleep cycles of 20–40 min.

There are several ways to assess fetal movements:
- Ask the patient to record daily how long it takes the fetus to make 10 movements. For most, this is usually achieved in about 2 hr; however, this is variable.
- Alternatively, ask the patient to record the number of fetal movements in 1 hr three times per week. A baseline is established in this way.
- For both of these strategies, a physician should be contacted if there is a change from the normal pattern or number of movements recorded.

NON-STRESS TEST (NST)

- The NST evaluates four components of the fetal heart rate (FHR) tracing:
- Baseline: Normally 110–160 beats/min.
- Variability: Beat-to-beat irregularity and waviness of the FHR. Presence of variability reflects an intact and mature brain stem and heart.
- Periodic changes: Transient accelerations or decelerations:
  - Early deceleration: Vagally mediated, caused by head compression usually at cervical dilation of 4–7 cm.
  - Variable deceleration: Caused by cord compression.
  - Late deceleration: Reflects hypoxemia.
  - Acceleration: At least two accelerations of at least 15 beats/min above baseline for 15 sec in a 20-min period. Presence of accelerations = fetal well-being. Reactive NST = two or more accelerations over 20 min.
  - Uterine contractions are also recorded to help interpret the NST.
- Preterm fetuses are frequently nonreactive:
  - 24–28 weeks: Up to 50% nonreactive.
  - 28–32 weeks: 15% nonreactive.
- An NST usually takes 20–40 min to complete. If the NST is nonreactive, the baby may be asleep. If this is suspected, ask the patient to eat or drink to make the baby active; if not reactive within 1–2 hours, then additional testing may need to be performed.

CONTRACTION STRESS TEST (CST)

The contraction stress test (CST) measures how the fetal heart rate (FHR) reacts to uterine contractions. The CST can be performed if the NST is nonreactive, although often a BPP will be performed instead as a means to evaluate fetal well-being. Because CSTs require uterine stimulation, they are potentially risky since contractions are induced. For this reason, the NST is usually the standard of care. The FHR and the contractions are recorded simultaneously. During a contraction, the blood flow to the placenta briefly ↓. A well-oxygenated fetus can compensate, and there are no decelerations in the FHR. If the fetus is already compromised with low levels of oxygen, the contraction may cause a late deceleration in FHR, which reflects hypoxemia in the fetus.

BPP > CST.

- Patient is placed in lateral recumbent position and contractions are stimulated.
    - Administration of oxytocin (pitocin).
    - Nipple stimulation (2-min self-stimulation through clothes every 5 min).
- Adequate contractions:
    - Occur three times in 10 min.
    - Lasting at least 40 sec.
    - Moderate to palpation.
- Interpreted as the presence or absence of late decelerations:
    - **Negative:** No late or significant variable decelerations.
    - **Positive:** Late decelerations following 50% or more of contractions.
    - **Equivocal:** Intermittent late decelerations or significant variable decelerations.
    - **Unsatisfactory:** Fewer than three contractions in 10 min.
- Contraindications:
    - Preterm labor patients at high risk of delivery.
    - Premature rupture of membranes (PROM).
    - History of extensive uterine surgery or previous cesarean delivery.
    - Known placenta previa.

EXAM TIP

A reactive NST has two or more accelerations over 20 min = fetal well-being.

ULTRASOUND (US)

- Standard US performed for:
    - Fetal number.
    - Presentation.
    - Fetal viability.
    - Gestational age assessment.
    - Amniotic fluid volume.
    - Fetal biometry.
    - Fetal anatomic survey.
    - Placental location.
- Limited—goal-directed US:
    - Presentation.
    - Placental location intrapartum.
    - Adjunct to invasive procedures.
- Specialized (Level II)—performed when high suspicion of anomaly:
    - Fetal Doppler.
    - Biophysical profile.

WARD TIP

When can a baby's heartbeat be detected with Doppler?
- 10–12 weeks of gestation.
- Fetal heart starts beating at 22–24 days.

BPP = NST + US exam
- NST
- Breathing
- movement
- tone
- AFI.

BIOPHYSICAL PROFILE (BPP)

- A biophysical profile (BPP) is the combination of the non-stress test and an ultrasound exam, for a total of five components:
  1. NST: Appropriate variation of fetal heart rate with a reactive NST.
  2. Breathing: ≥1 episode of rhythmic breathing movements of 30 sec or more within 30 min.
  3. Movement: ≥3 discrete body or limb movements within 30 min.
  4. Muscle tone: ≥1 episode of extension with return to flexion or opening/closing of a hand.
  5. Determination of amniotic fluid volume: Single vertical pocket of amniotic fluid measuring ≥2 cm is considered adequate* (or an amniotic fluid index >5 cm).
- Each category is given a score of 0 or 2 points:
  - 0: Abnormal, absent, or insufficient.
  - 2: Normal and present as previously defined.
  - Total possible score is 10 points.
  - Normal score: 8–10.
  - Equivocal: 6.
  - Abnormal: ≤4.

*In the presence of oligohydramnios (largest pocket of amniotic fluid ≤2 cm), further investigation is required.

MODIFIED BIOPHYSICAL PROFILE (mBPP)

- A modified biophysical profile (mBPP) includes two components: An NST and an amniotic fluid index (AFI).
- Normal amniotic fluid volume varies and ↑ with gestational age. The peak volume is 800–1000 mL at 36–37 weeks' gestation. In the late T2 or T3, amniotic fluid volume represents fetal urine output. If there is uteroplacental insufficiency and ↓ oxygenation to the fetus, the fetus preferentially shunts blood to the brain and heart, leaving the fetal kidneys underperfused. This results in ↓ fetal urine output and, as a result, ↓ amniotic fluid. Therefore, the AFI is used as a measure of chronic uteroplacental function.
- The AFI is the sum of amniotic fluid measured in four quadrants of the uterus via the US.
  - AFI 6–24 cm: Normal. Median AFI is 8–18 between weeks 20 and 35, after which values ↓.
  - AFI ≤5 cm: Abnormal (oligohydramnios).
  - AFI ≥25 cm: Abnormal (polyhydramnios).
- **Oligohydramnios:**
  - Most common cause: Ruptured membranes.
  - May be associated with uteroplacental insufficiency, and can see concurrent intrauterine growth restriction 60% of the time.
  - Evaluate for genitourinary malformations or other fetal anomalies.
- **Polyhydramnios:**
  - Many causes, including:
    - Fetal malformation (anencephaly, esophageal atresia).
    - Genetic disorders.
    - Maternal diabetes.
    - Multiple gestation.
    - Fetal anemia.
    - Viruses.
  - Associated with uterine overdistention, resulting in:
    - Preterm labor.
    - PROM.
    - Fetal malposition.
    - Uterine atony.

WARD TIP

mBPP = NST + AFI

WARD TIP

Most common cause of oligohydramnios = rupture of membranes.

DOPPLER VELOCIMETRY

- Doppler sonography is a noninvasive technique used to assess fetal hemodynamic vascular resistance by imaging specific fetal vessels:
    - Umbilical artery (UA) and umbilical vein.
    - Aorta.
    - Heart.
    - Middle cerebral artery (MCA).
- Commonly measured flow indices are:
    - Peak systolic frequency shift (S).
    - Peak diastolic frequency shift (D).
    - Mean peak frequency shift over the cardiac cycle (A).
    - Systolic to diastolic ratio (S/D).✶
    - Resistance index (S-D/S).✶
    - Pulsatility index (S-D/A).
- Flow velocity waveforms differ in normal-sized fetuses as compared to those suffering from growth restriction due to uteroplacental insufficiency:
    - Fetuses with normal growth: High-velocity diastolic flow.
    - Fetuses with restricted growth: ↓ velocity diastolic flow, ↑ flow resistance (↑ S/D) in umbilical artery and ↓ resistance (↓ S/D) in MCA.
    - Very severe intrauterine growth restriction: Diastolic flow may be absent or even reversed.
- Abnormal flow is usually the result of uteroplacental insufficiency, resulting in fetal hypoxia and acidosis. This may induce the phenomenon of brain sparing:
    - ↑ S/D in umbilical artery (↑ resistance).
    - ↓ S/D in MCA (↓ resistance).
    - Adaptive response to fetal hypoxemia.

> **EXAM TIP**
>
> "Brain sparing" may occur in hypoxic fetuses = ↑ S/D in umbilical artery + ↓ S/D in middle cerebral artery.

Screening for Congenital Abnormalities

Screening for fetal abnormalities can include testing during the first and second trimesters, and the tests can be noninvasive or invasive. Commonly used techniques are maternal serum screens, ultrasound, amniocentesis, chorionic villus sampling (CVS), and cordocentesis.

Cell-Free Fetal DNA (cfDNA)

- cfDNA is an optional serum screen performed after 10 weeks. It is a screening test and requires further invasive diagnostic tests if the results are abnormal.
- cfDNA screens for trisomy 21 (Down syndrome), trisomy 18, trisomy 13, and sex chromosome aneuploidies by using next-generation sequencing of cell-free fetal DNA (cfDNA) in the maternal circulation.
- The sensitivity is 98–99% for detection of T21.

FIRST-TRIMESTER SCREEN (FTS)

- The FTS is an optional noninvasive evaluation performed between weeks 11 and 13. It is a screening test and may require further diagnostic tests if the results are abnormal.
- The FTS combines a maternal blood screening test with a fetal US evaluation to identify risk for Down syndrome (trisomy 21). It can also detect Edwards syndrome (trisomy 18).

Down (Trisomy 21)
β-hCG ↑
PAPP-A ↓
Nuchal translucency ↑

A targeted US evaluates the fetus for congenital structural abnormalities that may correlate with abnormal serum screening findings.

Most neural tube defects are thought to be polygenic or multifactorial.

- The results of maternal hormone levels and fetal US, along with the mother's age, are combined to determine risk factors. The following is assessed in the FTS:
    - Maternal serum: Free or total β-hCG, PAPP-A.
    - US at 11–13 weeks' gestation: Nuchal translucency (NT)—measurement of fluid under the baby's skin at the level of the neck (see Figure 4-1).
    - In the case of Down syndrome, β-hCG will be ↑ and PAPP-A will be ↓.
- The FTS has a sensitivity of 85% for Down syndrome.

QUAD SCREEN

A 19-year-old Caucasian female, G1P0, at 16 weeks based on an unsure LMP has an ↑ risk for Down syndrome on her second-trimester quad screen. Her blood pressure is within normal limits, urine protein is negative, and fetal heart tones are 148 bpm. You palpate the fundal height 2 cm above the umbilicus. What is the most likely cause of the abnormal quad screen? What diagnostic tests can confirm the screening test?

Answer: The most common cause for the abnormal quad screen is incorrect dates. This patient's fundal height indicates that her pregnancy is further than what her LMP indicates. The next step is to perform an ultrasound to confirm the gestational age of the fetus and recalculate the quad screen. If the quad screen is abnormal with correct dating, the patient should undergo genetic counseling and be offered a genetic amniocentesis.

The quad screen is a screening test of maternal serum that evaluates the risk a patient has for delivering a baby with Down syndrome (trisomy 21), Edwards syndrome (trisomy 18), or NTDs. If the quad screen shows an ↑ risk for any of the screened conditions, further diagnostic tests may be performed to confirm the findings. See Table 4-2 for a summary of quad screen results.
- Ideally performed at 16–18 weeks' gestation (range is 15–21 weeks).
- Sensitivity: 81%.
- Evaluates four maternal serum analytes:
    - Maternal serum α fetoprotein.
    - Unconjugated estriol.

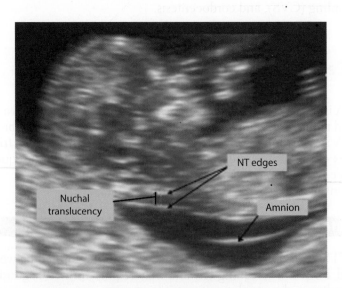

FIGURE 4-1. Nuchal translucency measurement. (Reproduced, with permission, from Cunningham FG, Leveno KJ, Bloom SL, et al. *Williams Obstetrics*, 23rd ed. New York: McGraw-Hill, 2010: 351.)

FTS / Down: ↑βhCG ↓PAPPA.
- edwards/patau = all ↓
Quad
- edwards = all ↓.
- Downs
↑B-hCG
↓estriol
↓MSAFP
↑inhibin A

TABLE 4-2. Quad Screen Summary

	Down (Trisomy 21)	Edwards (Trisomy 18)	NTD
uE3	↓	↓	Normal
AFP	↓	↓	↑
β-hCG	↑	↓	Normal
Inhibin A	↑	↓	Normal

AFP, α-fetoprotein; β-hCG, β-human chorionic gonadotropin; NTD, neural tube defect; uE3, unconjugated estriol.

- Human chorionic gonadotropin.
- Inhibin A.
- Abnormal quad screen → confirm dates (US) → genetic counseling + targeted US → diagnostic procedure (amniocentesis to obtain fetal cells) → karyotype analysis.
- Most common cause of abnormal quad screen: Incorrect dates.

EXAM TIP

If there is high α-fetoprotein at 16 weeks, a neural tube defect is a likely diagnosis, especially if the woman is older than 35. Low α-fetoprotein is associated with certain chromosomal defects (e.g., trisomy 21 or trisomy 18).

MATERNAL SERUM α-FETOPROTEIN (MSAFP)

- MSAFP is first produced in the yolk sac and then by the fetal gastrointestinal tract and liver.
- Normally, it passes by diffusion through the chorion and amnion. It begins to rise at 13 weeks and peaks at 32 weeks.
- In general, MSAFP levels >2.0–2.5 multiples of the mean (MOM) warrant further investigation, as they are suspicious of NTDs.
- MSAFP screening is most accurate between 16 and 18 weeks.
- High levels are associated with:
  - Underestimation of gestational age. *
  - NTDs.
  - Abdominal wall defects (gastroschisis and omphalocele).
  - Fetal death.
  - Placental abnormalities (e.g., abruption).
  - Multiple gestations.
  - Others: Low maternal weight, fetal skin defects, cystic hygroma, sacrococcygeal teratoma, oligohydramnios.
- Low levels are associated with:
  - Overestimation of gestational age.
  - Chromosomal trisomies: Down syndrome (trisomy 21), Edwards' syndrome (trisomy 18).
  - Fetal death.
  - Molar pregnancy.
  - High maternal weight.

WARD TIP

What can ultrasound determine?

- Diagnosis of early pregnancy.
- Determine if fetus is still viable in the setting of vaginal bleeding in early pregnancy.
- Determination of gestational age and assessment of fetal size.
- Diagnosis of fetal malformation (cleft lip, polydactyly, club foot, fetal sex, NTDs, abdominal wall defects, abdominal renal anomalies).
- Placental localization.
- Hydramnios and oligohydramnios.

UNCONJUGATED ESTRIOL (uE3)

Low levels are associated with:

- **Trisomy 21** (Down syndrome).
- **Trisomy 18** (Edwards syndrome).
- Possibly low in **trisomy 13** (Patau syndrome).

HUMAN CHORIONIC GONADOTROPIN (hCG)

- High levels are associated with Trisomy 21.
- Low levels are associated with Trisomy 18, anencephaly.

INHIBIN A

- This hormone is secreted by the placenta and granulosa cells in the female.
- High levels are associated with Trisomy 21.
- Low levels are associated with Trisomy 18.

SPECIALIZED (LEVEL II) ULTRASOUND

- Performed by maternal-fetal specialists.
- Evaluates the fetal anatomy for markers of aneuploidy.
- See Figures 4-2 through 4-10 for normal and abnormal US findings.

AMNIOCENTESIS

- Amniocentesis is the most frequently employed technique used to obtain fetal cells. A needle is placed through the maternal abdominal wall and uterus with ultrasound guidance (see Figure 4-11). Amniotic fluid is obtained for various purposes. Usually done at 15–20 weeks.
    - **Karyotype:** Fetal cells obtained via amniocentesis are cultured and an evaluation of the chromosomes is performed in the following circumstances:
        - Fetal anomaly suspected on US.
        - Abnormal serum genetic screen.
        - Family history of congenital abnormalities.
        - Indicated for patients ≥35 years of age because they have a higher risk of aneuploidy.
    - **Fetal lung maturity:** Usually done near term in order to deliver the baby.
    - **Others:** Rule out infection, check bilirubin.
- Risks:
    - Pain/cramping.
    - Vaginal spotting (resolves spontaneously).

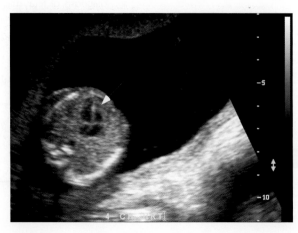

FIGURE 4-2. Normal four-chamber heart.

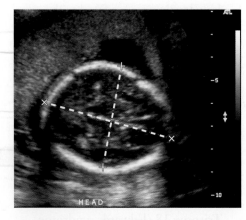

FIGURE 4-3. Measurement of biparietal diameter and head circumference.

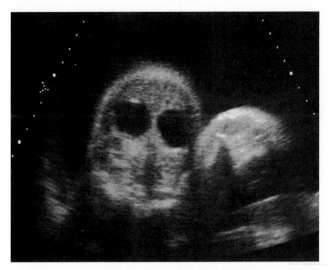

FIGURE 4-4.   Double-bubble sign of duodenal atresia (marker for Down syndrome). (Reproduced, with permission, from Cunningham FG, Leveno KJ, Bloom SL, et al. *Williams Obstetrics*, 23rd ed. New York: McGraw-Hill, 2010: 359.)

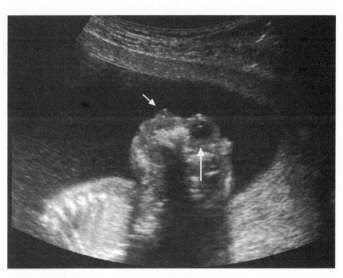

FIGURE 4-5.   Anencephaly. (Reproduced, with permission, from Cunningham FG, Leveno KJ, Bloom SL, et al. *Williams Obstetrics*, 23rd ed. New York: McGraw-Hill, 2010: 354.)

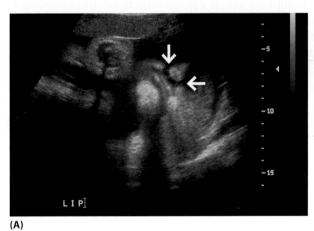

(A)

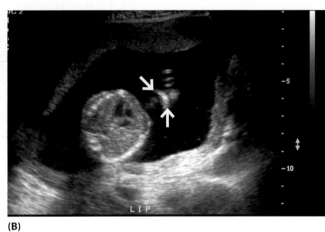

(B)

FIGURE 4-6.   (A). Cleft lip. (B). Normal lip.

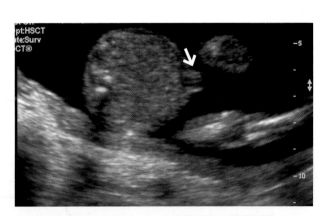

FIGURE 4-7.   Measurement of crown-rump length.

FIGURE 4-8.   Umbilical cord insertion.

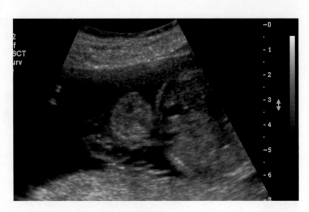

FIGURE 4-9.   Omphalocele.

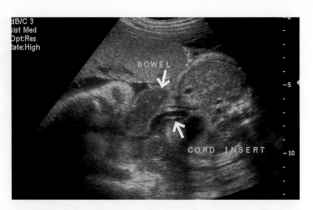

FIGURE 4-10.   Gastroschisis.

- Amniotic fluid leakage in 1–2% of cases.
- Symptomatic amnionitis in <1 in 1000 patients.
- **Rate of fetal loss is 1/300–1/500 and may be lower in experienced hands.**

CHORIONIC VILLUS SAMPLING (CVS)

- CVS is a diagnostic technique in which a small sample of chorionic villi is taken transcervically or transabdominally and analyzed (see Figure 4-12).
- Typically done between 9 and 12 weeks' gestation.
- Information on fetal karyotype.
- Biochemical assays or DNA tests can be done earlier than amniocentesis.

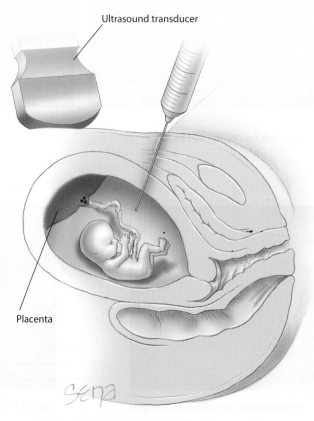

Ultrasound transducer

Placenta

FIGURE 4-11.   Amniocentesis. (Reproduced, with permission, from Cunningham FG, Leveno KJ, Bloom SL, et al. *Williams Obstetrics*, 23rd ed. New York: McGraw-Hill, 2010: 299.)

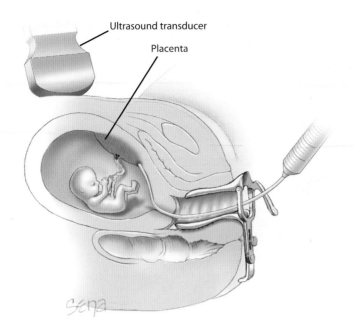

FIGURE 4-12. Transcervical chorionic villus sampling (CVS). (Reproduced, with permission, from Cunningham FG, Leveno KJ, Bloom SL, et al. *Williams Obstetrics*, 23rd ed. New York: McGraw-Hill, 2010: 300.)

- **Complications**—0.5–1%:
    - Preterm delivery.
    - PROM.
    - Fetal injury, especially limb abnormalities if performed before 9 weeks' gestation.

Differences Between CVS and Amniocentesis

- **CVS:**
    - Transvaginal or transabdominal aspiration of precursor cells in the intrauterine cavity.
    - Evaluates chromosomal abnormalities but does not evaluate NTDs.
    - Done at 9–12 weeks.
    - Higher risks (fetal loss has 1% risk, limb defects if done <9 weeks), diagnosis accuracy is comparable to amniocentesis.
- **Amniocentesis:**
    - Transabdominal aspiration of amniotic fluid using ultrasound-guided needle.
    - Evaluates chromosomal abnormalities.
    - Done at 15–20 weeks.
    - Indicated if >35-year-old mother at time of delivery.
    - Risks of fetal loss 1/300–1/500.

CORDOCENTESIS

- Cordocentesis is also known as percutaneous umbilical blood sampling (PUBS), fetal blood sampling, and umbilical vein sampling. It is a procedure in which a spinal needle is advanced transabdominally under US guidance into a cord vessel to sample fetal blood (see Figure 4-13). Typically performed after 17 weeks.
- Allows for rapid diagnosis because of the high number of nucleated cells (WBCs) collected which require no culturing.

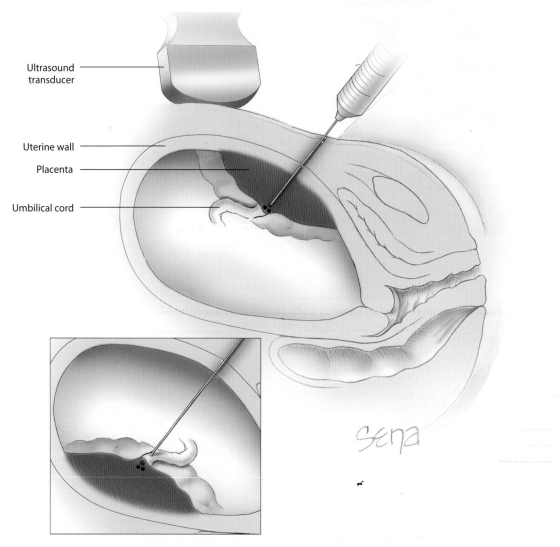

Ultrasound transducer

Uterine wall

Placenta

Umbilical cord

FIGURE 4-13. **Cordocentesis.** (Reproduced, with permission, from Cunningham FG, Leveno KJ, Bloom SL, et al. *Williams Obstetrics*, 23rd ed. New York: McGraw-Hill, 2010: 301.)

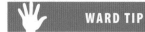
WARD TIP

Advanced maternal age (>35 years at delivery) is the most common indication for prenatal genetic testing.

INDICATIONS

- Fetal karyotyping because of fetal anomalies.
- To determine the fetal hematocrit in isoimmunization or severe fetal anemia.
- To assay fetal platelet counts, acid-base status, antibody levels, blood chemistries, etc.

GENETIC TESTING

Genetic testing is not required for every pregnancy, but current guidelines recommend offering all pregnant women genetic testing, regardless of risk status. There are specific circumstances where the risk of a genetic abnormality is particularly high, and where genetic testing should definitely be offered.

INDICATIONS

- Advanced maternal age.
- Previous child with abnormal karyotype.
- Known parental chromosome abnormality (balanced translocation or point mutation).
- Fetal structural abnormality on sonogram.
- Unexplained intrauterine growth retardation (IUGR).
- Abnormal quad screen.

TECHNIQUES

- **Fluorescent in situ hybridization (FISH):** A specific DNA probe with a fluorescent label that binds homologous DNA; allows identification of specific sites along a chromosome. **Looks for specific abnormalities. Very sensitive.**
- **Karyotyping:** Allows visualization of chromosome size, banding pattern, and centromere position. **Looks for all chromosomal abnormalities, but not as sensitive.**

Nutritional Needs of the Pregnant Woman

Proper nutritional habits are important for every woman; this is especially true for those who are pregnant. ↑ energy needs and specific vitamins are required by the mother to supply the appropriate nutrients essential to the normal development of the fetus. Without proper dietary control, certain common deficiencies and complications in both mother and baby may occur.

WEIGHT GAIN

- Weight gain for normal BMI: 25–35 lb.
- Weight gain of <15 lb (unless obese) can cause fetal IUGR.
- Weight gain of >40 lb ↑ morbidity.
- Target weight gain of 1–5 lb in T1; 3–4 lb/month in remaining pregnancy.

Risk factors for IUGR:
- Poor nutrition.
- Tobacco smoking. ⎤
- Drug use.   ⎥ drugs
- Alcoholism.   ⎦
- Severe anemia.   ⎤
- Thrombophilia.   ⎦ heme
- Prolonged pregnancy.
- Preeclampsia.
- Chromosomal abnormalities.
- Placental infarction/hematoma.
- Infections.
- Multiple gestations.

DIET

- The average woman must consume an additional **300 kcal/day** beyond baseline needs and an additional **500 kcal/day when breast-feeding**.
- High protein (70–75 g/day), low simple carbohydrates and fats, high fiber.

WARD TIP

Chromosomal abnormalities occur in 0.6% of all live births, account for 5% of stillbirths and 50–60% of spontaneous abortions.

WARD TIP

Body Mass Index (BMI)
BMI ≥30: Obese
25.0–29.9: Overweight
18.5–24.9: Normal
<18.5: Underweight

WARD TIP

Weight gain in pregnancy:
BMI >25: 15–25 lb
BMI normal: 25–35 lb
BMI <18: 30–40 lb

EXAM TIP

How do you monitor IUGR? Serial ultrasound.

WARD TIP

What should be taken to prevent NTDs? Folic acid 400 µg/day or 0.4 mg/day.

FOLIC ACID

 A 32-year-old Hispanic female, G3P2002, at 16 weeks presents for initial obstetric visit. She reports that the last child born 3 years ago has spina bifida. What is the amount of folic acid she should take?

Answer: Women with a previous child with an NTD should take 4 mg/day of folic acid starting at least 6 weeks before conception and continuing through 12 weeks of pregnancy.

- ↑ dietary folate is required to prevent NTDs.
- 400 µg/day is required. Ideal if started at least 6 weeks before pregnancy.
- If previous child with NTD, need folic acid 4 mg/day, starting 6 weeks prior to conception and through T1.

MINERALS

- **30-mg elemental iron per day is recommended in T2 and T3.** Total of 1-g iron is needed for pregnancy (500 mg for ↑ RBC mass, 300 mg for fetus, 200 mg for GI losses).
- The recommended dietary allowance (RDA) for calcium is ↑ in pregnancy to 1200 mg/day and may be met adequately with diet alone.
- The RDA for zinc is ↑ from 15 to 20 mg/day.

↑ Fe, Ca, Zn in pregnancy

VEGETARIANS

- **Lacto-ovovegetarians** in general have no nutritional deficiencies, except possibly iron and zinc.
- **Vegans** must consume sufficient quantities of vegetable proteins to provide all essential amino acids normally found in animal protein. Supplementation of zinc, vitamin B_{12}, and iron is necessary.

PICA

Occasionally seen in pregnancy, pica is the compulsive ingestion of nonfood substances with little or no nutritional value, such as ice, clay (geophagia), or starch (amylophagia).

Common Questions

Pregnancy is a complicated time for most women. Their bodies undergo a transformation which entails many physiologic adaptations. These changes may be alarming to some women, and as a physician, one must be able to discern between normal pregnant physiology and pathophysiologic changes, which may require further investigation or immediate attention in a hospital setting.

CAFFEINE IN PREGNANCY

- Contained in coffee, tea, chocolate, cola beverages.
- Ingestion of caffeine (>300 mg/day) may ↑ risk of early spontaneous abortion among nonsmoking women carrying fetuses of normal karyotype. This risk ↑ according to amount of caffeine ingested.

WARD TIP

The neural tube is nearly formed by the time of the first missed period. Starting folic acid supplementation when pregnancy is diagnosed is too late to prevent NTDs.

WARD TIP

Pregnant women develop iron deficiency anemia due to the ↑ hematopoietic demands of both mother and baby.

WARD TIP

Pica may occur during pregnancy, but all normal dietary and nutritional needs must be met and the substances consumed should be nontoxic (ice). Advise patients against the consumption of nonedible and possibly toxic items, such as dirt.

- Adverse maternal effects include:
  - Insomnia.
  - Acid indigestion.
  - Reflux.
  - Urinary frequency.

EXERCISE

- No data exist to indicate that a pregnant woman must ↓ the intensity of her exercise or lower her target heart rate.
- Women who exercised regularly before pregnancy should continue. Exercise may relieve stress, ↓ anxiety, ↑ self-esteem, modulate weight gain, and shorten labor.
- The form of exercise should be one with low risk of trauma, particularly abdominal (water exercises are ideal).
- Exercise that requires prolonged time in the supine position should be avoided in T2 and T3.
- Exercise should be stopped if patient experiences oxygen deprivation (manifested by extreme fatigue, dizziness, or shortness of breath).
- Contraindications to exercise include:
  - Evidence of IUGR.
  - Persistent vaginal bleeding.
  - Incompetent cervix.
  - Risk factors for preterm labor.
  - Rupture of membranes.
  - Pregnancy-induced hypertension/preeclampsia/eclampsia.

WARD TIP

Hyperemesis gravidarum: Excessive vomiting during pregnancy + dehydration + electrolyte imbalances. A **hypochloremic alkalosis** may occur. What is the treatment? IVF 5% dextrose, antiemetics.

NAUSEA AND VOMITING (N&V)

- Recurrent N&V in T1 occurs in 50% of pregnancies.
- If severe, can result in dehydration, electrolyte imbalance, and malnutrition.
- Management of mild cases includes:
  - Avoidance of fatty or spicy foods.
  - Eating small, frequent meals.
  - Inhaling peppermint oil vapors.
  - Drinking ginger teas.
  - Pyridoxine (vitamin B6) ± doxylamine (antihistamine)
- Management of severe cases includes:
  - IV fluids (usually with dextrose-containing fluid).
  - Discontinuation of vitamin/mineral supplements until symptoms subside.
  - Antihistamines. ⎤
  - Promethazine. ⎟
  - Metoclopramide. ⎟
  - Ondansetron.   ⎦

— obtain a UA as initial w/u in these patients to r/o ketosis

WARD TIP

Why is dextrose included in the IV fluid for hyperemesis gravidarum? The dextrose helps to ↓ the ketosis, which can cause a vicious cycle of nausea. Dextrose can help break the cycle.
"Morning sickness" can occur day or night.

HEARTBURN

- Occurs in 30% of pregnancies.
- **Etiology:**
  - Normal relaxation of lower esophageal sphincter (due to progesterone).
  - Mechanical forces.
- **Treatment:**
  - Elimination of spicy/acidic foods.
  - Small, frequent meals.

- Decreasing amount of liquid consumed with each meal.
- Limiting food and liquid intake a few hours prior to bedtime.
- Sleeping with head elevated on pillows.
- Utilizing liquid forms of antacids and H_2-receptor inhibitors.

CONSTIPATION

- Common in pregnancy (due to progesterone).
- **Management:**
  - Increasing intake of high-fiber foods.
  - Increasing liquids.
  - Use of psyllium-containing products (e.g., Metamucil).
  - Avoid enemas, strong cathartics, and laxatives.

VARICOSITIES

- Common in pregnancy, particularly in lower extremities and vulva.
- Can cause chronic pain and superficial thrombophlebitis.
- **Management:**
  - Avoidance of garments that constrict at the knee and upper leg.
  - Use of support stockings.
  - ↑ periods of rest with elevation of the lower extremities.

HEMORRHOIDS

- Varicosities of the rectal veins are common in pregnancy.
- **Management:**
  - Cool sitz baths.
  - Stool softeners.
  - ↑ fluid and fiber intake to prevent constipation.
  - Hemorrhoidal ointment to ↓ swelling, itching, and discomfort.
  - Topical anesthetic spray or steroid cream for the severe pain of thrombosed hemorrhoids.

LEG CRAMPS

- Occur in 50% of pregnant women, typically at night and in T3.
- Most commonly occur in the calves.
- Massage and stretching of the affected muscle groups is recommended.

BACKACHE

- Typically progressive in pregnancy (30–50%).
- **Management:**
  - Minimizing time standing.
  - Wearing a support belt over the lower abdomen.
  - Acetaminophen for pain as needed.
  - Exercises to ↑ back strength.
  - Supportive shoes and avoidance of high heels.
  - Gentle back massage.
  - Heating pad to back.

ROUND LIGAMENT PAIN

- Sharp, bilateral or unilateral groin pain.
- Frequently occurs in T2.
- May ↑ with sudden movement/change in position.

↑ movement
↓ rest.

SEXUAL INTERCOURSE

- There are no restrictions during the normal pregnancy.
- Nipple stimulation, vaginal penetration, and orgasm may cause release of oxytocin and prostaglandins, resulting in uterine contractions.
- Contraindications:
  - Ruptured membranes.
  - Placenta previa.
  - Preterm labor.

EMPLOYMENT

- Work activities that ↑ risk of falls/trauma should be avoided.
- Exposure to toxins/chemicals should be avoided.

TRAVEL

- The best time to travel is in T2. Patient is past possible complications of miscarriage in T1 and not yet encountered risk of preterm labor of T3.
- If prolonged sitting is involved, the patient should attempt to stretch her lower extremities and walk for 10 min every 2 hr. This is to avoid DVTs.
- The patient should bring a copy of her medical record.
- Wear seat belt when riding in car.
- Airplane travel in pressurized cabin presents no additional risk to the pregnant woman (if uncomplicated pregnancy). Air travel is not recommended after 35 weeks.
- In underdeveloped areas or when traveling abroad, the usual precautions regarding ingestion of unpurified water and raw foods should be taken. Appropriate vaccines should be given.

IMMUNIZATIONS (TABLE 4-3)

General principles:
- Delay vaccines until after the first trimester to avoid potential teratogenicity (except influenza, which may be given any time as the benefits outweigh the risks).
- Risk from vaccines is generally small. Always consider whether risk of the disease is worse than the risk of the vaccine.
- Live vaccines are not given in pregnancy.
- Viral vaccines may be safely given to the children of pregnant women.
- Immune globulins are safe in pregnancy and are recommended for women exposed to measles, hepatitis A and B, tetanus, varicella (chickenpox), and rabies.

WARD TIP

Ideally, women should avoid getting pregnant for 4 weeks after receiving live vaccines, such as measles, mumps, rubella (MMR), or varicella.

TABLE 4-3.   Vaccine Safety in Pregnancy

SAFE	NOT WELL STUDIED IN PREGNANT WOMEN, SO DEFER UNTIL FURTHER RECOMMENDATIONS ISSUED	ADMINISTER ONLY IF RISK OUTWEIGHS BENEFIT	UNSAFE (LIVE)
▪ Inactivated polio (IPV)	▪ Human papillomavirus (HPV)	▪ Yellow fever	▪ Oral polio (sabin)
▪ Inactivated typhoid	▪ Meningococcus (MPV4)	▪ Anthrax	▪ Oral typhoid
▪ Inactivated influenza	▪ Pneumococcus (PPV)	▪ Pertussis	▪ Intranasal influenza
▪ Diphtheria ✓	▪ Hepatitis A		▪ Measles, mumps, rubella (MMR)
▪ Tetanus ✓			▪ Varicella
▪ Rabies			▪ Bacillus Calmette-Guérin (BCG)
▪ Meningococcus (MPSV4)			▪ Shingles
▪ Hepatitis B			

(whole)
Inactivated vaccines

–Rabies
–influenza
–Polio (salk)/Pertussis
–Hep A

(subunit)
– Hep B
– HPV
– Influenza
– Pertussis (acellular)
– Anthrax

(toxoid)
– diphtheria
– tetanus.

Polysacc
–Pneumococcal – Hib
–Meningococcal – typhi

Cannot give:
–MMR
–varicella
–shingles
–polio (sabin)
–oral typhoid
–intranasal influenza.
–BCG

Notify the Physician

While many physiologic changes in pregnancy are uncomfortable, most are non-emergent. There are, however, some situations when a pregnant woman should contact her obstetrician immediately:

- Vaginal bleeding.
- Leakage of fluid from the vagina.
- Rhythmic abdominal cramping or back pain, >6/hr that does not improve with hydration and lying supine.
- Progressive and prolonged abdominal pain.
- Fever and chills.
- Dysuria or abnormally cloudy urine (indicative of a urinary tract infection).
- Prolonged vomiting with inability to hold down liquids or solids for >24 hr.
- Progressive, severe headache; visual changes; or generalized edema (pre-eclamptic symptoms).
- Seizure (eclampsia).
- Pronounced ↓ in frequency or intensity of fetal movements.

Complete listing of Live vaccines:
– MMR
–varicella
– Zoster
– sabin
– intranasal influenza
– Yellow fever
–Rotavirus
–BCG
–oral typhus.

Intrapartum

Three Stages of Labor

> A 25-year-old Hispanic female, G1P0, at 38 weeks presents to triage complaining of contractions that have been increasing in strength and frequency over a 12-hr period. She denies vaginal bleeding, leakage of fluid, and preeclampsia symptoms. She reports good fetal movement. Fetal heart rate is reassuring. She is contracting every 2 min on the monitor. Her cervical exam is 6 cm dilated, 50% effaced, 0 station, cephalic. What stage of labor is she in? If her labor progresses as expected, what should her cervical dilation be at the next vaginal exam in 2 hr?
>
> **Answer:** She is in the active phase of the first stage of labor. Since she is a primigravida, her cervix should dilate at a minimum of 1.2 cm/hr. So, in 2 hr, she should be 8.4 cm (or 8–9 cm) dilated.

Labor is defined as regular contractions that result in cervical change. The progression of labor is illustrated in Figure 5-1.

FIRST STAGE

- The first stage of labor begins with onset of uterine contractions of sufficient frequency, intensity, and duration to result in effacement and dilation of the cervix, and ends when the cervix is completely dilated to 10 cm.
- The first stage of labor consists of **two phases:**
  1. **Latent phase:** Begins with the onset of labor and ends at approximately 4–6 cm cervical dilation.
     - Nulliparous: Prolonged if >20 hr.
     - Multiparous: Prolonged if >14 hr.
  2. **Active phase:** Rapid dilation. Begins at 4–6 cm dilation and ends at 10 cm.
     - Active phase is further classified according to the rate of cervical dilation: **Acceleration phase, phase of maximum slope,** and **deceleration phase.**

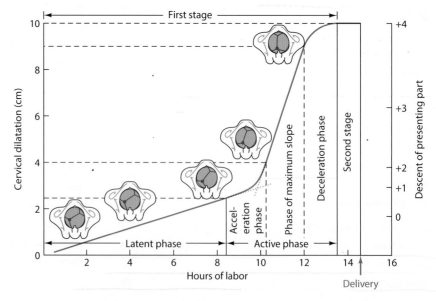

FIGURE 5-1.   Progression of labor. (Reproduced, with permission, from DeCherney AH, Pernoll ML. *Current Obstetrics & Gynecologic Diagnosis & Treatment.* Norwalk, CT: Appleton & Lange, 1994: 211.)

- Fetal descent begins at 7–8 cm of dilation in nulliparas and becomes most rapid after 8 cm.
- Average duration of cervical dilation from 4 to 10 cm (minimal normal rate):
  - Nulliparous: <1.2 cm/hr.
  - Multiparous: <1.5 cm/hr.

SECOND STAGE

The second stage of labor is the stage of **fetal expulsion.** It begins when the cervix is fully dilated and ends with the delivery of the fetus.

Average Pattern of Fetal Descent

- Nulliparous: <2 hr (3 with epidural).
- Multiparous: <1 hr (2 with epidural).

THIRD STAGE

The main event of the third stage is **placental separation**. It begins immediately after the delivery of the fetus and ends with the delivery of the fetal and placental membranes.
- **Duration:** Usually <10 min; considered prolonged if >30 min.
- The three signs of placental separation are:
  1. Gush of blood from vagina.
  2. Umbilical cord lengthening.
  3. Fundus of the uterus rises up and becomes firm.

True Labor Versus False Labor

FALSE LABOR (BRAXTON HICKS CONTRACTIONS)	TRUE LABOR
Occur at irregular intervals	Occur at regular intervals that shorten
Intensity remains the same	↑ in intensity
Discomfort in lower abdomen	Discomfort in back and lower abdomen
No cervical change	Cervix dilates
Relieved by medications	**Not** relieved by medications

Assessment of Patient in Labor

HISTORY

- Patients without prenatal care require a complete history and physical (H&P), and those with prenatal care require an update and focused physical. Prenatal record should be obtained when possible.

WARD TIP

If progress during the active phase is slower than these figures, evaluation for adequacy of uterine contractions, fetal malposition, or cephalopelvic disproportion should be done.

WARD TIP

Abnormalities of the second stage may be either protraction or arrest of descent (the fetal head descends <1 cm/hr in a nullipara and <2 cm/hr in a multipara).

WARD TIP

If 30 min have passed without placental expulsion, manual removal of the placenta may be required.

WARD TIP

What are the three signs of placental separation?
1. Gush of blood
2. Umbilical cord lengthening
3. Fundus of uterus rises and firms

- The following information should always be obtained from a laboring patient:
  - Time of onset and frequency of contractions.
  - Status of fetal membranes. Typical history for ruptured membranes: gush of fluid with continuous leakage. Color may be clear or yellow/green (meconium).
  - Presence/absence of vaginal bleeding. Bloody show is small amount of blood mixed with cervical mucus that is present with cervical dilation and effacement. It should be distinguished from vaginal bleeding.
  - Notation of fetal activity.
  - Symptoms of preeclampsia (headache, visual disturbances, right upper quadrant pain).
  - History of allergies.
  - How long ago patient consumed food or liquids and how much (mostly in case the patient needs to undergo a cesarean delivery).
  - Use of medications.

VAGINAL EXAM (VE)

- Perform a sterile **speculum** exam first if:
  - Rupture of membranes is suspected.
  - The patient is thought to be in preterm labor.
  - Bleeding suspicious for placenta previa is present.
- Otherwise, a sterile **digital** VE may be performed.

RUPTURE OF MEMBRANES

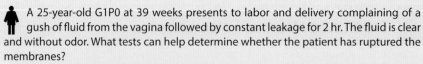
A 25-year-old G1P0 at 39 weeks presents to labor and delivery complaining of a gush of fluid from the vagina followed by constant leakage for 2 hr. The fluid is clear and without odor. What tests can help determine whether the patient has ruptured the membranes?
Answer: Perform a sterile speculum exam, testing for pooling, valsalva, ferning, and nitrazine. If these are positive, the membranes are likely ruptured and the fluid noted on the exam is likely amniotic fluid.

- Perform a sterile speculum exam:
  1. **Pooling:** The presence of fluid collection in the posterior fornix should be noted (positive pooling).
  2. **Valsalva:** Ask the patient to bear down and perform a Valsalva manuever. Note if fluid is seen to come through the cervical os (positive Valsalva).
  3. **Ferning:** Place a thin layer of the fluid on a slide. View the dried amniotic fluid under a microscope for a characteristic ferning pattern made by the crystallized sodium chloride in the amniotic fluid (positive ferning). Confirms ROM in 85–98% of cases (see Figure 5-2).
  4. **Nitrazine:** Place the vaginal fluid on nitrazine paper to assess the pH. If nitrazine paper turns blue, this indicates basic pH (positive nitrazine). Amniotic fluid has basic pH as compared to vaginal secretions that have acidic pH. Confirms ROM in 90–98% of cases.
- The presence of pooling, valsalva, ferning, and nitrazine indicates that the membranes are likely ruptured and the fluid noted on the exam is amniotic fluid.

FP nitrazine → Blood, Semen, TV.

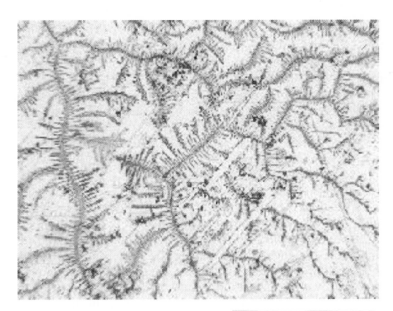

FIGURE 5-2.   Ferning pattern.

- Fluid should also be examined for meconium.
  - The presence of meconium in the amniotic fluid may indicate fetal stress.
  - Meconium staining is more common in term and postterm pregnancies than in preterm pregnancies.
  - **Meconium aspiration syndrome (MAS):** Fetal stress, like hypoxia, leads to meconium in the amniotic fluid. With further fetal gasping, the meconium is inhaled into the fetal lungs, causing lung damage. At birth, the infant will present with respiratory distress and can develop pulmonary hypertension. Intubation does not provide adequate oxygenation due to the lung injury and pulmonary hypertension. Infants with MAS may require extracorporeal membranous oxygenation (ECMO) which bypasses the lungs in order to provide oxygen to the baby.

CERVICAL EXAM

There are five parameters of the cervix that are examined: dilation, effacement, station, consistency, and position.

Dilation

Describes the size of the **opening** of the cervix at the external os.
- **Ranges:** Ranges from zero to 10 cm dilated (closed to completely dilated). The presenting part of a term-sized infant can usually pass through a cervix that is fully dilated.
- **Determination of dilation:** The index and/or the middle fingers are inserted in the cervical opening and are separated as far as the cervix will allow. The distance (cervical dilation) between the two fingers is estimated.

Effacement

Describes the **length of the cervix.** With labor, the cervix thins out and softens, and the length is reduced. The normal length is 3–4 cm.
- **Terminology:** When the cervix shortens by 50% (to around 2 cm), it is said to be 50% effaced. When the cervix becomes as thin as the adjacent lower uterine segment, it is 100% effaced. *(paper thin)*
- **Determination of effacement:** Palpate with finger and estimate the length from the internal to external os.

EXAM TIP

Vernix: The fatty substance consisting of desquamated epithelial cells and sebaceous matter that normally covers the skin of the term fetus.

EXAM TIP

Meconium: A dark green fecal material that collects in the fetal intestines and is discharged at or near the time of birth.

WARD TIP

Know this cervical exam stuff cold for the wards!

Station

Describes the degree of **descent** of the presenting part in relation to ischial spines, which are designated at 0 station.

- Terminology (two systems):
  1. The ischial spine is zero station, and the areas above and below are divided into thirds. Above the ischial spines are stations −3, −2, and −1, with −3 being the furthest above the ischial spines and −1 being closest. Positive stations describe fetal descent below the ischial spines. +3 station is at the level of the introitus, and +1 is just past the ischial spines.
  2. Very similar except that the areas above and below the ischial spines are divided by centimeters, up to 5 cm above and 5 cm below. Above are five stations or centimeters: −5, −4, −3, −2, and −1, with −5 being the 5 cm above the ischial spines and −1 being 1 cm above. Positive stations describe fetal descent below the ischial spines. +5 station is at the level of the introitus, and +1 is 1 cm past the ischial spines.
- If the fetus is vertex, the station should be determined by the location of the biparietal diameter (BPD), not the tip-top of the head, which may simply be caput and not the head at all. So when the BPD is at the level of the ischial spines, the station is 0.

endorsed by APGO.   →   *most commonly used*

Consistency

Breakdown of collagen bonds in the cervix changes the consistency of the cervix progressively from firm to medium to soft, in preparation for dilation and labor.

Position

Describes the location of cervix with respect to the fetal presenting part. It is classified as one of the following:

- **Posterior:** Difficult to palpate because it is behind the presenting part, and usually high in the pelvis.
- **Midposition.**
- **Anterior:** Easy to palpate, low in pelvis.

During labor, the cervical position usually progresses from posterior to anterior.

BISHOP SCORE

> A 26-year-old G2P1001 at 41 weeks presents to the hospital for an induction. Her dates are verified, and the infant is noted to be cephalic. Her cervical exam is 3 cm dilation, 70% effaced, −2 station, anterior position, and soft. What is her Bishop score? What is the likelihood of a successful vaginal delivery?
>
> **Answer:** Her Bishop score is 9 showing that she has a favorable cervix for induction of labor. Her chance of vaginal delivery is similar to those who present in spontaneous labor.

This is a scoring system that helps to determine the status of the cervix—favorable or unfavorable—for successful vaginal delivery.

- If induction of labor is indicated, the status of the cervix must be evaluated to help determine the method of labor induction that will be utilized. See Table 5-1 and section on Labor in chapter 5.
- A score of ≥6 indicates that the probability of vaginal delivery with induction of labor is similar to that of spontaneous labor.

TABLE 5-1. **Bishop Scoring System**

FACTOR	0 POINTS	1 POINT	2 POINTS	3 POINTS
Dilation (cm)	Closed	1–2	3–4	≥5
Effacement (%)	0–30	40–50	60–70	≥80
Station[a]	–3	–2	–1 to 0	+1 to +3
Consistency	Firm	Medium	Soft	—
Position	Posterior	Midposition	Anterior	—

[a] Station reflects –3 to +3 scale.

Assessment of the Fetus

LEOPOLD MANEUVERS

- Leopold maneuvers are begun in late pregnancy to determine which way the baby is presenting in the uterus (Figure 5-3). Consist of four parts:
  - **First maneuver** answers the question: "What fetal part occupies the fundus?"
  - **Second maneuver** answers the question: "On what side is the fetal back?"
  - **Third maneuver** answers the question: "What fetal part lies over the pelvic inlet?"
  - **Fourth maneuver** answers the question: "On which side is the cephalic prominence?"
- Four aspects of the fetus are described from the Leopold maneuvers:
  - Lie
  - Presentation
  - Position
  - Attitude

Lie

Lie describes the relation of the long axis of the fetus to that of the mother. A **longitudinal** (99% of term or near-term births) lie can be vertex (head first) or breech (buttocks first). The lie may be **transverse** or **oblique**.

Presentation/Presenting Part

Describes the portion of the fetus that is foremost within the birth canal. It is normally determined by palpating through the cervix on vaginal examination.

- If the lie is longitudinal, the presentation is either the head (cephalic), buttocks (breech), brow, or face. The most common type of presentation is the **vertex presentation** in which the posterior fontanel is the presenting part.
- If the lie is transverse, the shoulder, back, or abdomen may be the presenting part.

Position

Refers to the relation of the presenting part to the right (R) or left (L) side of the birth canal and its direction anteriorly (A), transversely (T), or posteriorly (P).

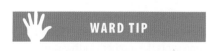

WARD TIP

Anterior fontanel: Larger diamond shape

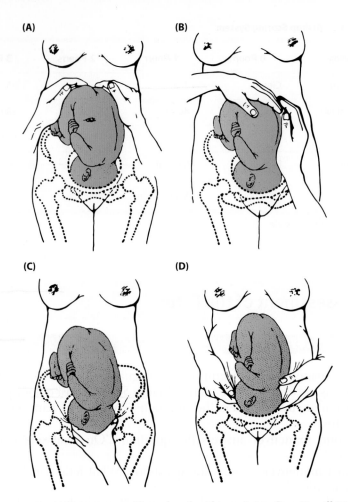

FIGURE 5-3.   Leopold maneuvers. (Reproduced, with permission, from Pernoll ML. *Benson & Pernoll's Handbook of Obstetrics and Gynecology*, 10th ed. New York: McGraw-Hill, 2001: 159.)

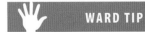

WARD TIP

Posterior fontanel: Smaller triangle shape

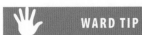

WARD TIP

Interpreting Fetal Positions
Imagine the mother lying in the dorsal lithotomy position (on her back, legs in stirrups) and the baby's occiput in relation to her body. You are at the end of the bed looking between mom's legs. Figure 5-4 represents the mother's birth canal with the fetal head in various positions.

- The top of the **fetal skull** is composed of five bones: two frontal, two parietal, and one occipital. The anterior fontanel lies where the two frontal and two parietal meet, and the posterior fontanel lies where the two parietal meet the occipital bone.
- For a cephalic presentation, the **occiput** is used as the reference point to determine the position:
  - Occiput anterior (OA).
  - Occiput posterior (OP).
  - Left occiput anterior (LOA).
  - Left occiput posterior (LOP).
  - Left occiput transverse (LOT).
  - Right occiput anterior (ROA).
  - Right occiput posterior (ROP).
  - Right occiput transverse (ROT).
- The **chin** is used as the reference point for face presentation. The **sacrum** is used as the reference point for breech presentation.

Attitude and Posture

In the later months of pregnancy, the fetus assumes a characteristic posture ("attitude/habitus"), which typically describes the position of the arms, legs, spine, neck, and face.

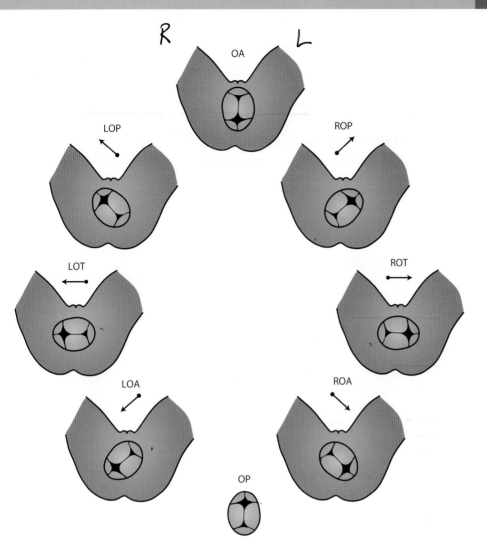

FIGURE 5-4. Vertex positions.

OA = desired position of the baby during birth.

NORMAL PRESENTATION

Vertex Presentation (Occiput Presentation)

Vertex presentation is **most common** (96% of term or near-term presentations). The head is flexed so that the chin is in contact with the chest. The **posterior fontanel** is the presenting part. This creates the shortest diameter of the fetal skull that has to pass through the pelvis.

MALPRESENTATIONS

Face Presentation

In face presentation (0.3% of presentations at or near term), the fetal neck is sharply extended so the occiput is in contact with the fetal back. The face is the presenting part. Diagnosis is made by palpation of the fetal face on vaginal exam.

Sinciput Presentation

The fetal head assumes a position between vertex presentation and face presentation so that the anterior fontanel presents first.

EXAM TIP

Ninety percent of babies presenting in the occiput posterior position spontaneously rotate to occiput anterior position.

Brow Presentation

The fetal head assumes a position such that the eyebrows present first. This forces a large diameter through the pelvis; usually, vaginal delivery is possible only if the presentation is converted to a face or vertex presentation.

Breech Presentations

In breech presentations, the presenting fetal part is the **buttocks**. Incidence: 3.5% at or near term but much greater in early pregnancy (14%). Those found in early pregnancy will often spontaneously convert to vertex as term approaches.

RISK FACTORS

- Low birth weight (20–30% of breeches).
- Congenital anomalies such as hydrocephalus or anencephaly.
- Uterine anomalies.
- Multiple gestation.
- Placenta previa.
- Hydramnios, oligohydramnios.
- Multiparity.

DIAGNOSIS

- Leopold maneuvers.
- Ultrasound.
- Vaginal exam.

TYPES OF BREECH (SEE FIGURE 5-5)

- **Frank breech (65%):** The thighs are flexed (bent forward) and knees are extended (straight) over the anterior surfaces of the body (feet are in front of the head or face).
- **Complete breech (25%):** The thighs are flexed (bent) on the abdomen and the knees are flexed (folded) as well.
- **Incomplete (footling) breech (10%):** One or both of the hips are not flexed so that a foot lies below the buttocks.

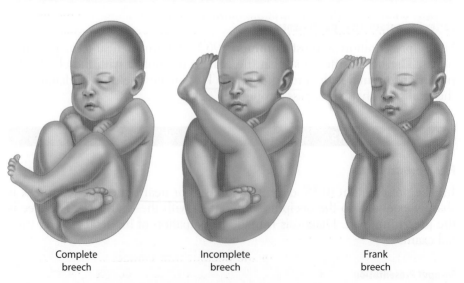

Complete breech   Incomplete breech   Frank breech

FIGURE 5-5.   Types of breech presentations. (Reproduced, with permission, from Ganti L. *Atlas of Emergency Medicine Procedures.* New York, NY: Springer Nature; 2016.)

MANAGEMENT OF BREECH FETUS

- Most frequently, the delivery is via cesarean.
- Frank breech positions with other ideal conditions may deliver vaginally.
- **External cephalic version:** Procedure that maneuvers the infant to a cephalic position by applying pressure through the maternal abdomen. Can be done only if breech is diagnosed before onset of labor and the gestational age is 35–37 weeks. The success rate is 50%, and the risks are placental abruption, fetal heart rate abnormalities, and reversion.

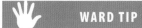

Complete and incomplete breeches are not delivered vaginally due to risk of umbilical cord prolapse.

Cardinal Movements of Labor

The cardinal movements of labor are movements of the fetal head that allow it to pass through the birth canal. The movements are as follows: engagement, descent, flexion, internal rotation, extension, and external rotation (restitution). Delivery of the shoulders follows (see Figure 5-6).

ENGAGEMENT

The descent of the biparietal diameter (the largest transverse diameter of the fetal head, 9.5 cm) through the plane of the pelvic inlet. Can occur in late pregnancy or in labor. Clinically if the presenting part is at 0 station, the head is thought to be engaged in the pelvis.

Engagement is determined by palpation of the presenting part of the occiput.

DESCENT

Occurs when the fetal head passes down into the pelvis. It occurs in a discontinuous fashion. The greatest rate of descent is in the deceleration phase of the first stage of labor and during the second stage of labor.

The fundal height ↓ at term due to engagement of the fetus.

FLEXION

Occurs when the chin is brought close to the fetal thorax. This passive motion facilitates the presentation of the smallest possible diameter of the fetal head to the birth canal.

INTERNAL ROTATION

Refers to turning of the head that moves the occiput gradually toward the symphysis pubis or less commonly toward the hollow of the sacrum.

EXTENSION

Extension moves the occiput toward the fetal back:
- Occurs after the fetus has descended to the level of the maternal vulva.
- This action brings the base of the occiput into contact with the inferior margin of the symphysis pubis, where the birth canal curves upward.
- The delivery of the fetal head occurs when it changes from the flexed to the extended position, curving under and past the pubic symphysis.

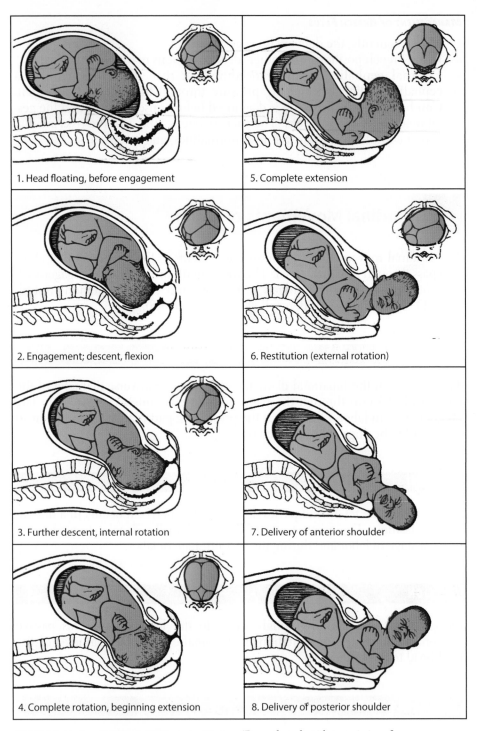

1. Head floating, before engagement

2. Engagement; descent, flexion

3. Further descent, internal rotation

4. Complete rotation, beginning extension

5. Complete extension

6. Restitution (external rotation)

7. Delivery of anterior shoulder

8. Delivery of posterior shoulder

FIGURE 5-6. **Cardinal movements of labor.** (Reproduced, with permission, from Cunningham FG, Leveno KJ, Bloom SL, et al. *Williams Obstetrics*, 22nd ed. New York: McGraw-Hill, 2005: 418.)

EXTERNAL ROTATION (RESTITUTION)

Occurs after delivery of the head, when the fetus resumes its normal "face-forward" position with the occiput and spine lying in the same plane. One shoulder is anterior behind the pubic symphysis, and the other is posterior.

EXPULSION

After external rotation, further descent brings the anterior shoulder to the level of the pubic symphysis. The shoulder is delivered under the pubic symphysis, and then the rest of the body is quickly delivered.

Normal Spontaneous Vertex Vaginal Delivery

DELIVERY OF THE HEAD

- Place fingers of one hand on the occiput as it is seen passing under the symphysis pubis to control the delivery of the head and avoid lacerations.
- Support the perineum with the other hand.
- With maternal effort, the infant's head will deliver and restitute either to the left or the right.
- Bulb suction the infant's mouth first, then the nares. Remember to squeeze the bulb first, place it inside the baby, then release. This may also be done after delivery.

CHECKING FOR NUCHAL CORD

- Occurs when loops of umbilical cord wrap around the fetal neck. To check for this condition, following delivery of the head, a finger should be passed along the fetal neck to ascertain the presence of the cord.
- If nuchal cord is present, a finger should be slipped under the cord and, if loose enough, the cord should be slipped over the infant's head.
- If the cord is wrapped tightly around the infant's neck, it should be cut between two clamps.

DELIVERY OF SHOULDERS

- Most frequently, the shoulders appear at the vulva just after external rotation and are delivered spontaneously.
- Occasionally, the shoulders must be extracted:
  - The sides of the head are grasped with both hands and *gentle* downward traction is applied until the anterior shoulder descends from under the pubic arch.
  - Next, *gentle* upward traction is applied to deliver the posterior shoulder.

DELIVERY OF THE INFANT

- The rest of the infant is delivered with maternal pushing.
- Support the infant's head with one hand by grasping the neck, taking care not to grasp the throat.
- Support the infant's buttocks as they are delivered with the other hand.
- Transfer the infant's buttocks in the crook of the elbow of the hand that is holding the head. This frees the other hand to suction the baby and clamp and cut the cord.
- Hand the baby to the nurse or pediatrician.

EXAM TIP

The anterior shoulder is the one closest to the superior portions of the vagina, while the posterior shoulder is closest to the perineum and anus.

EXAM TIP

Fundal pressure should never be used to relieve a shoulder dystocia.

WARD TIP

Squeeze the bulb between fingers first, then place in fetal mouth/nares.

APGAR
- Appearance (color)
- pulse
- Grimace
- activity (tone)
- respirations

WARD TIP

Know your Apgar scores: Assigns score of 0–2 for the following:
- Color
- Pulse
- Respirations
- Grimace
- Tone

WARD TIP

Signs of placental separation typically occur within 5 min of infant delivery.

DELIVERY OF THE PLACENTA

- Obtain arterial pH if indicated, and venous blood for fetal blood typing.
- Monitor for signs of placental separation:
  - There is often a sudden gush of blood.
  - Uterus becomes globular and firmer.
  - The uterus rises in the abdomen after the bulk of the separated placenta passes into the vagina.
  - The umbilical cord lengthens, indicating descent of the placenta.
- Apply pressure with one hand in the suprapubic region and apply gentle traction on the umbilical cord to guide placenta out.
- Once placenta is past the introitus, grasp with hands and gently remove membranes. Inspect the placenta for intact cotyledons and three-vessel cord.
- Perform fundal massage to help the uterus contract down and ↓ the bleeding.

INSPECTION

Inspect patient for any lacerations or extensions of episiotomy that may need to be repaired. Look at:
- Circumferential cervix.
- Vaginal walls.
- Labia.
- Perineum.

PERINEAL LACERATIONS

The perineum and anus become stretched and thin, which results in ↑ risk of spontaneous lacerations to the vagina, labia, perineum, and rectum.
- **First degree:** Involve the fourchette, perineal skin, and vaginal mucosa, but not the underlying fascia and muscle (skid mark).
- **Second degree:** First degree plus the fascia and muscle of the perineal body but *not* the anal sphincter.
- **Third degree:** Second degree plus involvement of the anal sphincter.
- **Fourth degree:** Extend through the rectal mucosa to expose the lumen of the rectum.

EPISIOTOMY

The incision of the perineum and/or labia to aid delivery by creating more room. Not performed routinely, but in special cases such as shoulder dystocia or operative vaginal deliveries. The classification of episiotomy is the same as perineal lacerations. The incision can be either midline or mediolateral (Figure 5-7).
1. **Midline:** The incision is made in the midline from the posterior fourchette. Most common. ↑ the risk of a fourth-degree laceration.
2. **Mediolateral:** The incision is oblique starting from 5 o'clock or 7 o'clock position of the vagina. Causes more bleeding and pain.

POSTDELIVERY HEMOSTASIS

After the uterus has been emptied and the placenta delivered, hemostasis must be achieved:
- The primary mechanism is myometrial contraction leading to vasoconstriction.

WARD TIP

Placental delivery should *never* be forced before placental separation has occurred; otherwise, uterine inversion may occur.

WARD TIP

There are two umbilical arteries and one umbilical vein in the cord.

WARD TIP

Proper repair of fourth-degree laceration is essential to prevent future fecal incontinence and rectovaginal fistula.

WARD TIP

Most common cause for postpartum hemorrhage = Uterine atony. Treat with uterotonics like pitocin, methergine, hemabate, misoprostol.

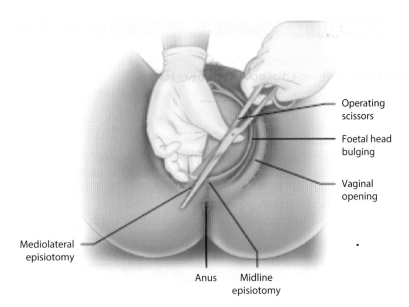

FIGURE 5-7. Episiotomy technique. (Reproduced, with permission, from Ganti L. *Atlas of Emergency Medicine Procedures*. New York, NY: Springer Nature; 2016.)

Labels: Operating scissors; Foetal head bulging; Vaginal opening; Mediolateral episiotomy; Anus; Midline episiotomy

- Fundal massage stimulates uterine contraction.
- Oxytocin (Pitocin) is administered in the third stage of labor. It causes myometrial contractions and reduces maternal blood loss.
- Postpartum hemorrhage: Often defined as >500 mL of blood loss for vaginal delivery and >1000 mL for cesarean delivery.

Management of Patients in Labor

VAGINAL EXAMS

Vaginal examinations should be kept to the minimum number required for the evaluation of a normal labor pattern, for example, every 4 hr in latent phase and every 2 hr in active phase. Sterile gloves and lubricant should be used.

MATERNAL VITAL SIGNS

Maternal blood pressure and pulse should be evaluated and recorded every 10 min.

OTHER CONSIDERATIONS

Usually, oral intake is limited to small sips of water, ice chips, popsicles, or hard candies.

Monitoring During Labor

During labor, uterine contractions and fetal heart rate are monitored closely.

EXAM TIP

Postpartum hemorrhage causes—
The 4 T's
Tissue: Retained placenta
Trauma: Instrumentation, lacerations, episiotomy
Tone: Uterine atony
Thrombin: Coagulation defects, DIC

WARD TIP

Inhalation anesthesia may be needed for cesarean delivery or for management of complications in the third stage of labor. Thus, consumption of foods or liquids is discouraged in order to avoid aspiration.

UTERINE CONTRACTIONS

Uterine activity is monitored by external or internal uterine monitors.
- **External monitors:** (tocodynamometer)
  - Accurately display the frequency of the contraction. Does not provide information about strength.
  - More commonly used unless more detailed information is needed.
- **Intrauterine pressure catheters:**
  - Record frequency, duration, and strength of the contraction.
  - Strength of contraction measured in **Montevideo units.**
    - Calculated by ↑ in uterine pressure above baseline multiplied by contraction frequency over 10 min.
    - If you have time, don't multiply—add every contraction.

FETAL HEART RATE

The **fetal heart rate (FHR)** can be assessed in two ways:
1. **Intermittent** auscultation with a fetal stethoscope or Doppler ultrasonic device.
2. **Continuous** electronic monitoring of the FHR and uterine contractions is most commonly used in United States. The standard fetal monitor tracing records the fetal heart rate on the top portion and the contractions on the bottom.
- **External (indirect) electronic FHR monitoring:** FHR is detected using a Doppler device placed on the maternal abdomen.
- **Internal electronic FHR monitoring:** A bipolar spiral electrode is attached to the fetal scalp, which detects the peak R-wave voltage of the fetal electrocardiogram. This is more invasive and is used if closer fetal monitoring is required.

"fetal scalp monitor"

Fetal Heart Rate Patterns

- The normal baseline for the fetal heart rate is 110–160 beats per minute (bpm).
- Baseline rate refers to the most common heart rate lasting ≥10 minutes.
- Periodic changes above and below termed **accelerations** (↑ in HR) and **decelerations** (↓ in HR).
- A **reassuring** fetal tracing has two accelerations of at least 15 bpm above the baseline, lasting for at least 15 sec, in 20 min. It indicates a well–oxygenated fetus with an intact neurological and cardiovascular system.

DEFINITIONS

- **Hypoxemia:** ↓ oxygen content in blood.
- **Hypoxia:** ↓ level of oxygen in tissue.
- **Acidemia:** ↑ concentration of hydrogen ions in the blood.
- **Acidosis:** ↑ concentration of hydrogen ions in tissue.
- **Asphyxia:** Hypoxia with metabolic acidosis. Goal of fetal monitoring during labor is to avoid metabolic acidosis and asphyxia, which can cause permanent neurological injury.

DECELERATIONS

A 32-year-old G2P1001 at 40 weeks presents to labor and delivery with contractions. She is noted to be 5 cm dilated, 50% effaced, −1 station, and cephalic. The monitor shows contractions every 2 min, and the FHR pattern shows a baseline of 150 bpm, minimal variability, and gradual decelerations that nadir after the peak of the contractions. No accelerations are noted. What is the most likely cause of the findings on the FHR? What is the next step in management?

Answer: Uteroplacental insufficiency is the most likely cause for this patient's late decelerations. The patient should be turned on her left side to maximize oxygenation to the fetus. Administer oxygen to the mother. If her membranes are ruptured, a fetal scalp electrode and an intrauterine pressure catheter (internal monitors) will help with the FHR monitoring. A search for the cause of uteroplacental insufficiency should be carried out.

Decelerations during labor have different interpretations depending on when they occur in relation to contractions. (See Table 5-2 and Figure 5-8.)

Early Decelerations

■ Early decelerations are *normal* and are due to **head compression** during contractions or during maternal expulsive efforts.
■ The nadir of the gradual deceleration corresponds to the peak of the contraction.
■ The effect is regulated by vagal nerve activation.
■ No intervention is necessary. They are clinically benign.

Late Decelerations

■ Late decelerations are *abnormal* and are due to **uteroplacental insufficiency** (blood without enough oxygen) during contractions.
■ They are a gradual decrease below the baseline with onset, nadir, and recovery occurring after uterine contraction onset, peak, and recovery, respectively.
■ Can follow epidural (hypotension) or uterine hyperstimulation.

TABLE 5-2.   Types of Decelerations

	EARLY DECELERATION	LATE DECELERATION	VARIABLE DECELERATION
Significance	Benign	Abnormal	Variable
Shape	U shaped	U shaped	Variable (often V or W shaped)
Onset	Gradual	Gradual	Abrupt
Depth	Shallow	Shallow	Variable
When	Nadir of decel = peak of ctx	Start and end after the uterine ctx Nadir of decel after peak of ctx	Variable
Why	Head compression	Uteroplacental insufficiency	Cord compression
Initial treatment	None required	O₂, lateral decubitus position, Pitocin off, close monitoring	Amnioinfusion

Ctx, contraction; decel, deceleration; **gradual**, baseline to nadir >30 sec; **abrupt**, baseline to nadir <30 sec.

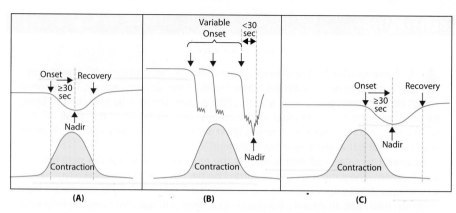

FIGURE 5-8. **Features of early (A), variable (B), and late (C) decelerations on fetal heart monitoring.** (Reproduced, with permission, from Cunningham FG, Leveno KJ, Bloom SL, et al. *Williams Obstetrics*, 22nd ed. New York: McGraw-Hill, 2005: 452–454.)

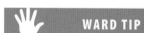

EXAM TIP

The left lateral recumbent position is best for maximizing cardiac output and uterine blood flow. (In the supine position, the vena cava and aortoiliac vessels may be compressed by the gravid uterus.)

WARD TIP

STOP when you see decelerations:
Sterile vaginal exam
Turn the patient to her left side
Give the patient **O**xygen
Pitocin off

MANAGEMENT

- Change maternal position to the left lateral recumbent position.
- Give oxygen by facemask.
- Stop oxytocin (Pitocin) infusion.
- Provide an IV fluid bolus.
- Consider tocolysis.
- Monitor maternal blood pressure. Treat hypotension with medications.
- Sterile vaginal exam to assess for change in fetal station or position.
- If repetitive (>50% of the contractions have late decelerations) and no other reassuring finding present, consider immediate delivery.

Variable Decelerations

- Variable decelerations are *abnormal* and reflect the fetal autonomic reflex response to umbilical cord compression.
- They can be seen with oligohydramnios or a nuchal cord.
- Abrupt deceleration that looks like a "v".
- They can occur at any time.

MANAGEMENT

- **Amnioinfusion:** Infuse normal saline into the uterus through the intrauterine pressure catheter to alleviate cord compression. Most commonly used for severe variable decelerations.
- Change maternal position to side/Trendelenburg position.
- Plan delivery of fetus soon if worsening or nonreassuring.

Prolonged Decelerations

Isolated decelerations with fall in baseline by ≥15 bpm that last 2–10 min. Causes include:
- Cervical examinations.
- Uterine hyperactivity.
- Maternal hypotension leading to transient fetal hypoxia.
- Umbilical cord compression.

MANAGEMENT

- Stop oxytocin and prostaglandins.
- Change maternal position.
- Administer IV fluids.

- Correct hypotension with vasopressors.
- Administer maternal O_2.
- Sterile vaginal exam to exclude cord prolapse, sudden cervical dilation, or fetal descent.

FETAL TACHYCARDIA

- Baseline HR >160 bpm for >10 min.
- Causes:
    - Fetal hypoxia.
    - Intrauterine infection. ⎤ * chorioamnonitis!
    - Maternal fever. ⎦
    - Drugs.

FETAL BRADYCARDIA

- HR <110 bmp.
- Causes:
    - Maternal beta-blocker therapy.
    - Hypothermia.
    - Hypoglycemia.
    - Fetal heart block.

SINUSOIDAL PATTERN

- Fluctuations in FHR baseline with regular amplitude and frequency.
- Associated with severe fetal anemia.

BEAT-TO-BEAT VARIABILITY (BTBV)

- **The single most important characteristic of the baseline FHR.**
- Variation of successive beats in the FHR BTBV is controlled primarily by the autonomic nervous system. ↑ in FHR is due to activation of the sympathetic nervous system. The ↓ in the FHR is due to the activation of the parasympathetic nervous system. The constant push and pull of the sympathetic and parasympathetic systems creates the BTBV, which indicates intact fetal CNS.
- At <28 weeks' gestational age, the fetus is neurologically immature; thus, ↓ variability is expected.
- Measured in a 10-minute window, with amplitude measured peak to trough in beats per minute (bpm).
    - Absent = amplitude undetectable.
    - Minimal = amplitude 0–5 bpm.
    - Moderate = amplitude 6–25 bpm.
    - Marked = amplitude >25 bpm.

Decreases in BTBV

Beat-to-beat variability ↓ with:
- Fetal acidemia.
- Fetal asphyxia.
- Maternal acidemia.
- Drugs (narcotics, magnesium sulfate [$MgSO_4$], barbiturates, etc.).
- Acquired or congenital neurologic abnormality.

WARD TIP

If an FHR of 160 bpm lasts for ≥10 min, then tachycardia is present.

WARD TIP

Scalp stimulation is done between decelerations to elicit a reactive acceleration and rule out metabolic acidosis.

WARD TIP

Internal FHR monitoring is the best way to determine BTBV.

Increases in BTBV

Beat-to-beat variability can ↑ with mild fetal hypoxemia, but may also be a normal variant.

Classification and Interpretation of FHR Patterns

- Three-tier FHR classification system:
  - Category I—normal FHR, minimal chance of fetal acidosis.
  - Category II—all patterns that are not Cat I or II. Risk of acidosis varies widely.
  - Category III—abnormal, associated with increased chance of fetal acidosis and/or hypoxia (Table 5-3).

Abnormal Labor Patterns

DYSTOCIA

A 32-year-old G3P2002 at 38 weeks is admitted for active labor. Two hours ago her cervical exam was 5 cm/80% effaced/–2 station. Her exam now is 6 cm/80% effaced/–2 station. What is her labor pattern? What is the next step in management?
Answer: She has a protracted active phase. Since she is a multipara, she should dilate 1.5 cm/hr at a minimum and should have been 8 cm over a span of 2 hr. The next step in management is to determine if there are adequate contractions, if the fetal size and position are amenable for a vaginal delivery, and whether the pelvis is adequate for a normal vaginal delivery.

TABLE 5-3. Classification of FHR Patterns

Cat I	ALL criteria must be present:
	■ Baseline rate: 110–160 bpm
	■ Moderate variability
	■ No late or variable decelerations
	■ ± early decelerations
	■ ± accelerations
Cat III	Either (1) or (2):
	1. Absent variability PLUS any of following:
	■ Recurrent late decelerations
	■ Recurrent variable decelerations
	■ Bradycardia
	2. Sinusoidal pattern
Cat II	Does not meet criteria for Cat I or Cat I
	Significance is indeterminate

TABLE 5-4.   Abnormal Labor Patterns

Labor Pattern	Nulliparas	Multiparas
Prolongation disorder (prolonged latent phase)	>20 hr	>14 hr
Protraction disorder		
1. Protracted active phase dilatation	<1.2 cm/hr	<1.5 cm/hr
2. Protracted descent	<1 cm/hr	<2 cm/hr
Arrest disorders		
1. Dilatation	>2 hr	>2 hr
2. Descent	>1 hr	>1 hr
3. Failure of descent (no descent in deceleration phase or second stage of labor)	>1 hr	>1 hr

[handwritten annotations:]
stage I problems
stage 2.
Abnormal Labor — protraction / arrest.

Dystocia literally means difficult labor and is characterized by abnormally slow or no progress of labor.

- **Prolonged latent phase** (see Table 5-4).
- **Active phase abnormalities:** May be due to cephalopelvic disproportion (CPD), excessive sedation, conduction analgesia, and fetal malposition (i.e., persistent OP).
- **Protraction disorders:** A slow rate of cervical dilation or descent.
- **Arrest disorders:** Complete cessation of dilation or descent (see Table 5-4).
- With the diagnosis of protraction or arrest disorder of labor, assess the following:
  - Contraction strength: Start or ↑ pitocin to obtain stronger contractions.
  - Fetal size and position: Baby too big to pass through pelvis? Position abnormal?
  - Pelvis: Does pelvimetry indicate adequate pelvis?

CAUSES

1. Abnormalities of the expulsive forces:
   - Uterine dysfunction can lead to uterine forces insufficiently strong or inappropriately coordinated to efface and dilate cervix.
   - Inadequate voluntary muscle effort during second stage of labor.
2. Abnormalities of presentation, position, or fetal development.
3. Abnormalities of the maternal bony pelvis.
4. Abnormalities of the birth canal.

Pelvic Shapes

See Table 5-5.

Induction of Labor

INDICATIONS

Medically indicated induction of labor is performed when the benefits of delivery to either the maternal or fetal status outweigh the risks of continuing the pregnancy.

EXAM TIP

Dystocia is the most common indication for primary cesarean delivery.

[handwritten:] consider membrane stripping!

WARD TIP

With the diagnosis of abnormal labor pattern, assess the three Ps:
- Power (contractions)
- Passenger (fetus)
- Pelvis

WARD TIP

In some cases, an immature fetus may be delivered due to maternal illness.

TABLE 5-5. Pelvis Shapes

	GYNECOID	ANDROID	ANTHROPOID	PLATYPELLOID
Frequency	In 50% of all females	One third of white women; one sixth of nonwhite women	One fourth of white women; one half of nonwhite women	Rarest, <3% of women
Inlet shape	Round	Heart shaped	Vertically oriented oval	Horizontally oriented oval
Sidewalls	Straight	Convergent	Convergent	Divergent, then convergent
Ischial spines	Not prominent (diameter ≥10 cm)	Prominent (diameter <10 cm)	Prominent (diameter <10 cm)	Not prominent (diameter >10 cm)
Sacrum	Inclined neither anteriorly nor posteriorly	Forward and straight with little curvature	Straight = pelvis deeper than other three types	Well curved and rotated backward; short = shallow pelvis
Significance	Good prognosis for vaginal delivery	Limited posterior space for fetal head → poor prognosis for vaginal delivery	Good prognosis for vaginal delivery; commonly seen with OP position	Poor prognosis for vaginal delivery

- **Maternal:**
  - Fetal demise.
  - Prolonged pregnancy.
  - Chorioamnionitis.
  - Severe preeclampsia/eclampsia.
  - Maternal conditions: Diabetes, renal disease, chronic pulmonary disease, chronic hypertension, antiphospholipid syndrome.
- **Fetal:**
  - Intrauterine growth retardation (IUGR).
  - Abnormal fetal testing.
  - Infection.
  - Isoimmunization.
  - Oligohydramnios.
  - Postterm.
  - Premature ROM.

CONTRAINDICATIONS

- **Maternal:**
  - Placenta or vasa previa.
  - Prior uterine surgery/malpresentation.

- - Classical cesarean delivery.
  - Active genital herpes infection.
  - Previous myomectomy.
- **Fetal:**
  - Acute distress.
  - Transverse fetal lie.
  - Cord prolapse.

CONFIRMATION OF FETAL MATURITY

Elective induction and/or cesarean should have fetal maturity documented by accurate dating criteria or amniocentesis. Elective indicates that there is no medical reason for delivery of fetus; it is more for convenience.

Dating Criteria

1. Documented fetal heart tones for 30 weeks by Doppler.
2. 36 weeks since a positive urine or serum pregnancy test.
3. Ultrasound of crown-rump length at 6–11 weeks dates the pregnancy and supports a gestational age of 39 weeks or more (gestational age is determined by the ultrasound).
4. Ultrasound at 12–20 weeks confirms a gestational age of 39 weeks or more determined by clinical history (LMP) and physical exam (ultrasound gestational age is consistent with LMP).

INDUCTION METHODS

Oxytocin

- A synthetic polypeptide hormone that stimulates uterine contraction.
- Acts promptly when given intravenously. Half-life about 5 min.

COMPLICATIONS

- Potent antidiuretic effects of oxytocin in high doses can cause water intoxication (i.e., hyponatremia), which can lead to convulsions, coma, and death. Oxytocin is related structurally and functionally to vasopressin or antidiuretic hormone.
- Risk of hyperstimulation: Frequent, strong contractions that cause an abnormality in the FHR.

oxytocin and ADH closely related in structure. can cause a hyponatremia.

Prostaglandins

- Misoprostol, a synthetic PGE$_1$ analog:
  - Can be administered intravaginally or orally.
  - Used for cervical ripening and induction.
- PGE$_2$ gel and vaginal insert:
  - Both contain dinoprostone.
  - Used for cervical ripening in women at or near term.

Mechanical

- Foley balloon: Passed through the internal cervical os into the extra-amniotic space, inflated and rested with traction on the internal os to cause dilation.
- Laminaria: Organic/synthetic material (i.e., seaweed) that slowly hygroscopically expands when placed in the cervix.

The term *cephalopelvic disproportion* (CPD) has been used to describe a disparity between the size of the maternal pelvis and the fetal head that precludes vaginal delivery. This condition can rarely be diagnosed with certainty and is often due to malposition of the fetal head (i.e., asynclitism).

Cephalopelvic disproportion (CPD) leads to failure to progress and cesarean delivery.

The most common reason for cesarean delivery (CD) = previous CD.

The skin incision on the maternal abdomen does not tell you the type of uterine incision the patient received. For example, a woman may have a midline skin incision but a low-transverse uterine incision.

Remember, if a young woman has an 18- or 20-week-size uterus but a negative pregnancy test, the most likely diagnosis is a fibroid uterus.

Cesarean Delivery (CD)

The birth of a fetus through incisions in the abdominal wall (laparotomy) and the uterine wall (hysterotomy).

TYPES (SEE FIGURE 5-9)

1. Low-transverse cesarean (LTC):
   - Horizontal incision made in lower uterine segment.
   - Most common type performed.
2. Classical:
   - Vertical incision made in the contractile portion of uterine corpus.
   - Performed when:
     - Lower uterine segment is not developed (i.e., extreme prematurity).
     - Fetus is transverse lie with back down.
     - Placenta previa.

INDICATIONS

- Prior cesarean (elective repeat, previous classical).
- Dystocia or failure to progress in labor.
- Breech presentation.
- Transverse lie.
- Concern for fetal well-being (i.e., nonreassuring fetal heart tones).
- Uterine malformations/scars.

Trial of Labor After Cesarean (TOLAC)

TOLAC is associated with a small but significant **risk of uterine rupture** with poor outcome for mother and infant:
- Classical uterine incision: 10% risk.
- Low-transverse incision: 1% risk.
- Maternal and infant complications are ↑ with a failed trial of labor followed by cesarean delivery.

CANDIDATES FOR TOLAC

- One LTC.
- Clinically adequate pelvis.

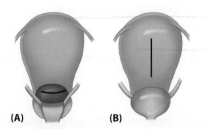

FIGURE 5-9.   Types of uterine incisions. (A) Low transverse. **(B)** Classical. (Reproduced, with permission, from Gabbe S, Niebyl J, Simpson J. *Obstetrics: Normal and Problem Pregnancies*, 5th ed. Philadelphia: Churchill Livingstone, 2007, Fig. 19-3. Copyright © Elsevier.)

- No other uterine scars or previous rupture.
- Physician immediately available throughout active labor capable of monitoring labor and performing an emergency CD.
- Availability of anesthesia and personnel for emergency CD.

CONTRAINDICATIONS TO TOLAC

- Prior classical or T-shaped incision or other transmyometrial uterine surgery.
- Contracted pelvis.
- Medical/obstetric complication that precludes vaginal delivery.
- Inability to perform emergency CD because of unavailable surgeon, anesthesia, sufficient staff, or facility.

Operative Vaginal Delivery

FORCEPS DELIVERY

Forceps are an important tool to allow for a vaginal delivery. The cervix must be fully dilated.

INDICATIONS

- Lack of progress in the second stage of labor.
- Fetal distress.
- Maternal factors: Exhaustion, heart disease, pulmonary edema, aneurysm, etc.
- After coming head for a breech delivery.

[handwritten margin note: lack of progress in 2nd stage of labor or maternal exhaustion]

CONTRAINDICATIONS

- Presenting part is not engaged.
- Position of head is not precisely known.
- Membranes are not ruptured.
- Cervix is not fully dilated.
- Presence of cephalopelvic disproportion.

VACUUM DELIVERY

- Same indications and contraindications as forceps.
- A safe, effective alternative to forceps delivery.
- A vertex fetus is required.
- Delivery should not be one that will require rotation or excessive traction.
- Prior scalp sampling is a contraindication.

ADVANTAGES

- Simpler to apply with fewer mistakes in application.
- Less force applied to fetal head.
- Less anesthesia is necessary (local anesthetic may suffice).
- No increase in diameter of presenting head.
- Less maternal soft-tissue injury.
- Less parental concern.

DISADVANTAGES

- Traction is applied only during contractions.
- Proper traction is necessary to avoid losing vacuum.

- Possible longer delivery than with forceps.
- Small ↑ in incidence of cephalohematomas.

Pain Control During Labor and Delivery

Three essentials of obstetric pain relief are simplicity, safety, and preservation of fetal homeostasis.

LOWER GENITAL TRACT INNERVATION

During the second stage of labor, much of the pain arises from the lower genital tract:

- Painful stimuli from the lower genital tract are primarily transmitted by the **pudendal nerve,** which passes beneath the posterior surface of the sacrospinous ligament (just as the ligament attaches to the ischial spine).
- The sensory nerve fibers of the pudendal nerve are derived from the ventral branches of the second, third, and fourth sacral nerves.

NONPHARMACOLOGICAL METHODS OF PAIN CONTROL

Women who are free from fear and who have confidence in their obstetrical staff require smaller amounts of pain medication:

- An understanding of pregnancy and the birth process.
- Appropriate antepartum training in breathing.
- Appropriate psychological support (e.g., by a friend or family member).
- Considerate obstetric care providers who instill confidence.

INTRAVENOUS ANALGESIA AND SEDATION

Pain relief with an opiate or opioid plus an antiemetic is typically sufficient, with no significant risk to the mother or infant:

- Discomfort is still felt during uterine contractions but is more tolerable.
- Slight ↑ in uterine activity.
- Does *not* prolong labor.

LOCAL ANESTHESIA

Administered before an episiotomy or after a delivery to repair a laceration.

REGIONAL ANESTHESIA

Nerve blocks that provide pain relief for women in labor and delivery without loss of consciousness.

Pudendal Block

- Local infiltration of the pudendal nerve with a local anesthetic agent (e.g., lidocaine) by obstetrician.
- Allows pinching of the lower vagina and posterior vulva bilaterally without pain.
- Effective, safe, and reliable method of providing analgesia for spontaneous delivery.

- Can be used along with epidural analgesia.
- **Complications:** Inadvertent intravascular injection will cause systemic toxicity, hematoma, infection.

Paracervical Block

- Agent is injected at the 3 o'clock and 9 o'clock positions around the cervix.
- Provides good relief of pain of uterine contractions during first stage of labor.
- Requires additional analgesia for delivery because the pudendal nerves are not blocked.
- **Complication:** Fetal bradycardia (usually transient).

Spinal (Subarachnoid) Block

- Introduction of local anesthetic into the subarachnoid space.
- Used for uncomplicated cesarean delivery and vaginal delivery.
- Provides excellent relief of pain from uterine contractions.
- Preceded by infusion of 1 L of crystalloid solution to prevent hypotension.
- Complications:
  - Maternal hypotension (common).
  - Total spinal blockade.
  - Spinal (postpuncture) headache—worse with sitting or standing.
  - Seizures.
  - Bladder dysfunction.
- Contraindications:
  - Severe preeclampsia: Hypotension from anesthesia can cause ischemic stroke.
  - Coagulation/hemostasis disorders.
  - Neurologic disorders.
  - Infection at the puncture site.
  - Surgical emergency.

Epidural Analgesia

- Injection of local anesthetic into the epidural or peridural space:
  - **Lumbar epidural analgesia:** Injection into a lumbar intervertebral space.
  - **Caudal epidural analgesia:** Injection through the sacral hiatus and sacral canal.
- Relieves pain of uterine contractions, abdominal delivery (block begins at the eighth thoracic level and extends to first sacral dermatome) or vaginal delivery (block begins from the tenth thoracic to the fifth sacral dermatome).
- Complications:
  - Inadvertent spinal blockade (puncture of dura with subarachnoid injection).
  - Ineffective analgesia.
  - Hypotension.
  - Seizures.
- Effects on Labor:
  - Longer second stage of labor (no significant impact on first stage of labor).
  - ↑ incidence of:
    - Chorioamnionitis.
    - Instrumental delivery.
    - Cesarean deliveries (although the incidence is higher, there is no causative link, and there may be other factors such as dysfunctional labor that contribute).
- Contraindications:
  - Same as spinal contraindications above.

WARD TIP

Always pull back on the syringe prior to injection of anesthetic to look for blood flow into the syringe; if present, you are in a vessel and must reposition your needle.

WARD TIP

When vaginal delivery is anticipated in 10 to 15 min, a rapidly acting agent is given through the epidural catheter to effect perineal analgesia.

* prolonged second stage
 - chorioamnionitis
 - instrumental deliv.
 - C/S.

WARD TIP

Prophylactic measures to avoid aspiration:
- Fasting for 6–8 hr.
- Administer antacids.
- Cricoid pressure before induction of anesthesia.

GENERAL ANESTHESIA

General anesthesia should not be induced until all steps preparatory to actual delivery have been completed, so as to minimize transfer of the agent to the fetus, thereby avoiding newborn respiratory depression.

CONCERNS

- **Fetal:** All anesthetic agents that depress the maternal CNS cross the placenta and depress the fetal CNS.
- **Maternal:** Induction of general anesthesia can cause aspiration of gastric contents, resulting in airway obstruction, pneumonitis, pulmonary edema, and/or death.

(handwritten notes)

active phase

protraction → cervical Δ slower than expected → oxytocin ± inadequate contractions

Arrest →
- no cervical Δ for ≥ 4 hrs w/ adequate contractions
- no cervical Δ for ≥ 6 hrs w/ inadequate contractions

CHAPTER 6

Postpartum

The Puerperium of the Normal Labor and Delivery

The **puerperium** is the period of confinement between birth and 6 weeks after delivery. During this time, the reproductive tract returns anatomically to a normal nonpregnant state.

UTERUS

Involution of the Uterine Corpus

Immediately after delivery, the fundus of the contracted uterus is slightly below the umbilicus. After the first 2 days postpartum, the uterus begins to shrink in size. Within 2 weeks, the uterus has descended into the cavity of the true pelvis. The contraction of the uterus immediately after delivery is critical for the achievement of hemostasis. "Afterpains" due to uterine contraction are common and may require analgesia. They typically ↓ in intensity by the third postpartum day.

Endometrial Changes

 A 27-year-old woman undergoes a spontaneous vaginal delivery and spontaneous placental delivery without lacerations. An hour later she has persistent vaginal bleeding. What is the likely diagnosis? What is the next step?
Answer: Most likely cause is uterine atony. Massage the fundus, which may feel boggy, and consider administration of uterotonics.

Within 2–3 days postpartum, the remaining decidua becomes differentiated into two layers:
1. Superficial layer becomes necrotic, sloughs off as vaginal discharge = *lochia*.
2. Basal layer (adjacent to the myometrium) becomes new endometrium.

Placental Site Involution

Within hours after delivery, the placental site consists of many thrombosed vessels. Immediately postpartum, the placental site is the size of the palm of the hand and rapidly ↓ in size.

Changes in Uterine Vessels

Large blood vessels are obliterated by hyaline changes and replaced by new, smaller vessels.

TABLE 6-1. Lochia

TYPE	DESCRIPTION	WHEN OBSERVED
Lochia rubra	Red due to blood in the lochia	Days 1–3
Lochia serosa	More pale in color	Days 4–10
Lochia alba	White to yellow-white due to leukocytes and reduced fluid content	Day 11 →

CERVIX

- The external os of the cervix contracts slowly and has narrowed by the end of the first week. The multiparous cervix takes on a characteristic fish mouth appearance.
- As a result of childbirth, the cervical epithelium undergoes much remodeling. Some women with cervical dysplasia will show regression after a vaginal delivery due to the remodeling of the cervix.

VAGINA

Gradually diminishes in size, but rarely returns to nulliparous dimensions:
- Rugae reappear by the third week.
- The rugae become obliterated after repeated childbirth and menopause.

PERITONEUM AND ABDOMINAL WALL

- The broad ligaments and round ligaments slowly relax to the nonpregnant state.
- The abdominal wall is soft and flabby due to the prolonged distention and rupture of the skin's elastic fibers; it resumes pre-pregnancy appearance in several weeks. However, the silver striae persist.

URINARY TRACT

- The puerperal bladder has an ↑ capacity and is relatively insensitive to intravesical fluid pressure. Hence, overdistention, incomplete bladder emptying, and excessive residual urine are common and can result in a urinary tract infection (UTI).
- Between days 2 and 5 postpartum, "puerperal diuresis" typically occurs to reverse the ↑ in extracellular water associated with normal pregnancy.
- Dilated ureters and renal pelves return to their pre-pregnant state 2–8 weeks postpartum.

HEMATOLOGY/CIRCULATION

- **Leukocytosis** occurs during and after labor (up to 30,000/µL).
- During the first few postpartum days, the **hemoglobin** and **hematocrit** fluctuate moderately from levels just prior to labor.
- **Plasma fibrinogen** and the **erythrocyte sedimentation rate** may remain elevated for ≥1 week postpartum.
- The **cardiac output** is higher than during pregnancy for ≥48 hours postpartum due to ↓ blood flow to the uterus (much smaller) and ↑ systemic intravascular volume.
- By 1 week postpartum, the **blood volume** has returned to the patient's nonpregnant range.

BODY WEIGHT

Most women approach their pre-pregnancy weight 6 months after delivery, but still retain approximately 1.4 kg of excess weight.
- Five to six kilograms are lost due to uterine evacuation and normal blood loss.
- Two to three kilograms are lost due to diuresis.

WARD TIP

At the completion of involution, the cervix does not resume its pregravid appearance:
- Before childbirth, the os is a small, regular, oval opening.
- After childbirth, the os is a horizontal slit.

WARD TIP

Instrument-assisted delivery and regional and general anesthesia are risk factors for postpartum urinary retention.

WARD TIP

All postpartum women who cannot void should be promptly catheterized.

EXAM TIP

The likelihood of cardiac overload is most likely in the immediate postpartum period, due to the autotransfusion of blood.

Routine Postpartum Care

IMMEDIATELY AFTER LABOR

First Hour

- Take blood pressure (BP) and heart rate (HR) at least every 15 min.
- Monitor the amount of vaginal bleeding.
- Palpate the fundus to ensure adequate contraction. If the uterus is relaxed, it should be massaged through the abdominal wall until it remains contracted. Massaging the uterus leads to ↑ release of oxytocin, which helps promote uterine contraction.

FIRST SEVERAL HOURS

Early Ambulation

Women are out of bed (OOB) within a few hours after delivery. Advantages include:
- **Reduced** frequency of puerperal venous thrombosis and pulmonary embolism.
- ↓ bladder complications.
- Less frequent constipation.

Care of the Vulva

The patient should be taught to cleanse and wipe the vulva from front to back (toward the anus).

If Episiotomy/Laceration Repair

- An ice pack should be applied for the first several hours to reduce edema and pain.
- At 24 hr postpartum, moist heat (e.g., via warm sitz baths) can ↓ local discomfort.
- The episiotomy incision is typically well healed and asymptomatic by week 3 of the puerperium.

Bladder Function

Ensure that the postpartum woman has voided within 4–6 hr of delivery. If not:
- This indicates further voiding trouble to follow.
- An indwelling catheter may be necessary.
- Bladder sensation and capability to empty may be diminished due to anesthesia.
- Consider a hematoma of the genital tract as a possible etiology.

THE FIRST FEW DAYS

Bowel Function

Encourage early ambulation and feeding to ↓ the possibility of constipation. Ask the patient about flatus.

If Fourth-Degree Laceration

Fecal incontinence may result, even with correct surgical repair, due to injury to the innervation of the pelvic floor musculature. Keep the patient on a stool softener and a low residue diet to avoid straining and ↓ risk of fistula formation. Avoid enemas or suppositories which can disrupt the repair.

WARD TIP

Hemostasis is obtained primarily by mechanical clamping of vessels by contracted myometrium.

EXAM TIP

Inadequate postpartum uterine contraction (= atony) is a major cause of early postpartum bleeding.

WARD TIP

Blood can accumulate within the uterus without visible vaginal bleeding: *Watch for:* Palpable uterine **enlargement** during the initial few hours postpartum.

WARD TIP

Sitz baths: Soaking the perineum in plain warm water or water with Epsom salts.

Discomfort/Pain Management

During the first few days of the puerperium, pain may result from:

- Afterpains: Contractions of the uterus as it involutes. Treat with nonsteroidal anti-inflammatory drugs (NSAIDs).
- Episiotomy/laceration pain: May require a narcotic medication, but NSAIDs or plain acetaminophen can help.
- Breast engorgement: Well-fitted with brassiere. NSAIDs.
- Postspinal puncture headache: Positional headache that is worse when upright, improved when lying down. Caffeine and hydration may help. Occasionally, patient may need a blood patch (performed by anesthesiologist).
- Constipation: Treat with stool softeners over 2–3 weeks. May discontinue iron supplementation if it worsens constipation.
- Urinary retention: May need intermittent bladder catheterizations. Evaluate the patient for causes and treat accordingly.

Abdominal Wall Relaxation

Exercise may be initiated any time after vaginal delivery and after abdominal discomfort has diminished after cesarean delivery.

Diet

- There are *no* dietary restrictions/requirements for women who have delivered vaginally. Two hours postpartum, the mother should be permitted to eat and drink. Those with an uncomplicated CD can be given clear liquids and regular diet as tolerated.
- Continue iron supplementation for a minimum of 3 months postpartum if tolerated.

Immunizations

- The non-isoimmunized D-negative mother whose baby is D-positive is given 300 µg of anti-D immune globulin within 72 hours of delivery.
- Mothers not previously immunized against/immune to rubella should be vaccinated prior to discharge. Rubella vaccine is not given during the pregnancy because it is a live attenuated virus.
- If the patient did not receive during pregnancy, she may be offered vaccinations against influenza and pertussis (tetanus-diphtheria toxoid, or Tdap).

WARD TIP

Kleihauer-Betke test detects fetal-maternal hemorrhage in Rh-negative mothers; 300 µg of anti-D immune globulin neutralizes 30 mL of fetal whole blood or 15 mL of Rh-positive RBCs.

WARD TIP

The uterine cavity is sterile before rupture of the amniotic sac.

Postpartum Infection

A 30-year-old G1P1001 is postpartum day 1 from a vaginal delivery over an intact perineum. On rounds, she reports lower abdominal pain. She reports no cough, back pain, leg pain, dysuria, or breast pain. She had a temperature of 100.1°F (37.8°C) 4 hr ago, and now has a temperature of 101.0°F (38.3°C). Her lungs are clear and her breasts are soft. There is no costovertebral angle tenderness (CVAT), suprapubic tenderness, or calf tenderness. She has fundal tenderness and foul-smelling lochia. She was admitted with ruptured membranes at 2 cm dilation and delivered after 20 hr in labor. Fetal heart tones were concerning for late decelerations, so she had internal monitors. She pushed for 3 hr before the infant was delivered. What is the most likely diagnosis? What risk factors did this patient have?

Answer: Endometritis. Fever, fundal tenderness, and foul-smelling lochia in the absence of other findings are consistent with endometritis. This patient's risk factors include prolonged rupture of membranes and internal monitors, and she likely had multiple vaginal exams during her long labor course.

WARD TIP

Cesarean delivery is an important risk factor for endometritis.

Pelvic infections are polymicrobial **ascending infections**. The bacteria responsible for pelvic infections are those that normally reside in the bowel and colonize the perineum, vagina, and cervix.

CAUSES

- **Gram-positive cocci:** Group A, B, and D streptococci.
- **Gram-positive bacilli:** *Clostridium* species, *Listeria monocytogenes.*
- **Aerobic gram-negative bacilli:** *Escherichia coli, Klebsiella, Proteus* species.
- **Anaerobic gram-negative bacilli:** *Bacteroides bivius, B. fragilis, B. disiens.*
- **Others:** *Mycoplasma hominis, Chlamydia trachomatis.*

RISK FACTORS

- Prolonged rupture of membranes >18 hr.
- Prolonged labor.
- Cesarean delivery
- Colonization of the lower genital tract with certain microorganisms (i.e., group B streptococci [GBS], *C. trachomatis, M. hominis,* and *Gardnerella vaginalis*).
- Preterm labor and birth.
- Multiple cervical exams.
- Manual extraction of placenta.
- Diabetes.
- Chorioamnionitis.
- Internal monitoring.

DIAGNOSIS

- Fever >100.4°F (38°C).
- Fundal tenderness.
- Rule out other sources of fever/infection (i.e., pyelonephritis, mastitis).

MANAGEMENT

Broad-spectrum antibiotics.

TYPES OF POSTPARTUM INFECTIONS

Endometritis (Metritis, Endomyometritis)

- A postpartum uterine infection involving the decidua, which may involve the myometrium and parametrial tissue.
- More common after cesarean delivery than vaginal delivery. Hypoxic tissue and foreign body (suture) with cesarean delivery increase risk for infection.
- Typically develops postpartum day 2–3.
- Treat with IV antibiotics until patient is afebrile for 24–48 hr.
- GBS colonization ↑ risk of endometritis.

Urinary Tract Infection

- Caused by catheterization, urinary stasis, birth trauma, conduction anesthesia, and frequent pelvic examinations.
- Presents with dysuria, frequency, urgency, and low-grade fever.
- Rule out pyelonephritis (costovertebral angle tenderness, pyuria, hematuria).
- Obtain a urinalysis and urinary culture (*E. coli* is isolated in 75% of postpartum women).
- Treat with appropriate antibiotics.

UTI → obtain UA + urine culture.

Cesarean Delivery: Surgical Site Infection (SSI)

 A 30-year-old G2P2002 is 2 weeks postoperative from a repeat cesarean delivery. She reports swelling around the incision site and ↑ tenderness. Her pain medications do not help. She reports a small amount of white malodorous drainage from the incision. She is tolerating her diet well and voiding spontaneously. On physical exam, she is afebrile. Her surgical site is indurated 2 cm around the incision and erythematous 3 cm around the incision. Purulent drainage is noted from a 1-cm opening at the right margin. What is the next step in management?

Answer: Next step is to differentiate whether this is a superficial or deep surgical site infection. The wound should be opened further and should be probed to evaluate whether the fascia is intact. Cultures should be obtained and the patient should receive antibiotics (usually IV).

DIAGNOSIS

- Fever, wound erythema and persistent tenderness, purulent drainage.
- Management: Obtain Gram stain and cultures from wound material.
- Wound should be drained, irrigated, and debrided.
- Antibiotics should be given along with:
  - Wet-to-dry packing if infection is superficial.
  - May need debridement if necrotic tissue is present. Consider necrotizing fasciitis.

Episiotomy Infection

- Look for pain at the episiotomy site, disruption of the wound, and a necrotic membrane over the wound.
- Rule out the presence of a rectovaginal fistula with a careful rectovaginal exam.
- Open, clean, and debride the wound to promote granulation tissue formation.
- Sitz baths are recommended.
- Reassess for possible closure after granulation tissue has appeared.

Discharge from Hospital

VAGINAL DELIVERY

One to two days postdelivery, if no complications. Return to the office at 4–6 weeks for postpartum exam.

CESAREAN DELIVERY

Two to three days postdelivery, if no complications. Return to the office in 2 weeks to check the incision if needed and 4–6 weeks for postpartum exam.

DISCHARGE INSTRUCTIONS

The patient should call the doctor or go to hospital if she develops:
- Fever >100.4°F (38°C).
- Excessive vaginal bleeding—soaking a pad an hour: Suspicious for retained placenta.
- Lower extremity pain and/or swelling: Suspicious for DVT.
- Shortness of breath: Suspicious for pulmonary embolus (PE).
- Chest pain—can occur with PE.

SSI
- superficial vs. deep.
- fascia intact?
- cultures
- broad spectrum Abx.

Postpartum intercourse

- After 6 weeks, intercourse may be resumed based on patient's desire and comfort. A vaginal lubricant may improve comfort.
- Dangers of premature intercourse:
  - Pain due to continued uterine involution and healing of lacerations/episiotomy scars.
- ↑ likelihood of hemorrhage and infection.

CONTRACEPTION

 A 25-year-old G1P1001 is postpartum day 2 from a vaginal delivery. She is overall healthy and is breast-feeding. She wants contraception that is easy to use. She reports that she had used a combination oral contraceptive pill prior to conceiving this baby and had no bad side effects. She is afraid of needles. What is the best contraceptive option for this patient?

Answer: Progestin-only pill. Progestin does not have an effect on breast milk, and it is easy to use.

- Do not wait until first menses to begin contraception; ovulation may come before first menses.
- Typically start contraceptive pills 2 weeks postpartum.
- See Contraception and Sterilization chapter.

Lactational Amenorrhea Method of Contraception

Lactational amenorrhea involves exclusive breast-feeding to prevent ovulation. It can be used as a contraceptive method. It is 98% effective for up to 6 months if:
- The mother is not menstruating.
- The mother is nursing >2–3 times per night, and more than every 4 hr during the day without other supplementation.
- The baby is <6 months old.

Oral Contraceptive Pills in Postpartum

- **Combined oral contraceptive pills** may reduce the amount of breast milk, and very small quantities of the hormones are excreted in the milk.
- **Progestin-only oral contraceptive pills** are 95% effective with typical use without substantially reducing the amount of breast milk. Need to take it the same time every day.

Depo-medroxyprogesterone

A progesterone-containing injection, given every 3 months, should not reduce breast milk production; 99% effective.

Intrauterine Device

May be inserted immediately postpartum (higher risk of expulsion) or interval insertion 6 weeks postpartum.

Implanon

A progestin-releasing implant that is placed in the arm; lasts for 3 years.

EXAM TIP

Nursing mothers rarely ovulate within the first 10 weeks after delivery. Non-nursing mothers typically ovulate 6–8 weeks after delivery.

Infant Care

Prior to discharge:

- Follow-up care arrangements should be made.
- All laboratory results should be normal, including:
  - Coombs' test.
  - Bilirubin.
  - Hemoglobin and hematocrit.
  - Blood glucose.
  - Maternal STD testing should be negative.
- Initial HBV vaccine should be administered.
- All screening tests required by law should be performed (e.g., testing for phenylketonuria [PKU] and hypothyroidism).
- Patient education regarding infant immunizations and well-baby care.

Breasts

DEVELOPMENT OF MILK-SECRETING MACHINERY

Progesterone, estrogen, placental lactogen, prolactin, cortisol, and insulin act together to stimulate the growth and development of the milk-secreting machinery of the mammary gland:

- Midpregnancy: Lobules of alveoli form lobes separated by stromal tissue, with secretion in some alveolar cells.
- T3: Alveolar lobules are almost fully developed, with cells full of protein-aceous secretory material.
- Postpartum: Rapid ↑ in cell size and in the number of secretory organelles. Alveoli distend with milk.

MILK DEVELOPMENT

- At delivery, the abrupt, large ↓ in progesterone and estrogen levels allow for milk production. All vitamins, except vitamin K, are found in human milk, necessitating neonatal administration of vitamin K to prevent hemorrhagic disease of the newborn.
- **Colostrum** can be expressed from the nipple by the second postpartum day and is secreted by the breasts for 5 days postpartum. It has more minerals and protein than breast milk. It has less sugar and fat when compared to breast milk. Antibodies in colostrum protect the infant against enteric organisms.

MATURE MILK AND LACTATION

- Colostrum is composed of protein, fat, carbohydrates (lactose), secretory IgA, and minerals.
- Milk comes in within the first week postpartum and is composed of protein, fat, carbohydrates (lactose), and water.
  - Protein: Colostrum > milk.
  - Fat: Milk > colostrum.
  - Carbs: Milk > colostrum.
- Colostrum is gradually converted to mature milk by 4 weeks postpartum. Subsequent lactation is primarily controlled by the repetitive stimulus of nursing and the presence of prolactin.

WARD TIP

Colostrum is a yellow-colored liquid secreted by the breasts that contains minerals, protein, fat, antibodies, complement, macrophages, lymphocytes, lysozymes, lactoferrin, and lactoperoxidase.

WARD TIP

Milk letdown may be provoked by the cry of the infant and suckling, and inhibited by stress or fright.

colostrum
↑ Ab (IgA)
↑ protein
↑ mineral

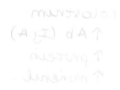

- Breast engorgement with milk is common on days 2–4 postpartum:
    - May be painful.
    - Often accompanied by transient temperature elevation.
    - May occur in non-breast-feeding women.
- Suckling stimulates the neurohypophysis to secrete oxytocin in a pulsatile fashion, causing contraction of myoepithelial cells and small milk ducts, which leads to milk expression.

LACTATION SUPPRESSION

A 26-year-old female who is 4 weeks postpartum presents with a 1-day history of fever of 100.9°F (38.3°C) and breast tenderness. She has been breast-feeding without problems and reports no other symptoms. Her left breast has a 4-cm area of induration and erythema at the 3 o'clock position that is tender to palpation. Milk expressed from that breast is white. What is the most likely diagnosis? What is the treatment?
Answer: Mastitis. Focal area of breast infection and fever approximately 1 month postpartum is consistent with mastitis. The patient should be started on dicloxacillin.

Women who do not want to breast-feed should wear a supportive bra, breast binder, or "sports bra." Pharmacologic therapy with bromocriptine is not recommended due to its associations with strokes, myocardial infarction, seizures, and psychiatric disturbances.

BREAST FEVER

Breast engorgement is a result of milk collecting in the breast.
- Occurs within 2–4 days of delivery. Seldom persists for >24 hr.
- Presents with **bilateral** painful, firm, globally swollen breasts.
- Rule out other causes of postpartum fever.
- Treat with supportive bra, 24 hr demand feedings, ice packs.
- **Mastitis** is an infection of the breast. It affects 1–2% of postpartum women. Approximately 3% of women with mastitis develop breast abscess.
    - Caused by:
        - *Staphylococcus aureus* from the infant's nasopharynx (40%), including MRSA. More likely to cause an abscess.
        - *Staphylococcus* coagulase negative, *Streptococcus viridans* (60%).
    - Presents approximately 4 weeks postpartum with fever, chills.
    - **Focal** area of erythema and induration with tenderness. No fluctuance.
    - May culture milk to identify the organism.
    - Treat with dicloxacillin for 7–10 days. Continue breast-feeding. Improves within 48 hr.
    - May continue breast-feeding.
- **Breast abscess** may follow mastitis:
    - Suspected when fever does not improve with antibiotic treatment within 48–72 hr.
    - A fluctuant, tender, palpable mass may be present.
    - Ultrasound can visualize the fluid collection.
    - Treat with broad-spectrum antibiotics and incision and drainage or ultrasound-guided needle aspiration.
    - In most cases, may continue breast-feeding or pumping breast milk.

BREAST-FEEDING

Human milk is the ideal food for neonates for the first 6 months of life.

Breast-fed infants are less prone to enteric infections than are bottle-fed babies.

Recommended Dietary Allowances

Lactating women need an extra 500 nutritious calories per day. Food choices should be guided by the Food Guide Pyramid, as recommended by the U.S. Department of Health and Human Services/U.S. Department of Agriculture.

Benefits

- Uterine involution: Nursing accelerates uterine involution (increases oxytocin).
- Immunity:
  - Colostrum and breast milk contain secretory IgA antibodies against *Escherichia coli* and other potential infections.
  - Milk contains memory T cells, which allows the fetus to benefit from maternal immunologic experience.
  - Colostrum contains interleukin-6, which stimulates an ↑ in breast milk mononuclear cells.
- Nutrients: All proteins are absorbed by babies, and all essential and nonessential amino acids available.
- Gastrointestinal (GI) maturation: Milk contains epidermal growth factor, which may promote growth and maturation of the intestinal mucosa.

Contraindications to Breast-Feeding

Mothers with the following infections:
- HIV infection.
- Breast lesions from active herpes simplex virus.
- Tuberculosis (active, untreated).
- Breast-feeding not contraindicated:
  - Cytomegalovirus (CMV): Both the virus and antibodies are present in breast milk.
  - Hepatitis B virus (HBV): If the infant receives hepatitis B immune globulin.
  - Hepatitis C: No documented evidence that breast-feeding spreads hepatitis C.
- **Medications:** Mothers ingesting the following contraindicated medications (not an exhaustive list):
  - Bromocriptine- and estrogen-containing oral contraceptives (OCPs) can suppress lactation.
  - Antineoplastic drugs such as cyclophosphamide (alkylating agent) or doxorubicin (anthracycline).
  - In most situations, the pros and cons of any medication must be weighed against the potential benefit to the mother, especially as it related to mental disorders.
- **Radiotherapy:** Mothers undergoing radiotherapy should not breastfeed. However, if the agent is being used as a diagnostic agent (i.e., CT with contrast), breast-feeding should be interrupted temporarily, but may be resumed after sufficient time (depends on dose administered).

WARD TIP

CMV, HBV, and HIV are excreted in breast milk.

EXAM TIP

A common misperception: Mothers who have a common cold should not breast-feed (false).

centra
- HIV, TB, HSV, ± HBV
- chemotherapeutic agents
- Bromocriptine, COCs.
- Radiotherapy.

EXAM TIP

What type of oral contraceptives is okay with breast-feeding? Progesterone-only OCPs.

EXAM TIP

Most drugs given to the mother are secreted in breast milk. However, the amount of drug ingested by the infant is typically small.

Postpartum Psychiatric Disorders

MATERNITY/POSTPARTUM BLUES

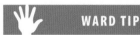 A 25-year-old G1P1001 presents 1 week postpartum with complaints of tearfulness, inability to sleep, fatigue, and decreased appetite. She has good support at home and is still very involved in taking care of her infant. What is the most likely diagnosis? What therapy should be offered?

Answer: Postpartum blues. She should be given supportive therapy with monitoring for more severe signs of depression.

Thirty percent of adolescent women develop postpartum depression.

A self-limited, mild mood disturbance due to biochemical factors and psychological stress:

- Affects 50% of women.
- Begins within 3–6 days after delivery.
- Usually resolves within 2 weeks.
- May be related to progesterone withdrawal.

SYMPTOMS

Similar to depression, but milder (see below).

TREATMENT

- Supportive—acknowledgment of the mother's feelings and reassurance.
- Monitor for the development of more severe symptoms (i.e., postpartum depression or psychosis).

POSTPARTUM DEPRESSION

WARD TIP

Criteria for Major Depression/ Postpartum Depression
Two-week period of depressed mood or anhedonia nearly every day plus four of the following. Symptoms must cause distress and not attributable to substance use or other medical condition.
1. Significant weight loss or weight gain without effort (or ↑ or ↓ in appetite).
2. Insomnia or hypersomnia.
3. Psychomotor agitation/retardation.
4. Fatigue or loss of energy.
5. Feelings of worthlessness/excessive or inappropriate guilt.
6. ↓ ability to concentrate/think.
7. Recurrent thoughts of suicide/death.

Similar to minor and major depression that can occur at any time:

- Classified as "postpartum depression" if it begins within 3–6 months after childbirth.
- Eight to fifteen percent of postpartum women develop postpartum depression within 2–3 months.
- Up to 70% recurrence.

SYMPTOMS

Symptoms are the same as major depression.

NATURAL COURSE

- Gradual improvement over the 6-month postpartum period.
- The mother may remain symptomatic for months to years.

TREATMENT

- Pharmacologic intervention is typically required:
  - Antidepressants.
  - Anxiolytic agents.
  - Electroconvulsive therapy.
- Mother should be co-managed with a psychiatrist or counselor (i.e., for psychotherapy to focus on any maternal fears or concerns).

POSTPARTUM PSYCHOSIS

- Mothers cannot discern real versus unreal (can have periods of lucidity). Hearing voices, seeing things.
- Occurs in 1–4 in 1000 births.
- Peak onset: 10–14 days postpartum, but may occur months later.

RISK FACTORS

- History of psychiatric illness.
- Family history of psychiatric disorders.
- Younger age.
- Primiparity.

COURSE

Variable and depends on the type of underlying illness; often 6 months.

TREATMENT

- Psychiatric care.
- Pharmacologic therapy.
- Hospitalization (in most cases).

seperate mem from baby!

Postpartum Thyroid Dysfunction

Postpartum thyroiditis is a transient lymphocytic thyroiditis in 5–10% of women during the first year after childbirth. The **two clinical phases** of postpartum thyroiditis are **thyrotoxicosis** and **hypothyroidism** (see Table 6-2).

TABLE 6-2. Thyrotoxicosis vs. Hypothyroidism

	THYROTOXICOSIS	HYPOTHYROIDISM
Onset	1–4 months postpartum	4–8 months postpartum
Mechanism	Destruction-induced hormone release	Thyroid insufficiency
Symptoms	Small, painless goiter Palpitations, fatigue	Goiter, fatigue, inability to concentrate
Treatment	β-blocker	Thyroxine for 6–12 months
Sequela	Two-thirds euthyroid One-third hypothyroid	One-third permanent hypothyroidism

NOTES

Medical Conditions in Pregnancy

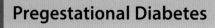

Pregestational Diabetes

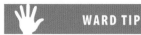

WARD TIP

Most common medical complication of pregnancy = diabetes (gestational + pregestational).

- Diabetes that existed before pregnancy:
  - Type 1 diabetes: Insulin deficiency due to destruction of pancreatic beta cells.
  - Type 2 diabetes: Defective insulin secretion or insulin resistance.
- Classes B through H in the White Classification (see Table 7-1).

DIAGNOSIS

- Classic symptoms:
  - Polyuria.
  - Polydipsia.
  - Unexplained weight loss.
- Fasting >126 mg/dL; random >200 mg/dL.

WARD TIP

Women with pregestational diabetes have higher maternal and fetal complications when compared to those with gestational diabetes.

MATERNAL COMPLICATIONS

- Gestational hypertension.
- Preeclampsia.
- Preterm delivery.
- Cesarean delivery.
- Polyhydramnios.
- Infections.
- Impaired wound healing.

TABLE 7-1. **Classification of Diabetes Complicating Pregnancy**

		PLASMA GLUCOSE LEVEL		
CLASS	ONSET	FASTING	2-HR POSTPRANDIAL	THERAPY
A₁	Gestational	<105 mg/dL	<120 mg/dL	Diet controlled
A₂	Gestational	>105 mg/dL	>120 mg/dL	Insulin
CLASS	AGE OF ONSET	DURATION (YR)	VASCULAR DISEASE	THERAPY
B	Over 20	<10	None	Insulin
C	10 to 19	10–19	None	Insulin
D	Before 10	>20	Benign retinopathy	Insulin
F	Any	Any	Nephropathy	Insulin
R	Any	Any	Proliferative retinopathy	Insulin
H	Any	Any	Heart	Insulin

(Reproduced, with permission, from Cunningham FG, Leveno KJ, Bloom SL, et al. *Williams Obstetrics*, 22nd ed. New York: McGraw-Hill. 2005: 1171.)

Handwritten notes (top right):
malfimatuns:
- NTD > cardiac > limb.
- macrosomnia / preterm.
- hypoglycemia territium
- polycythemia + hyperviscosity
- hyperbilirubinemia
- hypocalcemia
- NRDS.

FETAL COMPLICATIONS
- Preterm birth.
- Macrosomia.
- Fetal growth restriction.
- Congenital anomalies:
  - Caudal regression—absence of the sacrum with variable defects of the lower spine.
  - Cardiac anomalies.
  - Neural tube defects (NTDs).
  - ↑ risk of fetal anomalies in diabetes is due to poor glycemic control prior to conception and in early pregnancy (during organogenesis).
- Stillbirths—unexplained.
- Perinatal deaths.
- Neonatal hypoglycemia—chronic maternal hyperglycemia → hyperplasia of fetal β-islet cells → increased fetal insulin → rapid decline in fetal plasma glucose after delivery.
- Respiratory distress syndrome—likely due to earlier gestational age at delivery.
- Neonatal hypocalcemia.
- Neonatal hyperbilirubinemia.
- Polycythemia.

MANAGEMENT
Preconception
- Optimize glycemic control:
  - Preprandial: 70–100 mg/dL.
  - Postprandial: <140 mg/dL and <120 mg/dL at 1 and 2 hr, respectively.
  - Goal HbA$_{1C}$ is <6 mg/dL.
- HbA$_{1C}$ levels >10% significantly increase the risk of congenital malformations.
- Folic acid 0.4 mg/day during preconception and early pregnancy to ↓ risk of NTDs.
- Baseline 24-hr urine for total protein and creatinine clearance.
- Ophthalmologic exam.
- Electrocardiogram (ECG).
- Thyroid-stimulating hormone (TSH).

First Trimester
- Start individualized insulin regimen.
- Check fasting and 1-hr postprandial glucose.
- Viability ultrasound.
- Offer first trimester genetic screening (FTS or cfDNA).

Second Trimester
- 16–20 weeks: Offer quad screen if first trimester genetic screen not performed.
- 18–20 weeks: Targeted ultrasound (US) to evaluate for anomalies, then US every 4 weeks for growth.
- 20–22 weeks: Fetal echocardiogram looking for cardiac anomalies.

Third Trimester
- Antenatal testing at 32–34 weeks or when poor glycemic control.
- Consider amniocentesis for fetal lung maturity and delivery at 37 weeks if poor glycemic control.
- Consider delivery at 38 weeks without fetal lung maturity without amniocentesis if good glycemic control.
- Consider cesarean delivery if estimated fetal weight is >4500 g.
- Start insulin drip in labor for glycemic control.

WARD TIP

Diabetic ketoacidosis may be induced in patients with type 1 diabetes by:
- Corticosteroids (for lung maturity).
- β mimetics (for tocolysis).
- Hyperemesis gravidarum.
- Infections.

EXAM TIP

Gestational diabetes causes macrosomia, especially when fasting glucose is high. Pregestational diabetes causes growth restriction especially due to concurrent maternal vascular disease.

WARD TIP

Insulin requirements ↑ during the second trimester due to the antagonistic effect of pregnancy hormones. Immediately following delivery, insulin requirements dramatically ↓.

Thyroid Disease

Thyroid hormone is essential for the normal development of the fetal brain and mental function. The incidence of hyperthyroidism, hypothyroidism, and thyroiditis is each about 1%.

- TSH:
  - Essential for diagnosis of thyroid dysfunction in pregnancy.
  - Unchanged in pregnancy.
  - Does not cross the placenta.
- Free thyroxine (T_4): Unchanged in pregnancy.
- Thyroid-binding globulin ↑ in pregnancy.

HYPERTHYROIDISM

> A 32-year-old G2P1001 at 16 weeks presents with complaints of palpitations, nervousness, insomnia, and fatigue. Physical exam demonstrates a fine tremor in her hand, and pulse of 120 beats/min. What is the most likely diagnosis? What is the best treatment?
>
> **Answer:** She has symptoms most consistent with hyperthyroidism. Although this patient has many symptoms that are normal for pregnancy, she should be screened for thyroid disorder with TSH and free T_4. Hyperthyroidism should be treated with PTU or methimazole in pregnancy.

- Thyrotoxicosis complicates 1 in 2000 pregnancies.
- Graves' disease is the most common cause of thyrotoxicosis in pregnancy.

TREATMENT

- Ablation with radioactive iodine **contraindicated.**
- Propylthiouracil (PTU):
  - Drug of choice for treatment during the first trimester of pregnancy.
  - Risk of liver failure has decreased use outside of T1.
  - Inhibits conversion of T_4 to T_3.
  - Small amount transfers across the placenta.
- Methimazole:
  - Readily crosses placenta.
  - Associated with aplasia cutis and other teratogenic effects in fetus.
  - Currently used after T1, once organogenesis complete.
- Thyroidectomy:
  - Rarely necessary during pregnancy.
  - For women who fail medical management.

COMPLICATIONS

- Women who remain hyperthyroid despite treatment have higher incidence of preeclampsia, heart failure, and adverse perinatal outcomes (stillbirth, preterm labor).
- Neonatal thyrotoxicosis: 1% risk due to placental transfer of thyroid-stimulating antibodies.
- Fetal goiter/hypothyroid—from propylthiouracil (PTU).
- **Thyroid storm:** An acute, life-threatening, hypermetabolic state in patients with thyrotoxicosis. Often associated with heart failure. Treatment in intensive care unit (ICU) setting:
  - PTU orally or nasogastric tube.
  - β-blocker to control tachycardia.
  - Sodium iodide inhibits release of T_3 and T_4 (lithium if iodine allergic).
  - Dexamethasone blocks peripheral conversion of T_4 to T_3.

WARD TIP

Free T_4 and TSH do not change in pregnancy and are the most sensitive markers to detect thyroid disease.

WARD TIP

In normal pregnancy, total T_3, T_4, and thyroid-binding globulin (TBG) are elevated, but free thyroxine levels do not change = euthyroid.

(handwritten notes:)

(T1)   (T2, T3)
PTU → methimazole

Thyroid storm:

    — Fever
- tachycardia (>140) out of proportion to fever.
- AMS
- vomiting, diarrhea
- arrhythmias

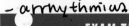

EXAM TIP

Hyperthyroidism (↑ free T_4, ↓ TSH) may be noted in hyperemesis gravidarum and gestational trophoblastic disease.

HYPOTHYROIDISM

- Hashimoto's thyroiditis is the most common cause of hypothyroidism during pregnancy.
- Subclinical hypothyroidism is more common than overt hypothyroidism.
  - Overt hypothyroidism is diagnosed by ↑ TSH and ↓ free T_4.
  - Subclinical hypothyroidism is an ↑ TSH with normal free T_4.
- Diagnosis may be difficult, as many of the symptoms of hypothyroidism (weight gain, fatigue, constipation, etc.) are also symptoms of pregnancy.
- The American College of Obstetricians and Gynecologists recommends **against** routine prenatal screening for subclinical hypothyroidism.

TREATMENT

Levothyroxine replacement:

- TSH is monitored every 8 weeks after the initiation of treatment or a change in dose.
- TSH is monitored every trimester if no change in medication is needed due to increased thyroxine requirements in advancing pregnancy.
- Usually requires 20% increase in dose once pregnancy is diagnosed.

COMPLICATIONS

- Preeclampsia.
- Placental abruption.
- Cardiac dysfunction.
- Low birth weight.
- Still births.

EXAM TIP

Hypothyroidism: ↑ TSH, ↓ Free T4
Subclinical Hypothyroidism:
↑ TSH, normal free T4

WARD TIP

Overt hypothyroidism is often associated with infertility and higher miscarriage rates.

Chronic Hypertension

A 37-year-old G3P2002 at 37 weeks by an unsure last menstrual period (LMP) presents to triage complaining of a severe headache for 1 day that is unrelieved with acetaminophen. Her pregnancy has been complicated by chronic hypertension that has been well controlled with Aldomet (methyldopa). Her blood pressures are normally 140/90. She had no proteinuria during her prenatal visits. She reports no visual changes, right upper quadrant pain, contractions, vaginal bleeding, or leakage of fluid. She reports good fetal movement. Her blood pressure is 180/110 and 175/100. She has 3+ proteinuria. Fetal heart rate is reassuring. What is the most likely diagnosis?

Answer: Chronic hypertension with superimposed preeclampsia. Women with chronic hypertension are at high risk for developing preeclampsia; worsening blood pressure and proteinuria can indicate the development of superimposed preeclampsia.

- Hypertension prior to 20th week of gestation.
- Prevalence is markedly ↑ in obese and diabetic patients.

PRECONCEPTION

Evaluate for renal and cardiac function:

- Echocardiography: Women with left ventricular hypertrophy or cardiac dysrhythmias indicate long-standing or poorly controlled hypertension leading to ↑ risk for congestive heart failure (CHF) in pregnancy.
- Serum creatinine and proteinuria: Abnormal results indicate risk for adverse pregnancy outcome.

WARD TIP

Poorly controlled hypertension and presence of end organ damage = ↑ adverse outcomes in pregnancy.

WARD TIP

Blood pressure is dynamic during pregnancy. It normally ↓ in T_2. If a patient with chronic hypertension is seen for the first time in T_2, she may appear normotensive.

COMPLICATIONS

- Superimposed preeclampsia: Development of preeclampsia in the setting of chronic hypertension. Infant may require delivery for maternal indications, even if premature.
- Abruptio placenta: ↑ risk with severe hypertension. Smoking compounds the risk.
- Fetal growth restriction: Directly related to the severity of hypertension.
- Preterm delivery.

MANAGEMENT

- Fetus should undergo testing to assess for adequate perfusion.
- Fetus should receive ultrasounds to monitor growth.
- Unless other complications develop, patients with chronic hypertension should deliver at term.
- Vaginal delivery is preferred to cesarean.

MEDICATIONS

- Labetalol: α- and β-adrenergic blocker.
- α-Methyldopa: Generally not used outside obstetrics.
- Hydralazine: Vasodilator.
- Nifedipine: Calcium channel blocker. Also used for tocolysis in preterm labor.
- Angiotensin-converting enzyme (ACE) inhibitors/angiotensin receptor blockers (ARBs): Not given due to teratogenic potential (hypocalvaria and renal defects).

Cardiovascular Disease

- Pregnancy-induced hemodynamic changes have profound effects on underlying heart disease. Cardiac output ↑ by 50% in midpregnancy.
- Need to monitor for CHF.
- Some congenital heart lesions are inherited. There is a 4% risk of congenital heart disease in the infant of a woman with a particular defect.
- Pain control:
  - Essential during labor and delivery to decrease the cardiac workload.
  - Continuous epidural anesthesia is recommended.
  - General anesthesia can cause hypotension.
- Vaginal delivery (spontaneous, forceps, vacuum) desired over cesarean delivery.

MITRAL STENOSIS (MS)

- ↑ preload due to normal ↑ in blood volume results in left atrial overload. ↑ pressure in the left atrium is transmitted into the lungs, resulting in **pulmonary hypertension (HTN)**.
- Tachycardia associated with labor and delivery exacerbates the pulmonary HTN because of decreased filling time. May lead to pulmonary edema.
- Twenty-five percent of women with mitral stenosis have cardiac failure for the first time during pregnancy.
- Fetus is at risk for growth restriction.
- **Peripartum period is the most hazardous time.**

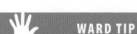

- Labetalol
- Nifedipine
- α-methyldopa
- Hydralazine

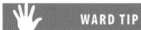

MITRAL VALVE PROLAPSE

- Normally asymptomatic.
- Systolic click on physical exam.
- Generally safe pregnancy.

AORTIC STENOSIS

- Similar problems with mitral stenosis.
- Avoid tachycardia and fluid overload.

EISENMENGER SYNDROME AND CONDITIONS WITH PULMONARY HYPERTENSION

- Extremely dangerous to the mother.
- This condition may justify the termination of pregnancy on medical grounds.
- Maternal mortality can be as high as **50%,** with death usually occurring postpartum.

Pulmonary Disease

The adaptations to the respiratory system during pregnancy must be able to satisfy the ↑ O_2 demands of the hyperdynamic circulation and the fetus. Advanced pregnancy may worsen the pathophysiological effects of many acute and chronic lung diseases.

ASTHMA

- Asthmatics have a small but significant ↑ in pregnancy complications.
- Fetal growth restriction ↑ with the severity of asthma.
- Arterial blood gases analysis provides objective information as to severity of asthma.

EPIDEMIOLOGY

- One to four percent of pregnancies are complicated by asthma.
- The impact of pregnancy on asthma is variable; roughly 1/3 improve, 1/3 worsen, and 1/3 stay the same.

TREATMENT

- Generally, asthma is exacerbated by respiratory tract infections, so killed influenza vaccine should be given.
- Pregnant asthmatics can be treated with β-agonists, epinephrine, and inhaled steroids (same medications used outside of pregnancy).

PNEUMONIA

COMPLICATIONS

- Premature rupture of membranes.
- Preterm delivery due to acidemia.

WARD TIP

Think: **PPSS**
Prolapse—okay to be **P**regnant
Stenosis—**S**ick in pregnancy

WARD TIP

F-series prostaglandins exacerbate asthma, so avoid in pregnancy.

WARD TIP

Severe pneumonia is a common cause of acute respiratory distress syndrome (ARDS).

MANAGEMENT

- **Any pregnant woman suspected of having pneumonia should undergo chest radiography (CXR) with an abdominal shield (indications are the same as in non-pregnant patients).**
- Abnormalities seen on CXR may take up to 6 weeks to resolve.
- Pneumococcal vaccine is not recommended for healthy pregnant patients. Use in patients who are immunocompromised or have severe cardiac/renal/pulmonary disease.
- Influenza vaccine is recommended for prevention in all trimesters.
- Antibiotics similar to nonpregnant women. For uncomplicated community-acquired pneumonia, treat with a beta-lactam (ceftriaxone, cefotaxime, ampicillin-sulbactam) plus azithromycin.
- Vancomycin is added for community-acquired methicillin-resistant *Staphylococcus aureus* (MRSA).

Renal and Urinary Tract Disorders

Pregnancy causes hydronephrosis (dilatation of renal pelvis, calyces, and ureters; R > L):
- Pregnant uterus compresses the lower ureter.
- Hormonal milieu ↓ ureteral tone (progesterone).
- Urinary stasis and ↑ vesicoureteral reflux lead to increased risk of pyelonephritis.

ASYMPTOMATIC BACTERIURIA

- Five percent incidence.
- If untreated, 25% will develop pyelonephritis.
- Routine screening at the first prenatal visit recommended.

PYELONEPHRITIS

> A 23-year-old G3P2002 at 25 weeks presents to triage with fever, nausea, and vomiting for 1 day. She complains of back pain and lower abdominal pain. She has a fever of 101.2°F (38.4°C), clear lungs, and right costovertebral tenderness. Fetal heart rate is reassuring. The monitor shows contractions every 2 min. Cervix is closed/thick/high. Urine dip shows many bacteria, leukocytes, nitrites, and ketones. What is the most likely diagnosis? What is the next step in management?
> **Answer:** The clinical presentation is most consistent with pyelonephritis. She should be admitted to the hospital and given IV hydration and IV antibiotics.

- Acute pyelonephritis is the most common serious medical complication of pregnancy.
- Unilateral, right-sided >50% of cases.
- *Escherichia coli* cultured 80% of cases.
- Bacteremia in 15–20% of women with acute pyelonephritis.

COMPLICATIONS

- Renal dysfunction: ↑ creatinine.
- Pulmonary edema: Endotoxin-induced alveolar injury.
- ARDS.
- Hemolysis.
- Preterm labor.

WARD TIP

Pregnant women with asymptomatic bacteriuria should be treated because of their ↑ risk of developing pyelonephritis.

WARD TIP

Hydronephrosis: Usually R > L

WARD TIP

Highest incidence of asymptomatic bacteriuria: African-Americans with sickle-cell trait.

WARD TIP

Most common cause of septic shock in pregnancy: Urosepsis.

DIFFERENTIAL DIAGNOSIS
- Preterm labor.
- Chorioamnionitis.
- Appendicitis.
- Placental abruption.

MANAGEMENT
- Hospitalization.
- IV antibiotics, usually cephalosporins (pending sensitivity studies).
- .IV hydration for adequate urinary output.
- Long-term antibiotic suppression for remainder of pregnancy is warranted.

Gastrointestinal Disorders

During advanced pregnancy, gastrointestinal (GI) symptoms become difficult to assess, and physical findings are often obscured by the enlarged uterus.

DIFFERENTIAL DIAGNOSIS OF ACUTE ABDOMEN

- Pyelonephritis.
- Appendicitis.
- Pancreatitis.
- Cholecystitis.
- Ovarian torsion.
- Ectopic pregnancy (early pregnancy).
- Labor.

APPENDICITIS

- Appendicitis is the most common surgical condition in pregnancy (occurs in 1 in 2000 births).
- Incidence is same throughout pregnancy, but rupture is more frequent in third trimester (40%) than first (10%).
- Symptoms of appendicitis, such as nausea, vomiting, and anorexia, may also be a part of normal pregnancy complaints, making diagnosis difficult.
- Uterus displaces the appendix superiorly and laterally. Pain may not be located at McBurney's point (RLQ).
- Physical exam may be obscured from the enlarging uterus.

COMPLICATIONS
- Abortion.
- Preterm labor.
- Maternal-fetal sepsis → neonatal neurologic injury.

TREATMENT
- Appendectomy.
- Laparoscopy (early pregnancy when uterus is small).
- Laparotomy in later pregnancy.

CHOLELITHIASIS AND CHOLECYSTITIS

- Incidence of cholecystitis is 1 in 1000 pregnancies (more common than nonpregnant).
- Same clinical picture as nonpregnant.

EXAM TIP

Most common cause of persistent pyelonephritis despite adequate therapy: Nephrolithiasis.

WARD TIP

Increased estrogen in pregnancy → increased cholesterol saturation in bile → increased biliary stasis and gallstones.

WARD TIP

Most common indications for surgery in pregnancy:
- Appendicitis
- Adnexal masses
- Cholecystitis

- Medical management unless common bile duct obstruction or pancreatitis develops, in which case a cholecystectomy should be performed.
- High risk of preterm labor.

Seizure Disorder

COMPLICATIONS

- Women with epilepsy taking anticonvulsants during pregnancy have double the general population risk of fetal malformations and preeclampsia.
- Women with a seizure disorder have an ↑ risk of birth defects even when they do not take anticonvulsant medications.
- Pregnant epileptics are more prone to seizures due to the associated stress and fatigue of pregnancy.
- The fetus is at risk for megaloblastic anemia.

TREATMENT

- Management of the epileptic female should begin with pre-pregnancy counseling.
- Anticonvulsant therapy should be reduced to the minimum dose of the minimum number of anticonvulsant medications.
- Folic acid supplementation should be taken by those women taking anticonvulsants.
- Once pregnant, the fetus should be screened for NTDs and congenital malformations.
- Blood levels of anticonvulsant medications should be checked at the beginning of pregnancy to determine the drug level that controls epileptic episodes successfully.

Thromboembolic Disorders

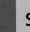 A 27-year-old G1 at 26 weeks presents with swelling of the left leg and thigh since the previous night. She reports no trauma, dyspnea, or chest pain. She is afebrile and in no apparent distress. Her left calf measures 4 cm more than the right and is tender to palpation. The fetal status is reassuring. What is the most likely diagnosis?
Answer: Deep vein thrombosis.

DEEP VEIN THROMBOSIS (DVT)

SIGNS AND SYMPTOMS

- Calf/leg swelling.
- Calf pain.
- Palpable cord in calf.

DIAGNOSIS (FIGURE 7-1)

- Venography: Gold standard. Many complications, time consuming, cumbersome.
- Impedance plethysmography: Better for larger veins.
- Compression ultrasonography: Test most often used currently.

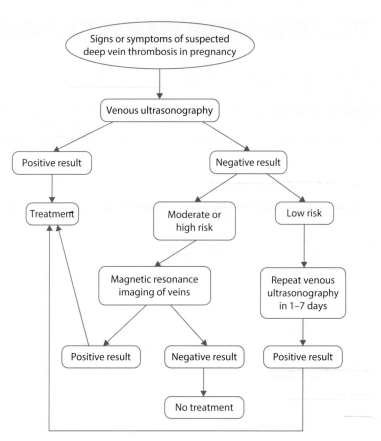

D-dimer ↑ in infections, malignancy, pregnancy, post-op; d-dimer is not useful in pregnancy.

FIGURE 7-1. **Diagnosis of Deep Venous Thrombosis.** (Reproduced, with permission, from Silver R, Lockwood C. *Clinical Updates in Women's Health Care: Thrombosis, Thrombophilia, and Thromboembolism*, Vol. XV, No. 3. American College of Obstetricians and Gynecologists, May 2016. Figure 4.)

COMPLICATIONS

Pulmonary embolism develops in about 25% of patients with untreated DVT.

TREATMENT

- Anticoagulation with unfractionated or low-molecular-weight heparin (LMWH) during pregnancy.
- Heparin should be suspended during labor and delivery (ideally 12–24 hr before onset of labor if known) and restarted after 12–48 hr, depending on the degree of trauma to the genital tract.
- Okay to convert to warfarin postpartum (do **not** use warfarin when pregnant), or continue LMWH.
- Anticoagulation ↓ the risk of pulmonary embolism to <5%.

PULMONARY EMBOLISM (PE)

- **Symptoms:** Dyspnea, chest pain, cough, syncope, hemoptysis.
- **Signs:** Tachypnea, tachycardia, apprehension, rales, hypoxemia.
- **Diagnosis:** CT pulmonary angiography or lung scintigraphy (ventilation/perfusion or V/Q scan) *→ preferred; CT ↑ radiation exposure.*
- **Complications** include maternal death.
- **Treatment:** Anticoagulation with heparin/LMWH.
- Half of women presenting with a DVT will have a "silent" PE.

WARD TIP

Warfarin is a teratogen, so not used in pregnancy. Can breast-feed with it postpartum.

WARD TIP

Pulmonary embolus may originate in the iliac veins rather than the calf in pregnancy.

WARD TIP

Antithrombin deficiency: Most thrombogenic of the heritable coagulopathies.

THROMBOPHILIAS

- ↑ risk of thrombus formation and associated complications.
- **Antithrombin III deficiency:** The most thrombogenic of the heritable coagulopathies.
- **Protein C deficiency:** 6- to 12-fold ↑ risk of first venous thromboembolism (VTE) in pregnancy.
- **Protein S deficiency:** Two- to sixfold ↑ risk of first VTE in pregnancy.
- **Factor V Leiden mutation:**
  - Most common heritable thrombophilia; 5–8% of the general population.
  - Heterozygous inheritance.
  - Four- to eightfold ↑ risk of first VTE in pregnancy.
- **Antiphospholipid antibodies:** Commonly seen in patients with lupus. See section Antiphospholipid Syndrome.
- **Prothrombin G20210A mutation.**
- **Hyperhomocysteinemia.**

WARD TIP

Most common thrombophilia: Factor V Leiden mutation, often diagnosed when an asymptomatic woman starts combination oral contraceptive pills and develops a blood clot.

EXAM TIP

How do you treat a pregnant woman with a deep vein thrombosis (DVT)? Heparin or low-molecular-weight heparin. **Do not use** coumadin.

COMPLICATIONS

- Preeclampsia/eclampsia.
- HELLP syndrome (hemolysis, elevated liver enzymes, low platelets).
- Fetal growth restriction.
- Placental abruption.
- Recurrent abortion.
- Stillbirth.

TREATMENT

Heparin or LMWH.

Sickle Cell Disease

- Red cells with hemoglobin S undergo sickling with ↓ oxygen leading to cell membrane damage.
- One in 12 African-Americans are carriers.
- **Sickle-cell crisis:** Pain due to ischemia and infarction in various organs. Infarction of bone marrow causes severe bone pain.
- Crisis more common in pregnancy.
- Acute chest syndrome: Pleuritic chest pain, fever, cough, lung infiltrates, hypoxia.

PREGNANCY COMPLICATIONS

- Thromboses (cerebral vein thrombosis, DVT, PE).
- Pneumonia.
- Pyelonephritis.
- Sepsis syndrome.
- Gestational HTN, preeclampsia, or eclampsia.

functional asplenia → encapsulated organisms

DELIVERY COMPLICATIONS

- Placental abruption.
- Preterm delivery.
- Fetal growth restriction.
- Stillbirth.

MANAGEMENT

- Supplementation with 4 mg/day of folic acid to accommodate for rapid cell turnover.
- IV hydration and pain control for crises.
- Administer oxygen via nasal cannula to ↓ sickling.
- Prophylactic blood transfusions throughout pregnancy are **controversial.**

Anemia

- Physiologic Anemia during pregnancy is due to a greater expansion of plasma volume relative to increase in RBC mass (hemodilution).
- Anemia during pregnancy also occurs due to iron deficiency.
- The CDC defines anemia during pregnancy as a hemoglobin <11 g/dL.

INCIDENCE

Sixteen to twenty-nine percent of pregnant women become anemic during T3.

COMPLICATIONS

- Preterm delivery.
- Intrauterine growth restriction (IUGR).
- Low birth weight.

TREATMENT

Two hundred milligrams of elemental iron daily from either ferrous sulfate, fumarate, or gluconate.

WARD TIP

The two most common causes of anemia during pregnancy and the puerperium are iron deficiency and acute blood loss.

Antiphospholipid Syndrome

DIAGNOSIS

Clinical Criteria

- Arterial and venous thrombosis.
- Pregnancy morbidity:
  - At least one otherwise unexplained fetal death at or beyond 10 weeks.
  - At least one preterm birth before 34 weeks.
  - At least three consecutive spontaneous abortions before 10 weeks.
- Puerperium:
  - Fe deficiency.
  - Acute blood loss.

[handwritten margin notes:]
- ≥1 fetal death >10 weeks
- ≥3 spontaneous abortus <10 weeks
- preterm birth before 34 weeks.

Laboratory Criteria

- Lupus anticoagulant.
- Medium to high titers of anticardiolipin antibody.
- Anti-β_2 glycoprotein.
- Each of these findings must be present in plasma, on at least two occasions >12 weeks apart.

MANAGEMENT

Ranges from no treatment to daily low-dose aspirin to heparin, depending on the patient's past history of thrombosis and pregnancy morbidity.

Systemic Lupus Erythematosus

COMPLICATIONS

Significant ↑ in maternal morbidity/mortality and other complications:

- Preeclampsia.
- Preterm labor.
- Fetal growth restriction.
- Anemia.
- Thrombophilia.
- Neonates may have symptoms of lupus for several months after birth.
- **Congenital heart block** may be seen in the offspring of women with anti-Ro (SS-A) and anti-La (SS-B).

MANAGEMENT

- Patients should be counseled to get pregnant while their disease is in remission.
- Monitor for disease flares and hypertensive episodes.
- Unless there is evidence of fetal compromise, the pregnancy should progress to term.
- High-dose methylprednisolone can be given for a lupus flare.
- Azathioprine is an immunosuppressant that can be used safely in pregnancy.
- Cyclophosphamide, methotrexate, and mycophenolate mofetil should be avoided, or at least not started until after 12 weeks' gestation. The risks and benefits should always be weighed.

EXAM TIP

Presence of anti-Ro (SS-A) and anti-La (SS-B) is associated with fetal congenital heart block.

— IV methyl prednisolone for flairs
— Azathioprine for meunt.

WARD TIP

Rule of thumb for pregnant patients with lupus: one-third get better, one-third get worse, and one-third remain the same.

Pruritic Urticarial Papules and Plaques of Pregnancy (PUPPP)

INCIDENCE

- The most common pruritic dermatosis in pregnancy.
- Incidence is 1/160–1/300 singleton pregnancies, 8- to 12- fold ↑ with multiples.
- Seldom occurs in subsequent pregnancies.

CLINICAL SIGNS AND SYMPTOMS

- Intensely pruritic cutaneous eruption that usually appears late in pregnancy.
- Usually starts as erythematous papules within stria with periumbilical sparing.
- Begins on the abdomen and spread to arms and legs. Coalesces to form urticarial plaques. The face, palms, and soles are usually spared.

TREATMENT

- Oral antihistamines and topical steroids are the mainstays of treatment.
- May require systemic corticosteroids for severe pruritus.
- Rash usually disappears shortly before or a few days after delivery.

↑ risk w/ multifetal gestation!

Cancer Therapy During Pregnancy

SURGERY

As long as the reproductive organs are not involved, surgery is generally well tolerated by both the mother and fetus during pregnancy and should not be delayed.

RADIATION

- Therapeutic radiation can cause significant complications in the fetus, such as carcinogenesis, cell death, and brain damage.
- The most susceptible period is during organogenesis.
- The site of the tumor is important. Radiation to head and neck cancers can be done more safely than radiation to abdominal tumors.

CHEMOTHERAPY

- Risks to the fetus include malformations, growth restriction, intellectual disability, and the risk of future malignancies.
- Risk is highest during organogenesis. Few adverse outcomes are seen if chemotherapeutic agents are used after T1.

NOTES

CHAPTER 8

Obstetric Complications

Hypertension in Pregnancy

HYPERTENSIVE DISEASES OF PREGNANCY

A 28-year-old G2P1001 at 37 weeks complains of severe headaches and black spots in her vision. Her blood pressures are 165/95 and 163/96 and she has 4+ protein on urine dipstick. Her cervical exam is closed, thick, and high. The fetal heart tones are reassuring and she has no contractions. The ultrasound (US) shows a fetus that is appropriate for 37 weeks, with normal amniotic fluid index (AFI), and in cephalic position. What is the next best step?
Answer: This patient has signs and symptoms of severe preeclampsia and should be delivered immediately, especially when term. Vaginal delivery is usually attempted. Patients with preeclampsia can have a seizure at any point before, during, or after labor, so seizure prophylaxis with magnesium sulfate is indicated.

Hypertensive disorders of pregnancy include chronic hypertension (HTN), chronic HTN with superimposed preeclampsia, gestational hypertension, and preeclampsia. Eclampsia is the development of grand mal seizures in a woman with preeclampsia. HELLP (hemolysis, elevated liver enzymes, low platelets) is likely a severe form of preeclampsia, but this relationship is controversial because it may be seen in the absence of hypertension or proteinuria. These disorders may all be a spectrum of the same disease process that manifest at different levels of severity at different gestational ages.

Hypertension-related deaths in pregnancy account for 15% of maternal deaths (second after pulmonary embolism).

There are four categories of HTN in pregnancy:
1. **Preexisting or chronic HTN during pregnancy:**
   - Preexisting HTN begins prior to pregnancy or before 20 weeks.
   - Defined as a sustained systolic BP ≥140 mm Hg and/or diastolic BP ≥90 mm Hg documented on more than one occasion *prior* to the 20th week of gestation, HTN that existed before pregnancy, or HTN that persists >12 weeks after delivery.
   - Usually not associated with significant proteinuria or end-organ damage if well controlled.
2. **Gestational hypertension**:
   - Hypertension without proteinuria or other signs/symptoms of preeclampsia.
   - A sustained or transient systolic blood pressure (BP) ≥140 mm Hg and/or diastolic BP ≥90 mm Hg occurs after 20 weeks.
3. **Preeclampsia:**
   - Defined as new onset HTN with either proteinuria or end-organ dysfunction (or both) after 20 weeks (proteinuria no longer required to diagnose preeclampsia with severe features).
   - **Criteria for diagnosis of preeclampsia:**
     - Systolic BP ≥140 mm Hg or diastolic BP ≥90 mm Hg twice at least 4 hr apart. AND
     - Proteinuria: 1+ on dipstick or ≥300 mg/24 hr or protein (mg/dL)/creatinine (mg/dL) ratio ≥0.3.
     - In pregnant patients with new onset HTN without proteinuria, a new finding of any of the following is diagnostic of preeclampsia:
       - Thrombocytopenia (platelet <100,000/mL).
       - Serum creatinine >1.1 mg/dL or doubling of serum creatinine.
       - LFTs at least twice the normal concentration.

- Pulmonary edema.
- Cerebral or visual symptoms (headache, scotomata).
- **Preeclampsia with severe features** is defined by the presence of one of the following:
    - Severe BP elevation: systolic BP ≥160 mmHg or diastolic BP ≥110 mmHg at least 4 hr apart.
    - Neurologic dysfunction: headache, scotomata, altered mental status.
    - Renal abnormality: serum creatinine >1.1 mg/dL or doubling of serum creatinine.
    - Hepatic abnormality: Epigastric or right upper quadrant pain (hepatocellular ischemia and edema that stretches Glisson's capsule), ↑ aspartate transaminase (AST), alanine transaminase (ALT) ≥ twice the normal level, or both.
    - Pulmonary edema.
    - Thrombocytopenia (<100,000 platelets/μL).
4. **Superimposed preeclampsia:**
    - Preeclampsia in patients with chronic HTN in pregnancy.
    - Defined by new onset of either proteinuria or end-organ dysfunction after 20 weeks in a woman with chronic HTN.
    - For women with chronic HTN who have preexisting proteinuria, superimposed preeclampsia is defined by worsening HTN or development of severe features (see above).
    - Twenty-five percent of patients with chronic HTN in pregnancy develop preeclampsia.

PATHOPHYSIOLOGY

Vasospasm in various organs (brain, kidneys, lungs, uterus) causes most of the signs and symptoms of preeclampsia; however, the cause of the vasospasm is unknown.

The pathophysiology of preeclampsia has many factors that are poorly understood. However, one contributing factor is the method of development of placental vasculature in early pregnancy.

COMPLICATIONS

- Placental abruption.
- Eclampsia with possible intracranial hemorrhage.
- Coagulopathy.
- Renal failure.
- Hepatic subcapsular hematoma.
- Uteroplacental insufficiency.

TREATMENT

See Figure 8-1 for a management algorithm.
- The only cure for preeclampsia and its variants is **delivery** of the fetus.
- Preexisting chronic HTN in pregnancy: Antihypertensive medications versus close observation.
- **Magnesium sulfate (MgSO₄)** is given for **seizure prophylaxis** when the decision is made to deliver fetus or when expectantly managing a patient with severe preeclampsia. It is **not** a treatment for HTN.
- **Preeclampsia management:**
    - Preterm: Close monitoring for worsening maternal or fetal disease.
        - Antenatal testing: (non-stress tests [NSTs] and/or biophysical profiles [BPPs]) to ensure fetal well-being.
        - Bed rest is not necessary, although ↓ physical activity is recommended.
        - Administer steroids if indicated for fetal lung maturity.
        - Deliver based on gestational age, and maternal and fetal condition.

WARD TIP

In 2013, the American College of Obstetricians and Gynecologists (ACOG) removed massive proteinuria (5 g/24 hr), fetal growth restriction, and oliguria as criteria for preeclampsia with severe features.

WARD TIP

Preeclampsia is usually asymptomatic; it is critical to pick it up during routine prenatal visits.

WARD TIP

The only definitive treatment for preeclampsia is delivery.

WARD TIP

Magnesium toxicity (7–10 mEq/L) is associated with loss of patellar reflexes, respiratory depression, and cardiac arrest. Treat with calcium gluconate 10% solution 1 g IV.

WARD TIP

Magnesium sulfate prevents seizures in preeclampsia; does not treat HTN.

WARD TIP

When patients are given MgSO₄ for seizure prophylaxis, they must be closely monitored for magnesium toxicity by obtaining magnesium levels and watching for hyporeflexia.

WARD TIP

HTN may be absent in 20% of women with HELLP syndrome and severe in 50%.

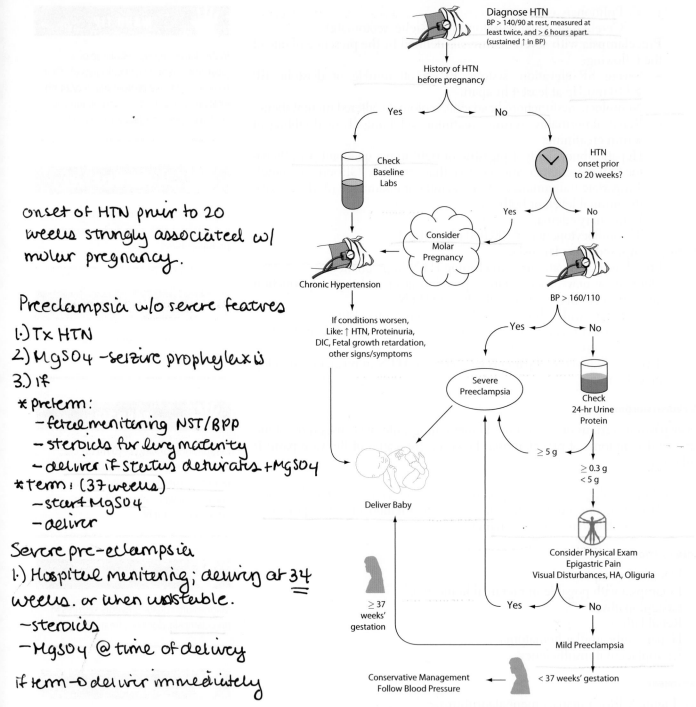

onset of HTN prior to 20
weeks strongly associated w/
molar pregnancy.

Preeclampsia w/o severe features

1.) Tx HTN
2.) MgSO4 – seizure prophylaxis
3.) if
* preterm:
  – fetal monitoring NST/BPP
  – steroids for lung maturity
  – deliver if status deteriorates + MgSO4
* term: (37 weeks)
  – start MgSO4
  – deliver

Severe pre-eclampsia
1.) Hospital monitoring; deliver at 34
weeks. or when unstable.
  – steroids
  – MgSO4 @ time of delivery

if term → deliver immediately

FIGURE 8-1. Management of hypertension in pregnancy. (Reproduced, with permission, from Lindarkis NM, Lott S. *Digging Up the Bones: Obstetrics and Gynecology*. New York, NY: McGraw-Hill Education, 1998: 60.)

- Term: delivery.
  - Vaginal delivery is usually attempted via induction of labor; cesarean delivery for other obstetric indications.
  - Start MgSO₄ for seizure prophylaxis.
- **Management of severe preeclampsia:**
  - Preterm: Close monitoring in hospital, and in general, deliver by 34 weeks or when the maternal or fetal condition is unstable.
    - Delivery may not be in the best interest of the premature baby, but may be indicated to prevent worsening maternal disease.

- Vaginal delivery is usually attempted via induction of labor; cesarean delivery for other obstetric indications.
- Start $MgSO_4$ for seizure prophylaxis.
- Administer steroids for fetal lung maturity.
- Term patients with severe preeclampsia should be delivered.

HELLP SYNDROME

- HELLP syndrome is likely a manifestation of severe preeclampsia with:
  - **H**emolysis.
  - **E**levated **L**iver enzymes.
  - **L**ow **P**latelets.
- It is associated with high morbidity, and immediate delivery is indicated. It may occur with or without HTN.

ECLAMPSIA

Defined as seizure or coma without another cause in a patient with preeclampsia. Eclampsia → hemorrhagic stroke → death.

TREATMENT

- Airway, breathing, and circulation (ABCs).
- Rule out other causes: Head trauma is a possible confounder; others include cerebral tumors, cerebral venous thrombosis, drug overdoses, epilepsy, and cerebrovascular accidents.
- Control seizures with magnesium sulfate (the only anticonvulsant used).
- Delivery is the only definitive treatment; expectant management is not appropriate.
  - Induction of labor may be appropriate to accomplish vaginal delivery, and factors such as gestational age, cervical exam, fetal position, and parity should be considered when deciding mode of delivery.
  - Control BP with hydralazine or labetalol.

RISK FACTORS FOR HYPERTENSIVE DISEASES IN PREGNANCY

- Nulliparity.
- Age >40 years.
- Family history of preeclampsia in first degree relative.
- Chronic HTN.
- Chronic renal disease.
- Antiphospholipid syndrome.
- Diabetes mellitus.
- Multiple gestation.
- History of preeclampsia in prior pregnancy.

ANTIHYPERTENSIVE AGENTS USED IN PREGNANCY

Short-Term Control

- **Hydralazine:** IV or PO, direct vasodilator. Side effects: systemic lupus erythematosus (SLE)-like syndrome, headache, palpitations.
- **Labetalol:** IV or PO, nonselective β_1 and α_1 blocker. Side effects: headache and tremor.

Long-Term Control

- **Methyldopa:** PO, false neurotransmitter. Side effects: postural hypotension, drowsiness, fluid retention.
- **Nifedipine:** PO, calcium channel blocker. Side effects: edema, dizziness.

WARD TIP

Objectives in management of severe preeclampsia:
1. Prevent eclampsia which can cause intracranial hemorrhage and damage to other vital organs
2. Deliver a healthy infant

WARD TIP

Diuretics are not used in pregnancy because they ↓ plasma volume and this may be detrimental to fetal growth. Salt restriction also ↓ plasma volume and is not recommended.

WARD TIP

Angiotensin-converting enzyme (ACE) inhibitors are contraindicated because they are teratogenic. Use other classes of antihypertensives to control HTN in pregnancy.

EXAM TIP

Eclampsia:
- 60% of seizures are before labor.
- 20% of seizures are during labor.
- 20% of seizures are postdelivery (most occur within one week of delivery).

Gestational Diabetes Mellitus

 A 33-year-old G4P3003 at 26 weeks undergoes the 50-g glucose challenge test. The result is 160 mg/dL. What is the next step in management?
Answer: She should undergo the 3-hr glucose tolerance test since her 1-hr result was >140 mg/dL.

- **Pregestational diabetes (DM):** Patient diagnosed with DM prior to pregnancy.
- **Gestational diabetes (GDM):** Patient develops diabetes only during pregnancy.
  - Prevalence in 6–7% of population.
  - White Classification A1: Controlled with diet.
  - White Classification A2: Requires insulin or oral agents.

SCREENING

When obtaining a patient's history, look for risk factors for gestational diabetes or undiagnosed type 2 diabetes. This will direct screening. If patient is suspected of having type 2 diabetes, order HbA1c at first visit.
- See Chapter 7 regarding Pregestational Diabetes.
- **Risk factors:**
  - Age >35.
  - Prior pregnancy with gestational diabetes.
  - Family history of diabetes in a first degree relative.
  - Obesity (BMI >30).
  - Previous infant >4000 g (8¾ lb).
  - History of stillbirth or child with cardiac defects (poor obstetrical outcome).
  - Race: Black, Hispanic, Native American.
- Screening for GDM:
  - Two-step approach:
    - Most widely used.
    - First step is glucose challenge to identify patients at high risk.
    - Second step is diagnostic test.
  - One-step approach.
    - One step diagnostic test; omits screening.

TWO-STEP APPROACH

- **Glucose challenge test** at 24–28 weeks:
  - Give 50-g glucose load (nonfasting state).
  - Draw glucose blood level 1 hr later.
  - If ≥140, a 3-hr glucose tolerance test (GTT) is then administered to diagnose GDM.
  - If >200, patient is diagnosed with GDM and a diabetic diet is initiated.
- **3-hr GTT**—if glucose challenge test is ≥140 and <200:
  - Fast at least 8 hr.
  - Draw fasting glucose level.
  - Give 100-g glucose load.
  - Draw glucose levels at 1 hr, 2 hr, and 3 hr.
  - Diagnosis of GDM made if two or more values are equal to or greater than those listed (see Table 8-1). Either criterion can be used to make the diagnosis.

EXAM TIP

What is a major fetal complication of gestational diabetes mellitus? Macrosomia

if pt obese, test for diabetes at first visit.

EXAM TIP

Diabetes is the most common medical complication of pregnancy.

EXAM TIP

Gestational diabetes probably results from human placental lactogen secreted during pregnancy, which has large glucagon-like effects.

WARD TIP

If a pregnant woman has an abnormal 1-hr glucose challenge test, then check a 3-hr GTT.

TABLE 8-1.   Diagnosis of Gestational Diabetes

Diagnosis of Gestational Diabetes with 2-hr 75-g glucose load GTT International Association of Diabetes and Pregnancy Study Groups (IADPSG) and American Diabetes Association (ADA) Criteria	
Fasting	≥92 mg/dL
OR	
One hour	≥180 mg/dL
OR	
Two hour	≥153 mg/dL

ONE-STEP APPROACH

- Administer a 75-g 2-hr oral GTT.
- Fast at least 8 hr.
- Draw fasting glucose level.
- Give 75-g glucose load.
- Draw glucose levels at 1 hr and 2 hr.
- Diagnosis of GDM made if one of the three values is elevated (see Table 8-1).

MATERNAL EFFECTS

- Four times ↑ risk of preeclampsia.
- ↑ risk of bacterial infections.
- Higher rate of cesarean delivery.
- ↑ risk of polyhydramnios.
- ↑ risk of birth injury.
- ↑ lifetime risk of type 2 diabetes.

> **EXAM TIP**
>
> Thirty percent of women with gestational diabetes develop diabetes mellitus in later life.

FETAL EFFECTS

- ↑ risk of perinatal death.
- Fetal anomalies not ↑ in gestational diabetes (as opposed to pregestational diabetes).
- Hyperinsulinemia → fetal macrosomia → birth injury (shoulder dystocia).
  - Hyperglycemia affects most fetal organs except brain.
  - Excessive fat on shoulders and trunk.
- Metabolic derangements at birth (hypoglycemia, hypocalcemia).

> **EXAM TIP**
>
> The CNS anomaly most specific to DM is **caudal regression**.

MANAGEMENT

The key factors involved in successful management of these high-risk pregnancies include:

- A glucose control log should be checked at each prenatal visit.
- Maintain fasting glucose <95 and 2-hr postprandial (breakfast, lunch, dinner) glucose <135.
- If A1 with continued ↑ in glucose, start oral hypoglycemic agent (glyburide, metformin) or insulin.
- If A2 with continued ↑ in glucose, ↑ insulin or oral agent dose.
- If A2 on oral agent with continued ↑ in glucose, switch to insulin.
- Fasting glucose most important for fetal and maternal effects.
- **At 32–34 weeks for A2 gestational diabetics:**
  - Fetal testing (BPP or twice weekly NST with amniotic fluid index).
  - US for growth in the late third trimester and possibly early third trimester as clinically indicated and depending on glycemic control.

- For A1 well-controlled GDM:
  - US for growth 36–39 weeks.
  - Need for antenatal testing is controversial.
- **Delivery:**
  - A1 GDM: Await labor. Antenatal testing is controversial. Deliver no later than 41 weeks.
  - A2 GDM:
    - If glucose is well controlled, deliver at 39 weeks to decrease risk of stillbirth.
    - If glucose is poorly controlled, deliver as clinically indicated before 39 weeks.
  - Maintain euglycemia during labor (insulin drip for A2).
  - May offer cesarean delivery (to avoid birth trauma or shoulder dystocia) if fetal weight ≥4500 g. → C/S .

Shoulder Dystocia

> A 25-year-old G1P0 presents in labor. She has a protracted labor course and pushes for 3 hr. The head delivers and then retracts into the perineum (i.e., turtle sign). The infant's anterior shoulder does not deliver with gentle downward traction. What is the diagnosis? What is the next step in management?
> **Answer:** Shoulder dystocia. The next step is to call for help (nursing, anesthesia, pediatrics) and prepare to perform additional maneuvers.

Shoulder dystocia is diagnosed when the anterior fetal shoulder is lodged behind the pubic symphysis after the fetal head has been delivered, and gentle downward traction fails to accomplish delivery. The fetal head retracts against the perineum, forming the "turtle sign." The incidence is 0.2–3% of births, and it is considered to be an obstetric emergency. If infant is not delivered quickly, it may suffer neurologic injury or death from hypoxia.

RISK FACTORS

- Shoulder dystocia cannot accurately be predicted by either risk factors or imaging studies predicting fetal weight.
- Maternal factors:
  - Obesity.
  - Multiparity.
  - Gestational diabetes.
  - Advanced maternal age (>35).
- Fetal factors:
  - Post-term pregnancy (>42 weeks).
  - Macrosomia.
  - Male gender.
- Intrapartum factors:
  - Prolonged first and/or second stage of labor.
  - Operative vaginal delivery.
  - History of shoulder dystocia.

COMPLICATIONS

- Brachial plexus nerve injuries.
- Fetal humeral/clavicular fracture.
- Hypoxia/death.

WARD TIP

Shoulder dystocia = obstetric emergency

WARD TIP

Shoulder dystocia management—
HELPERR
Call for **H**elp
Episiotomy
Legs up (McRoberts maneuver)
Pressure suprapubically
Enter vagina for shoulder rotation
(Woods screw or Rubin)
Reach for posterior arm
Return head into vagina for cesarean delivery (Zavanelli).

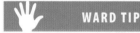
G = Gaeslies

TREATMENT

Several maneuvers can be performed to dislodge the shoulder:

- **McRoberts maneuver:** Maternal thighs are sharply flexed against maternal abdomen. This flattens the sacrum and the symphysis pubis and may allow the delivery of the fetal shoulder. Performed at the same time as suprapubic pressure. (See Figure 8-2.)
- **Suprapubic pressure** slightly superior to the symphysis pubis and in the direction of the desired shoulder rotation. (NOTE: NOT fundal pressure!)
- **Woods screw maneuver:** Pressure is applied to the anterior surface of the posterior shoulder to rotate the posterior shoulder and "unscrew" the anterior shoulder. (See Figure 8-3.)
- **Rubin maneuver:** Pressure is applied to the most accessible part of the fetal shoulder and rotated toward the chest. (See Figure 8-4.)

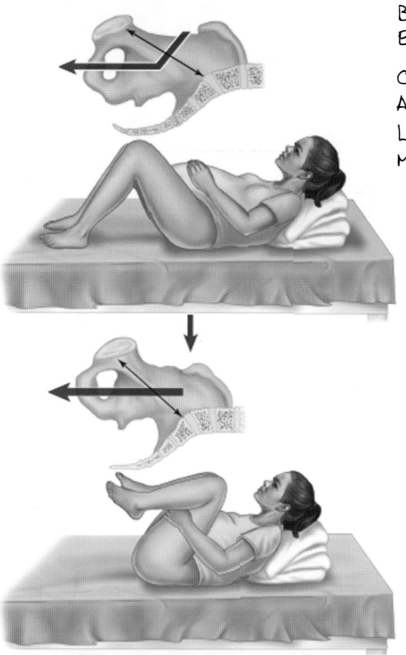

(handwritten notes:)
Breathe, do not push
Elevate legs (mcroberts)

Call for help.
Apply suprapubic pressure.
Large vaginal opening –epis.
Maneuvers.
- deliver posterior shoulder
- rotate posterior shoulder (woodscrew)
- adduct posterior fetal shoulder (rubin)
- Gaskin–mum on hands and knees.
- Zavnelli–replace fetal head for

FIGURE 8-2.   McRoberts maneuver for shoulder dystocia. (Reproduced, with permission, from Ganti L. *Atlas of Emergency Medicine Procedures.* New York, NY: Springer Nature; 2016.)

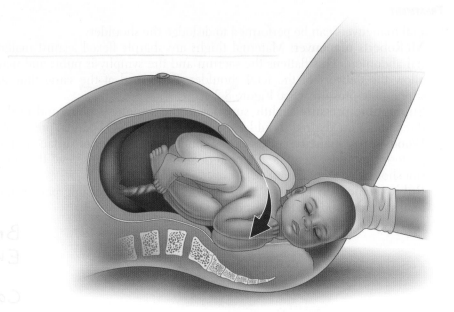

FIGURE 8-3. **Ruben maneuver for shoulder dystocia: pressure is applied to the most accessible part of the fetal shoulder and rotated toward the chest.** (Reproduced, with permission, from Ganti L. *Atlas of Emergency Medicine Procedures.* New York, NY: Springer Nature; 2016.)

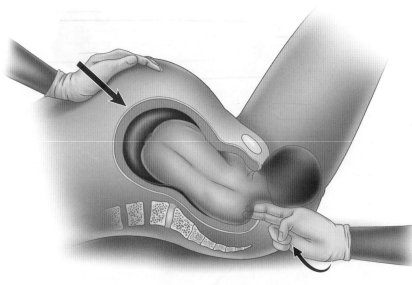

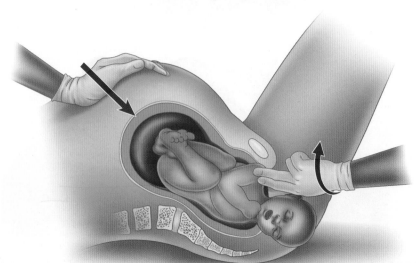

FIGURE 8-4. **Woods corkscrew maneuver for shoulder dystocia: pressure is applied to the clavicle of the posterior arm, enabling rotation and dislodgement of the anterior shoulder.** (Reproduced, with permission, from Ganti L. *Atlas of Emergency Medicine Procedures.* New York, NY: Springer Nature; 2016.)

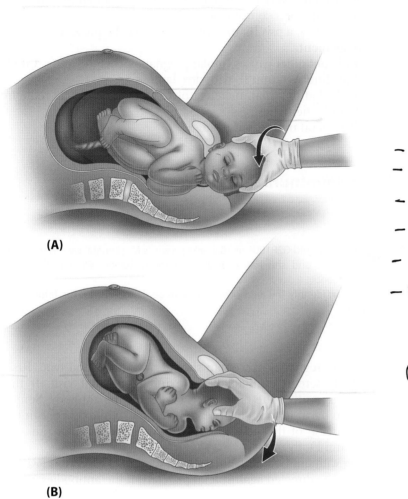

- Breathe, do not push.
- Elevate legs (mcroberts)
- Call for help.
- Apply suprapubic press
- Largen vaginal open (epi)
- Maneuvers.
  1.) delivery posterior shoulder
  2) posterior shoulder rotation (wood screw, Rubin)
  3.) hands + knees (Gaskin)
  4.) Replace fetus in prep for a C/S. (Zavanelli)

FIGURE 8-5. **Zavanelli maneuver: the fetal head is rotated into the direct occiput anterior position, flexed, and pushed back into the birth canal.** (Reproduced, with permission, from Ganti L. *Atlas of Emergency Medicine Procedures*. New York, NY: Springer Nature; 2016.)

- **Posterior arm delivery:** Hand is inserted into vagina and posterior arm is pulled across chest, delivering posterior arm and shoulder. This creates a shorter distance between the anterior shoulder and posterior axilla, allowing the anterior shoulder to be delivered.
- **Zavanelli maneuver:** If the above measures do not work, the fetal head can be returned to the uterus by reversing the cardinal movements of labor. At this point, a cesarean delivery can be performed. (See Figure 8-5.)
- Maneuvers that do not require direct contact with the fetus should be done first because they have lower morbidity for the fetus.

> **WARD TIP**
>
> Do not apply fundal pressure in shoulder dystocia. It causes further impaction of the shoulder behind the symphysis pubis.

Hyperemesis Gravidarum

- Severe vomiting that results in:
  - Weight loss.
  - Dehydration.
  - Metabolic derangements.

- Due to high levels of human chorionic gonadotropin (hCG), estrogen, progesterone, or a combination.
- In some cases, a psychiatric component may be present.
- **Management:**
    - Rule out other causes (molar pregnancy, thyrotoxicosis, GI etiology).
    - First line: Vitamin B$_6$ with doxylamine.
    - IV hydration, thiamine/electrolyte replacement, acid reducing medications, antiemetics.
    - Parenteral nutrition if needed.

Isoimmunization

 A 29-year-old G2P1001 at 16 weeks presents for prenatal care. Her blood type is A negative and she has a positive antibody screen. What is the next step in management?

Answer: Identify the antibody. Some can be dangerous for the fetus and some are benign.

- In each pregnancy, a woman should have her blood type, Rh status, and antibody screen evaluated at the initial prenatal visit. If the antibody screen is positive, the next step is to identify the antibody. Some antibodies pose no harm to the fetus (i.e., anti-Lewis), while others can cause hemolytic disease of the newborn (HDN) and can be fatal (i.e., anti-D, anti-Kell, anti-Duffy).
- Along with antibodies to antigens on fetal red blood cells (RBCs), antibodies may be directed against fetal platelets. If the antibodies are not harmful to the fetus, no further workup needs to be done. If antibodies are known to cause harm to the fetus, next step is to determine the titer of the antibodies. A **critical titer**, usually 1:16 at most institutions, is the titer associated with a significant risk for HDN. Fetal surveillance with possible therapeutic interventions may be needed (see Figure 8-6).

ANTI-D ISOIMMUNIZATION

An understanding of D (or Rho) RBC antigen compatibility is a crucial part of prenatal care. If a mother and developing child are incompatible, very serious complications can cause fetal death. This section will review the appropriate screening and therapy for anti-D isoimmunization.

What Is Rh or D?

- The surface of the human RBC may or may not have a Rho (Rh) antigen. If a patient with blood type A has a Rho antigen, the blood type is A+. If that person has no Rho antigen, the blood type is A–. In the following discussion, the Rh antigen will be referred to as D.
- Half of all antigens on fetal RBCs come from the father, and half come from the mother. That means that the fetus may have antigens to which the mother's immune system is unfamiliar.

The Problem with D Sensitization

- If the mother is D negative and the father is D positive, there may be a chance that the baby may be D positive.

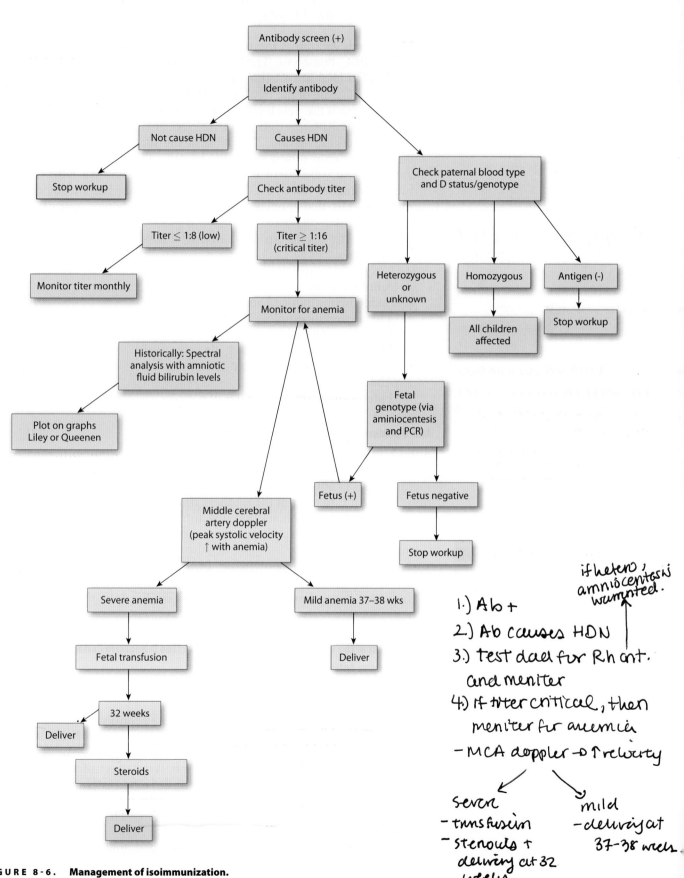

FIGURE 8-6.   Management of isoimmunization.

- If the mother is D negative and her fetus is D positive, she may become sensitized to the D antigen and develop antibodies against the baby's RBCs.
- These antibodies cross the placenta and attack the fetal RBCs, resulting in fetal RBC hemolysis. The hemolysis results in significant fetal anemia, resulting in fetal heart failure and death. This disease process is known as hemolytic disease of the newborn (HDN).
- Sensitization is the development of maternal antibodies against D antigens on the fetus RBC. Sensitization may occur whenever fetal blood enters the maternal circulation. The fetus of the pregnancy when sensitization occurred usually suffers no harm because the maternal antibody titers are low. The subsequent pregnancies with a D-positive fetus are at significantly higher risk of HDN because the mother has already developed memory cells that quickly produce anti-D antibodies against the fetus RBCs.
- The following conditions can cause fetal-maternal bleeding, and lead to sensitization:
    - Chorionic villus sampling.
    - Amniocentesis.
    - Spontaneous/induced abortion.
    - Threatened/incomplete abortion.
    - Ectopic pregnancies.
    - Placental abruption/bleeding placenta previa.
    - Vaginal or cesarean delivery.
    - Abdominal trauma.
    - External cephalic version.

Anti-D Immune Globulins (IgG) (Brand Name: RhoGAM)

Anti-D immune globulins are collected from donated human plasma. When a mother is given a dose of anti-D IgG, the antibodies bind to the fetal RBCs that have the D antigen on them and clear them from the maternal circulation. The goal is to prevent the mother's immune system from recognizing the presence of the D antigen and forming antibodies against it.

- Give to D-negative mothers, who have not formed antibodies against D antigen.
- **Not** indicated for patients who already have anti-D antibodies and are sensitized.
- Indicated for patients who might be sensitized to other blood group antigens.

Management of the Unsensitized D-Negative Patient (The D-Negative Patient with a Negative Antibody Screen)

1. Antibody screen should be done at the initial prenatal visit and again at 28 weeks.
2. If antibody screen negative, the fetus is presumed to be D positive, and one dose of anti-D IgG immune globulin is given to the mother at 28 weeks to prevent development of maternal antibodies. Anti-D immune globulins last for ~12 weeks, and the highest risk of sensitization is in T3.
3. At birth, the infant's D status is tested. If the infant is D negative, no anti-D IgG is given to the mother. If the infant is D positive, anti-D IgG is given to the mother within 72 hr of delivery. The dose of anti-D IgG is determined by KB test.
4. Administration of anti-D IgG at 28 weeks' gestation and within 72 hr of birth reduces sensitization to 0.2%.

Management of the Sensitized D-Negative Patient (Antibody Screen Positive for Anti-D Antibody)

> 🧍 A 35-year-old G4P2012 at 26 weeks is diagnosed with anti-Kell antibodies with the titer of 1:32. Amniocentesis shows that the fetus is positive for the Kell antigen. In addition to antenatal (i.e., biophysical profile), what other testing is critical for this fetus?
> **Answer:** The fetus should be monitored with middle cerebral artery Dopplers, which indicate the severity of anemia.

1. If antibody screen at initial prenatal visit is positive, and is identified as anti-D,
2. Check the antibody titer. Critical titer is 1:16.
   - If titer remains stable at <1:16, the likelihood of hemolytic disease of the newborn is low. Follow the antibody titer every 4 weeks.
   - If the titer is ≥1:16 and/or rising, the likelihood of hemolytic disease of the newborn is high. Amniocentesis is done.
3. Amniocentesis:
   - Fetal cells are analyzed for D status.
   - Historically, amniotic fluid was analyzed by spectral analysis, which measured the light absorbance by bilirubin (delta OD 450). Absorbance measurements were plotted on a Liley graph to predict the severity of disease. The preferred method now is to perform middle cerebral artery (MCA) Dopplers to assess for anemia.
4. Serial US monitoring for:
   - Anatomy scan for hydrops fetalis.
   - MCA Doppler for presence or severity of anemia (see Figure 8-7). Consider blood transfusion to fetus if very premature.
5. Delivery:
   - Mild anemia: Induction of labor at 37–38 weeks.
   - Severe anemia: Deliver at 32–34 weeks.
     - Most babies >32 weeks do well in the neonatal intensive care unit (NICU).
     - Weigh risks for continued cord blood sampling and transfusions with neonatal risks of preterm delivery.
     - Administer steroids to mother to enhance fetal lung maturity.

Hemolytic Disease of the Newborn
Hemolytic disease of the newborn (HDN)/fetal hydrops occurs when the mother lacks an antigen present on the fetal RBC → fetal RBCs in maternal circulation trigger an immune response → maternal antibodies lyse fetal RBCs → fetal anemia → fetal hyperbilirubinemia + kernicterus + heart failure, edema, ascites, pericardial effusion → death.

Fetal hydrops = collection of fluid in two or more body cavities:
- Scalp edema
- Pleural effusion
- Pericardial effusion
- Ascites

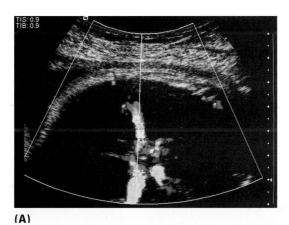
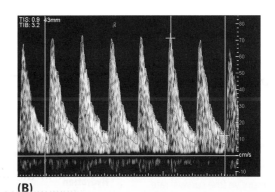

(A)   **(B)**

FIGURE 8-7. **Middle cerebral artery. (A) Doppler. (B) Waveform.** (Reproduced, with permission, from Cunningham FG, Leveno KJ, Bloom SL, et al. *Williams Obstetrics*, 23rd ed. New York, NY: McGraw-Hill, 2010: 365.)

With the use of anti-D immune globulin, there is an ↑ of isoimmunization caused by minor antigens acquired by incompatible blood transfusion. Some minor antigens cause HDN, and some do not. Those that do cause HDN are managed the same way as anti-D isoimmunized mothers. Kell isoimmunization is an exception because:

- It is less predictable and results in more severe anemia than alloimmunization due to other erythrocyte antigens.
- Maternal Kell antibody titers and amniotic fluid delta OD_{450} are not predictive of the severity of fetal anemia as with anti-D sensitization.
- MCA Dopplers are accurate in predicting severe anemia with Kell isoimmunization.

Preterm Labor

CRITERIA

Gestational age (GA) <37 weeks with regular uterine contractions and progressive cervical change.

RISK FACTORS

- Previous history of preterm delivery.
- Polyhydramnios.
- Multiple gestations.
- Substance abuse.
- Systemic infection (pyelonephritis, appendicitis, etc.).
- Vaginal infections (bacterial vaginosis, chlamydia).
- Placental abruption.
- History of cervical surgery.

ASSESSMENT

- Evaluate for causes such as infection (gonococcus, bacterial vaginosis), abruption.
- Confirm GA of fetus (i.e., by US).
- Predictors of preterm labor:
  - Transvaginal cervical length measurement:
    - >30 mm: Low risk of preterm delivery.
    - <20 mm (especially with funneling): High risk of preterm delivery.
  - Fetal fibronectin assay:
    - Vaginal swab of posterior fornix prior to digital exam.
    - If negative, 99% predictability for no preterm delivery within 1 week.
    - Can be especially helpful predicting risk of preterm delivery in women with cervical length <30 mm but >20 mm.

high negative predictive value. ←

Hydration

Not proven to reduce preterm labor, but hydration may decrease uterine irritability. Dehydration causes antidiuretic hormone (ADH) secretion, and ADH mimics oxytocin, which causes uterine contractions.

WARD TIP

Braxton Hicks contractions (irregular, nonrhythmic, usually painless contractions that begin at early gestation and ↑ as term approaches) may make it difficult to distinguish between true and false labor.

EXAM TIP

Most infants born after 34 weeks' gestation will survive (the survival rate is within 1% of the survival rate beyond 37 weeks).

Tocolytic Therapy

Tocolysis is the pharmacologic inhibition of uterine contractions. Tocolytic drugs have not been shown to decrease neonatal morbidity or mortality, but may prolong gestation for 2–7 days to allow time for administration of steroids and transfer to a facility with a neonatal ICU. It is used when fetus is <34 weeks' gestation.

Tocolytic Agents

- **Magnesium sulfate:** Suppresses uterine contractions.
  - Unknown mechanism of action: Competes with calcium, inhibits myosin light chain.
  - Maternal side effects: Flushing, lethargy, headache, muscle weakness, diplopia, dry mouth, pulmonary edema, cardiac arrest. Toxicity is treated with calcium gluconate.
  - Fetal side effects: Lethargy, hypotonia, respiratory depression.
  - Contraindications: Myasthenia gravis.
- **Nifedipine:** Oral calcium channel blocker.
  - Maternal side effects: Flushing, headache, dizziness, nausea, transient hypotension.
  - Fetal side effects: None yet noted.
  - Contraindications: Maternal hypotension, cardiac disease; use with caution with renal disease. Avoid concomitant use with magnesium sulfate.
- **Ritodrine, terbutaline, β-agonist:** β_2-receptor stimulation on myometrial cells →↑ cyclic adenosine monophosphate (cAMP) →↓ intracellular Ca →↓ contractions:
  - Maternal side effects: Pulmonary edema, tachycardia, headaches.
  - Fetal side effect: Tachycardia.
  - Contraindications: Cardiovascular disease, hyperthyroidism, uncontrolled diabetes mellitus.
- **Indomethacin,** prostaglandin inhibitors: For <32 weeks.
  - Maternal side effects: Nausea, heartburn.
  - Fetal side effects: Premature constriction of ductus arteriosus, pulmonary HTN, reversible ↓ in amniotic fluid.
  - Contraindications: Renal or hepatic impairment, peptic ulcer disease.

Corticosteroids

- Indicated for patients in preterm labor from 24 to 34 weeks.
- Actions: Accelerate fetal lung maturity (↓ RDS), and reduce intraventricular hemorrhage.

Neuroprotection

If at high risk for imminent delivery, administer magnesium sulfate for neuroprotection between 24 and 32 weeks. The dosing regimen is different than that given for tocolysis. Give 4 g bolus followed by 1 g/hr maintenance.

Assessing Fetal Lung Maturity

An amniocentesis may be performed to assess fetal lungs for risk of RDS. Fetal lungs are mature if:
- Phosphatidylglycerol is present in amniotic fluid.
- Surfactant-albumin in amniotic fluid at a ratio >55.
- Lecithin-sphingomyelin in amniotic fluid at a ratio >2.

EXAM TIP

Tocolytics have not been proven to prolong pregnancy.

WARD TIP

Contraindications to tocolysis—
BAD CHU
- **B**leeding (severe) from any cause
- **A**bruptio placentae
- **D**eath of fetus/life-incompatible anomaly
- **C**horioamnionitis
- **H**ypertension (i.e., preeclampsia)
- **U**nstable maternal hemodynamics

WARD TIP

Maternal corticosteroid administration with:
- Preterm labor 24–34 weeks
- Preterm premature rupture of membranes (PPROM) 24–32 weeks

Fetal benefits:
- ↓ respiratory distress syndrome (RDS).
- ↓ intraventricular hemorrhage.

tocolytics can lead / precip. pulmonary edema.

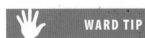

<20 mm (2 cm)
Cervix is short → give
progesterone to prevent
Preterm delivery

Hx of preterm
labor?

no → TVUS-CL
yes → progesterone + TVUS-CL

TVUS-CL:
normal → none —
short → progest.

progesterone + TVUS-CL:
normal → serial TVUS-CL to 24 wks
short (<20mm) → cerclage → serial TVUS until 24 weeks

Prevention of Preterm Labor

Progesterone supplementation has been shown to decrease the risk of preterm birth in women with:

- A history of term singleton preterm delivery.
- A shortened cervix on ultrasound during current pregnancy.

Progesterone relaxes the myometrium and suppresses cytokine production. It may be started between 16 and 20 weeks and continued through 36 weeks. Preparations include:

- 17α-hydroxyprogesterone caproate 250 mg IM every week.
- Micronized progesterone tablet 100–200 mg per vagina each evening.

Premature Rupture of Membranes

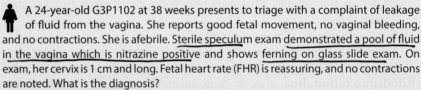

A 24-year-old G3P1102 at 38 weeks presents to triage with a complaint of leakage of fluid from the vagina. She reports good fetal movement, no vaginal bleeding, and no contractions. She is afebrile. Sterile speculum exam demonstrated a pool of fluid in the vagina which is nitrazine positive and shows ferning on glass slide exam. On exam, her cervix is 1 cm and long. Fetal heart rate (FHR) is reassuring, and no contractions are noted. What is the diagnosis?

Answer: Premature rupture of membranes (PROM) is diagnosed when the membranes rupture prior to the onset of labor. Rupture of membranes is confirmed by the sterile speculum exam. Based on the cervical exam and the absence of contractions, the patient is not in labor. Considering that the fetus is term, the next step should be induction of labor in order to prevent chorioamnionitis.

Premature rupture denotes spontaneous rupture of fetal membranes before the onset of labor. This can occur at term (PROM) or preterm (PPROM).

- **ROM:** Rupture of membranes.
- **PROM:** Premature rupture of membranes (ROM before the onset of labor).
- **PPROM:** Preterm (<37 weeks) premature rupture of membranes.
- **Prolonged rupture of membranes:** Rupture of membranes present for >18 hr.

WARD TIP

PPROM: Most common diagnosis associated with preterm delivery.

EXAM TIP

Prolonged rupture of membranes may be due to premature rupture (PROM) or an abnormally long labor (not PROM).

ETIOLOGY

- Unknown but hypothesized:
  - Vaginal and cervical infections.
  - Incompetent cervix.
  - Nutritional deficiencies.

COMPLICATIONS

- Prematurity: If PROM occurs at <37 weeks, the fetus is at risk of being born prematurely with its associated complications.
- Pulmonary hypoplasia: If PROM occurs at <24 weeks → oligohydramnios → **pulmonary hypoplasia.** *Survival at this age is low.*
- Chorioamnionitis.
- Placental abruption.
- Neonatal infection.
- Umbilical cord prolapse.
- Preterm labor.

MANAGEMENT OF ALL PROM PATIENTS

- Avoid vaginal exams if possible to ↓ risk of chorioamnionitis.
- Evaluate patient for chorioamnionitis: Fever >100.4°F (38°C), leukocytosis, maternal/fetal tachycardia, uterine tenderness, malodorous vaginal discharge.
- If chorioamnionitis present, delivery is performed regardless of GA, and broad-spectrum antibiotics (ampicillin, gentamicin) are initiated.

uterine discharge (foul) + uterine tenderness
- fever
- maternal/fetal tachy
- leukocytosis

SPECIFIC MANAGEMENT FOR PROM AT TERM

Ninety percent of term patients go into spontaneous labor within 24 hr after rupture:

- Patients in active labor should be allowed to progress.
- If labor is not spontaneous, it should be induced. Cesarean delivery should be performed for obstetric indications.

WARD TIP

Nitrazine test may be falsely positive if contaminated with blood or semen.

SPECIFIC MANAGEMENT OF PPROM

> An 18-year-old G1P0 at 30 weeks presents to triage with complaints of clear fluid leaking from her vagina. Her exam is positive for pooling, ferning, and nitrazine. The cervix is visually closed on sterile speculum exam. FHR is reassuring, and no contractions are noted. The US shows a breech singleton fetus. What is the next step in management?
>
> **Answer**: The patient has preterm premature rupture of membranes (PPROM). She should be admitted to the hospital. Steroids should be administered to ↓ the risk of RDS in the fetus, and antibiotics should be given to ↑ the latency period.

- Fifty percent of preterm patients go into labor within 24 hr after rupture.
- Management strategy balances the risks of premature birth against the risks of complications such as infection, abruption, and cord accident.
- Consider amniotic fluid assessment for fetal lung maturity from vaginal pool specimen, and deliver if mature.
- US to assess GA, anomalies, presentation, and AFI.
- Monitor in hospital for infection, abruption, fetal distress, and preterm labor.
- If <34 weeks' gestation, give steroids to ↓ the incidence of RDS.
- If delivery is thought to be imminent, administer magnesium sulfate for neuroprotection.
- Antibiotic coverage to prolong latency period (time between ROM and onset of labor).
- Fetal testing to ensure fetal well-being.
- Delivery:
  - If infection, abruption, fetal distress noted.
  - At 34 weeks' gestation. At this GA, most babies have low risk of RDS, and risks of complications such as infection outweigh risks of prematurity.

>37 weeks
- delivery (induction)
- GBS prophylaxis
34-36 6/7
- delivery
- GBS prophylaxis
- ± corticosteroids
32-33 6/7
- corticosteroids
- latency antibiotics (amp-gent)
24-31 6/7
- corticosteroids
- MgSO4
- Abx (amp-gent)
<23 6/7 (PPPROM)
- counseling on outcomes.

WARD TIP

Golden rule: **Never** do a digital vaginal exam in third-trimester bleeding until placenta previa is ruled out.

Third-Trimester Bleeding

INCIDENCE

Occurs in 2–5% of pregnancies.

WORKUP

- History, including trauma.
- Vitals: Signs of hypovolemia include hypotension and tachycardia.

■ Labs: Complete blood count (CBC), coagulation profile, type and cross-match, urinalysis, drug screen.
■ US to look for placenta previa, as well as monitoring for fetal well-being.
■ See Figure 8-8 for management of third-trimester bleeding.
■ Determine whether blood is maternal, fetal, or both:
  Apt test: Put blood from vagina in tube with KOH: Turns brown for maternal; turns pink for fetus.

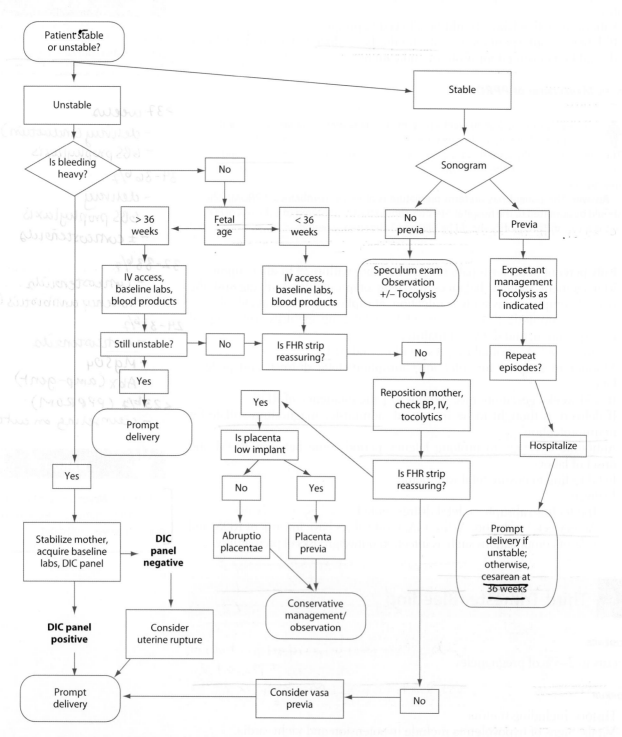

FIGURE 8-8. **Management of third-trimester bleeding.**

- **Kleihauer-Betke test:** Take blood from mother's arm and determine percentage of fetal RBCs in maternal circulation: >1% = fetal bleeding. Maternal cells are washed out (ghost cells); fetal cells are bright red (due to fetal hemoglobin). This is the test most commonly used.
- **Wright's stain:** Vaginal blood; nucleated RBCs indicate fetal bleed.

DIFFERENTIAL

- **Obstetric causes:**
  - Placental abruption.
  - Placenta previa.
  - Vasa previa/velamentous insertion.
  - Uterine rupture.
  - Circumvillate placenta.
  - Extrusion of cervical mucus ("bloody show").
- **Nonobstetric causes:**
  - Cervicitis.
  - Polyp.
  - Neoplasm.

PLACENTAL ABRUPTION (ABRUPTIO PLACENTAE)

> A 32-year-old G2P1001 at 34 weeks is brought to triage after a motor vehicle accident. She was a restrained driver who was rear-ended while going 65 miles per hour on the freeway. The airbags were deployed. She has dark-red vaginal bleeding and severe abdominal pain. Her vitals are stable. On exam, her abdomen is firm and tender. FHR shows a baseline of 130, ↓ variability, no accelerations, and late decelerations. Contractions are seen on the monitor. US shows a fundal grade 2 placenta. What is the most likely diagnosis?
>   **Answer:** Placental abruption.

Premature separation of placenta from uterine wall before the delivery of baby (see Figure 8-9).

INCIDENCE

0.5–1.3%; severe abruption can lead to death (0.12%).

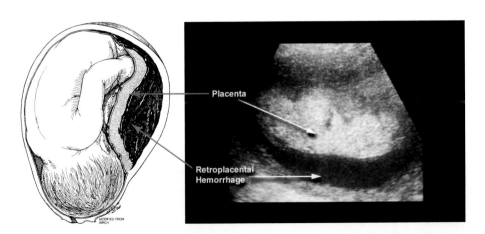

FIGURE 8-9. **Placental abruption.** (Courtesy of SUNY at Buffalo School of Medicine, Residency Program in Emergency Medicine.)

RISK FACTORS

- Trauma (motor vehicle accident, domestic violence).
- Previous history of abruption.
- Preeclampsia (and chronic HTN).
- Smoking.
- Cocaine abuse.
- High parity.

CLINICAL PRESENTATION

> A 28-year-old woman at 35 weeks' gestation is brought in by ambulance following a car accident. She is complaining of severe abdominal pain, and on exam she is found to have vaginal bleeding. An US shows a fundal placenta and a fetus in the cephalic presentation. What is most likely the cause?
>
> **Answer:** Placental abruption. Microangiopathic hemolytic anemia seen on maternal blood smear. What is occurring? Disseminated intravascular coagulation (DIC). What is the next step? Transfuse blood products (PRBCs, platelets, FFP) and expedite a vaginal delivery. Want to avoid major surgery in the setting of DIC.

- Vaginal bleeding (can be mild or life-threatening).
- Constant and severe abdominal pain.
- Irritable, tender, and typically hypertonic uterus.
- Evidence of fetal distress (if severe).
- Maternal shock.
- Disseminated intravascular coagulation. → tissue factor is exposed.

DIAGNOSIS

- Retroplacental hematoma on US supports diagnosis, but is not always seen.
- Clinical findings most important.

MANAGEMENT

- Correct shock (IV fluids, packed RBCs, fresh frozen plasma, cryoprecipitate, platelets).
- Maternal oxygen administration.
- Expectant management or delivery: Close observation of mother and fetus with ability to intervene immediately.
- If there is fetal distress, perform cesarean delivery. Otherwise may be candidate for vaginal delivery.

> **WARD TIP**
>
> Up to 20% of placental abruptions can present without vaginal bleeding because bleeding is concealed.

PLACENTA PREVIA

A condition in which the placenta is implanted in the immediate vicinity of the cervical os. It can be classified into four types:

- **Complete placenta previa:** The placenta covers the entire internal cervical os (see Figure 8-10).
- **Partial placenta previa:** The placenta partially covers the internal cervical os.
- **Marginal placenta previa:** One edge of the placenta extends to the edge of the internal cervical os.
- **Low-lying placenta:** Within 2 cm of the internal cervical os.

INCIDENCE

0.5–1%.

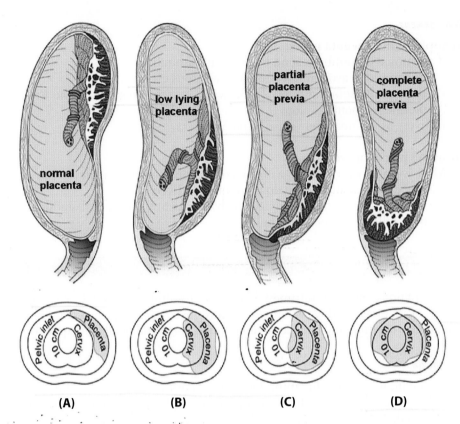

FIGURE 8-10. **(A) Normal placenta. (B) Low implantation. (C) Partial placenta previa. (D) Complete placenta previa.** (Reproduced, with permission, from DeCherney AH, Nathan L. *Current Obstetric & Gynecologic Diagnosis & Treatment*, 9th ed. New York, NY: McGraw-Hill, 2003.)

ETIOLOGY

Unknown, but associated with:
- Multiparity.
- Advanced maternal age.
- Previous abortions.
- Previous history of placenta previa.
- Multiple gestation.
- Previous cesarean delivery.
- Infertility treatment.

CLINICAL PRESENTATION

- **Painless** vaginal bleeding in second or third trimester.
- If patient has not had a second-trimester ultrasound, do not perform digital vaginal exam until ultrasound demonstrates placental location.

DIAGNOSIS

- **Transabdominal US** (95% accurate). **Transvaginal ultrasound** helps to further define placental location.
- **Magnetic resonance imaging (MRI) findings:** MRI is a good imaging modality to diagnose placenta previa, but its cost and limited availability make it mostly useful when placenta accrete is suspected.

EXAM TIP

Third trimester bleeding:
  Painless bleeding = previa
  Painful bleeding = abruption

EXAM TIP

US reveals an anterior placenta previa in a patient with two prior cesarean deliveries. What are you suspicious of? Placenta accreta

MANAGEMENT

Asymptomatic placenta previa:

- If diagnosed at routine second-trimester ultrasound:
    - Recommend avoid intercourse and vigorous exercise.
    - Repeat ultrasound around 28–32 weeks to see if resolves as the lower uterine segment develops.
- Delivery by cesarean between 36 and 37 weeks.

Bleeding placenta previa:

- Most women who present with bleeding due to placenta previa can be managed conservatively and do not require delivery.
- Severe bleeding should be managed by correcting shock and stabilizing mother, followed by cesarean delivery.

FETAL VESSEL RUPTURE

Two conditions cause third-trimester bleeding resulting from fetal vessel rupture: (1) vasa previa and (2) velamentous cord insertion. These two conditions often occur together and can cause fetal hemorrhage and death very quickly.

Vasa Previa

- A condition in which the unprotected fetal cord vessels pass over the internal cervical os, making them susceptible to rupture when membranes are ruptured.
- **Prevalence:** 1/2500 deliveries, and higher with use of fertility treatments.

Velamentous Cord Insertion

- Fetal vessels insert in the membranes and travel unprotected to the placenta, with no protection from Wharton's jelly. This leaves them susceptible to tearing when the amniotic sac ruptures.
- **Prevalence:** 1% of singletons, 10% of twins.

CLINICAL PRESENTATION

Vaginal bleeding with fetal distress.

MANAGEMENT

Correction of shock and immediate delivery (usually cesarean delivery).

UTERINE RUPTURE

The disruption of the uterine musculature through all of its layers, usually with part of the fetus protruding through the opening.

COMPLICATIONS

- Maternal: Hemorrhage, hysterectomy, death.
- Fetal: Permanent neurologic impairment, cerebral palsy, death.

RISK FACTORS

Prior uterine scar from a cesarean delivery is the most important risk factor:
- Vertical scar: 10% risk due to scarring of the active, contractile portion of the uterus.
- Low transverse scar: <1% risk.
- Can occur in the setting of trauma.

WARD TIP

Sinusoidal heart rate pattern = fetal anemia (from any cause).

EXAM TIP

Risk of uterine rupture in patients desiring trial of labor after cesarean (TOLAC):
- <1% if previous low transverse cesarean × 1.
- <2% if previous low transverse cesareans × 2.
- ~10% if previous classical cesarean. Classical uterine scar is a contraindication for TOLAC.

PRESENTATION AND DIAGNOSIS

- Nonreassuring fetal heart tones or bradycardia: Most suggestive of uterine rupture.
- Sudden cessation of uterine contractions.
- "Tearing" sensation in abdomen.
- Presenting fetal part moves higher in the pelvis.   *loss of fetal station*
- Vaginal bleeding.
- Maternal hypovolemia from concealed hemorrhage.

MANAGEMENT

- Immediate laparotomy and delivery.
- May require a cesarean hysterectomy if uterus cannot be reconstructed.

> **EXAM TIP**
>
> The biggest risk for uterine rupture is a prior cesarean delivery.

OTHER OBSTETRIC CAUSES OF THIRD-TRIMESTER BLEEDING

Extrusion of cervical mucus ("bloody show"): A consequence of effacement and dilation of the cervix, with tearing of the small vessels leading to small amount of bleeding that is mixed with the cervical mucus. Benign finding. Often used as a marker for the onset of labor.

Abnormalities of the Third Stage of Labor

A 37-year-old G6P6006 with a history of asthma and chronic hypertension undergoes a spontaneous vaginal delivery of a 4500-g infant. After the placenta delivers spontaneously, profuse vaginal bleeding was noted from the vagina. Pitocin is given, fundal massage is performed, and large clots are removed from the uterus. No lacerations are noted. Estimated blood loss is 700 cc. What is the most likely cause of the bleeding? What is the next step in management?

Answer: Uterine atony is the most likely cause for this patient's postpartum hemorrhage. Prostaglandin F2α (asthma) and methergine (hypertension) are contraindicated due to her medical conditions. The next best agent is misoprostol.

> **EXAM TIP**
>
> One unit of blood PRBCs contains ≈ 250 mL/unit.

EARLY POSTPARTUM HEMORRHAGE (PPH)

- Excessive bleeding that makes patient symptomatic and/or results in signs of hypovolemia.
- Blood loss >500 mL in vaginal delivery; >1000 mL for cesarean delivery (difficult to quantify).
- During first 24 hr: "**Early**" PPH.
- Between 24 hr and 6 weeks after delivery: "**Late**" PPH.
- The most common cause of early PPH is uterine atony (the uterus does not contract as expected). Normally when the uterus contracts, it compresses blood vessels and prevents bleeding. Other causes of postpartum hemorrhage are summarized in the mnemonic CARPIT.

> **EXAM TIP**
>
> Incidence of excessive blood loss following vaginal delivery is 5–8%.

> **EXAM TIP**
>
> Most common cause of early PPH = uterine atony.

RISK FACTORS

- Blood transfusion/hemorrhage during a previous pregnancy.
- Prolonged labor.
- Retained placenta/membranes.
- Multiparity.
- Overdistended uterus: macrosomia/twins/polyhydramnios.

- Operative vaginal delivery (vacuum, forceps).
- Chorioamnionitis.

MANAGEMENT (examine: uterine atony → placenta → lac retures)

1. Manually compress and massage the uterus—controls most cases of hemorrhage due to atony.
2. Start two large-bore IVs and infuse isotonic crystalloids. Type and cross blood. Monitor vitals, including ins and outs.
3. Carefully explore the uterine cavity to ensure that all placental parts have been delivered and that the uterus is intact.
4. Inspect the cervix and vagina for trauma/lacerations.
5. If uterus is boggy, suspect atony:
   - Give additional dilute oxytocin.
   - Methergine—contraindicated: HTN.
   - Prostaglandin F2α—contraindicated: Asthma.
   - Misoprostol.
   - ↓ uterine pulse pressure:
     - Uterine artery embolization.
     - Surgical exploration: Hypogastric artery ligation, uterine artery ligation, ligation of utero-ovarian ligament, uterine compression suture (B-Lynch stitch). → done at the time of laparotomy!
   - Hysterectomy.
6. Consider coagulopathy if persistent bleeding with above management.
   - Red top tube for clot retraction test. Normal coags if clot forms <8 min. Coagulopathy if no clot >12 min.
   - Uterine packing until fresh frozen plasma and/or cryoprecipitate available.
   - Hysterectomy (additional surgery) should be avoided in setting of coagulopathy.

PLACENTAL ATTACHMENT DISORDERS

Abnormal implantation of the placenta in the uterus can cause retention of the placenta after delivery and heavy bleeding.

TYPES

- **Placenta accreta:** Placental villi attach directly to the myometrium rather than to the decidua basalis (see Figure 8-11).
- **Placenta increta:** Placental villi invade the myometrium.
- **Placenta percreta:** Placental villi penetrate through the myometrium. May invade the bladder.

ETIOLOGY

Placenta accreta, increta, and percreta are associated with:
- Placenta previa.
- Previous cesarean delivery (↑ number, ↑ risk).
- Previous dilation and curettage (D&C).
- Grand multiparity.

MANAGEMENT

All of these conditions result in hemorrhage in the third stage of labor. Treatment of choice: hysterectomy.

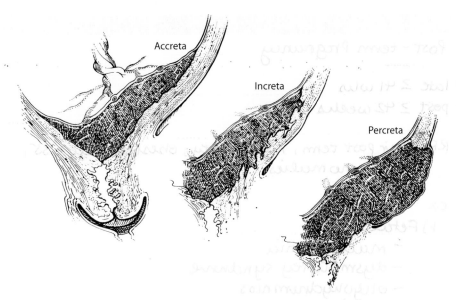

FIGURE 8-11. **Placenta accreta, increta, and percreta.** (Reproduced, with permission, from Cunningham FG, Leveno KJ, Bloom SL, et al. *Williams Obstetrics*, 22nd ed. New York, NY: McGraw-Hill, 2005: 831.)

UTERINE INVERSION

This medical emergency may result from excessive cord traction during placental delivery, and can also be a result of abnormal placental implantation. Morbidity results from shock and sepsis.

INCIDENCE

One in 2200 deliveries.

MANAGEMENT

- Call for help.
- Administer anesthesia.
- Large-bore IV.
- Do not remove placenta until the uterus has been replaced.
- Stop uterotonic medications and give uterine relaxants.
- Immediately try to replace inverted uterus by pushing on the fundus toward the vagina.
- Oxytocin is given after uterus is restored to normal configuration and anesthesia is stopped.

WARD TIP

If a mass is palpated in the vagina immediately after the placenta delivers, suspect uterine inversion.

WARD TIP

Never pull excessively on the cord to deliver the placenta. Gentle traction will be sufficient in a normally implanted placenta.

NOTES

* Post-term Pregnancy

- late ≥ 41 wks
- post ≥ 42 weeks

- RF: prior post term, nulliparity, obesity, age ≥ 35, fetal anomalies

- cx
  1.) Fetal
     - macrosomnia
     - dysmaturity syndrome
     - oligohydramnios
     - Demise
  2.) Maternal
     - obstetric lacerations
     - c/s
     - PPH

- mgmt:
     - fetal monitoring (NST)
     - Delivery prior to 43 weeks gestion

* IUGR

- US shows fetal weight <10%ile for GA

1st trimester	2nd/3rd trimester.
- chromosomal	- Uteroplacental insuff.
- congenital infection	- maternal malnutrition
→ features: global growth lag.	→ "Head sparing" growth lag.

- mgmt:
  1.) weekly BPP
  2.) Serial umbilical artery Doppler US.
  3.) Serial Growth US.

* short interpregnancy period: < 6 - 18 months btwn delivery + next preg.
     cx: PPROM, maternal anemia, preterm delivery, low birth weight

Infections in Pregnancy

Immune System in the Developing Embryo, Fetus, and Newborn

Infant cell-mediated and humoral immunity begins to develop at 9–15 weeks. The initial fetal response to infection is the production of immunoglobulin M (IgM). Passive immunity is provided by transplacental crossing of IgG from the mother. After birth, breast-feeding provides some protection that wanes after 2 months. Infections diagnosed in neonates less than 72 hr of age are usually acquired in utero or during delivery. Infections after this time are acquired after birth (see Table 9-1).

[handwritten notes in left margin:]
Toxo
Other: Syphilis, Parvo, Listeria, Varicella.
Rubella
CMV
HIV, HBV, HSV

note: HBV @ time of birth!

TABLE 9.1.   Perinatal Infections

INTRAUTERINE[a]	VIRAL	BACTERIAL	PROTOZOAN
Transplacental	Varicella-zoster	*Listeria*	Toxoplasmosis
	Coxsackievirus	Syphilis	Malaria
	Parvovirus		
	Rubella		
	Cytomegalovirus		
	HIV		
	Hepatitis		
Ascending infection	HSV	GBS	
		Coliforms, GC/	
		chlamydia	
INTRAPARTUM[b]			
Maternal exposure	HSV	Gonorrhea	
	Papillomavirus	*Chlamydia*	
	HIV	GBS	
	HBV	TB	
External contamination	HSV	*Staphylococcus*	
		coliforms	
NEONATAL			
Human transmission	HSV	*Staphylococcus*	
Respirators and		*Staphylococcus*	
catheters		coliforms	

[handwritten note with arrow pointing to HBV row:]
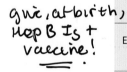
give, at birth,
Hep B Ig +
vaccine!

[a]Bacteria, viruses, or parasites may gain access transplacentally or cross the intact membranes.

[b]Organisms may colonize and infect the fetus during L&D.

GBS, group B Streptococcus; GC, gonococcus; HBV, hepatitis B virus; HIV, human immunodeficiency virus; HSV, herpes simplex virus; TB, tuberculosis.

Varicella-Zoster

A 25-year-old G1P0 at 15 weeks reports that she came in contact with a child that had chickenpox 2 days ago. She does not recall ever having chickenpox or the vaccine. What is the next step?

Answer: She should be tested for the presence of varicella antibodies. Many people are immune to chickenpox, but do not recall ever having it or being vaccinated. If testing indicates that she lacks the antibodies, she should receive the varicella immunoglobulin within 96 hr. If she has the varicella antibodies, nothing further needs to be done.

- More severe in adults; even more severe in pregnancy.
- Can cause **pneumonia**; treat with IV acyclovir.
- Varicella vaccine introduced in 1995 has decreased the incidence of the disease.
- Confirm presence of antibodies if immunity is uncertain. Ideally assess at first prenatal visit.
- Post-exposure prophylaxis with **VZIG** (varicella-zoster immune globulin) within 10 days of exposure is indicated for those who are exposed and susceptible.

FETAL EFFECTS

- Early pregnancy: Transplacental infection causes congenital malformations.
  - Chorioretinitis.
  - Cerebral cortical atrophy.
  - Hydronephrosis.
  - Cutaneous and bony leg defects.
- Late pregnancy: Lower risk of congenital varicella infection.
- Before/during labor:
  - Much higher risk to infant due to absence of protective maternal antibodies.
  - Neonates develop disseminated disease that can be fatal.
  - If maternal infection 5 days before or after delivery, give infant VZIG for passive immunity.

VACCINE

- Live attenuated: **Not** recommended for pregnant women or newborn.
- Not secreted in breast milk, so can give postpartum.

WARD TIP

Varicella infection can cause maternal pneumonia in pregnancy.

Influenza

Not usually life-threatening, but pulmonary involvement can be serious. Pregnant women with influenza are more likely to develop severe illness, to be hospitalized, and to require ICU admission.

FETAL EFFECTS

Possible neural tube defects (NTDs) due to high fever if exposed in early pregnancy.

I G's: To Be Healed
Very Rapidly before
Dying
— Tetanus
— Botulinism
— HBV
— varicella
— Rabies
— Diphtheria

3 bacteria	3 virus
-tetanus	-HBV
-botulinism	-varicella
-diphtheria	-Rabies

Flu like Sx

Fever
headache
chills
fatigue
myalgia
arthralgias

TREATMENT

- Neuraminidase inhibitors oseltamivir or zanamivir recommended for treatment and prophylaxis.
- Pregnancy category C drugs.

VACCINE

- Inactivated vaccine recommended for all pregnant women at any gestational age (GA) during flu season.
- [Live attenuated intranasal vaccine not recommended for pregnant women.]

Parvovirus (B19)

A 30-year-old G2P1001 at 24 weeks presents with a bright red rash on both of her cheeks that started yesterday. She reports a two-day history of fever of 100.4°F (38°C) and lethargy. On physical exam, she is afebrile and has a fine erythematous, lacelike rash on her arms. What is the most likely diagnosis? What is the risk to the fetus?
Answer: Flulike symptoms, slapped cheek rash, and fine reticular rash (erythema infectiosum) are a classic presentation for parvovirus infection. The fetus is at risk for aplastic anemia, which can cause nonimmune hydrops and fetal death.

- Causes **erythema infectiosum** or **fifth disease**.
- Transmitted via respiratory or hand-to-mouth contact.
- Infectivity highest before clinical illness.
- Highest infection in women with school-aged children and day care workers (not teachers).
- Flulike symptoms are followed by bright-red rash on the face—**slapped-cheek** appearance. Rash may become lacelike, spreading to trunk and extremities.
- Twenty to thirty percent of adults are asymptomatic.
- IgM is produced 10–12 days after infection and persists for 3–6 months.
- IgG present several days after IgM appears. IgG persists for life and offers natural immunity against subsequent infections.

FETAL EFFECTS

Acute infection
  — IgM if immunocompetent, NAAT
    if immuno compromised

- Abortion, fetal death.
- Nonimmune hydrops: 1% of infected women, due to fetal aplastic anemia.

MANAGEMENT

Prerus infection: IgG Ab.
reactivation: NAAT.

- After exposure, check IgM and IgG.
- If IgM+, then perform ultrasound (US) for hydrops.
- Middle cerebral artery Doppler evaluates for anemia.
- Sample fetal blood for degree of anemia.
- Consider transfusion.
- Delivery based on GA and severity of disease.

PREVENTION

None.

Rubella (German Measles)

Mild infection in adults caused by an RNA virus.

FETAL EFFECTS

- One of the most teratogenic infections, worse during organogenesis.
- Congenital rubella syndrome: → *cataracts, sensorineural deafness, PDA.*
  - Cataracts, congenital glaucoma (blindness).
  - **Hearing loss:** Most common single defect.
- Central nervous system (CNS) defects: Microcephaly, intellectual disability.
- Newborns shed virus for many months; susceptible infants and adults at risk.

PRENATAL DIAGNOSIS

Rubella RNA in chorionic villi, amniotic fluid, and fetal blood can confirm fetal infection.

VACCINE

Live attenuated vaccine should be avoided 1 month before and during pregnancy. Can be given postpartum.

Cytomegalovirus (CMV)

- Most common cause of perinatal infection in the developed world.
- Spread via body fluids and person-to-person contact.
- Fetal infection via intrauterine, intrapartum, or postpartum infection (breast-feeding).
- Day care centers are common source of infection.

MATERNAL INFECTION

- Most asymptomatic.
- Fifteen percent of adults have mononucleosis-type symptoms (fever, pharyngitis, lymphadenopathy, polyarthritis).
- Primary infection → virus latent → periodic reactivation and shedding.
  - Primary infections cause severe fetal morbidity in fetus.
  - Infections from reactivation have few sequelae.
- Maternal immunity does not prevent:
  - Recurrence.
  - Reactivation.
  - Exogenous infection.
  - Congenital infection.
  - Infection from a different strain.

CONGENITAL INFECTION

Five percent of infected infants have this syndrome:

- **Intracranial calcifications.**
- **Chorioretinitis.**
- Microcephaly.
- Intellectual disability and motor retardation.
- Hemolytic anemia.
- Sensorineural deficits.

PRENATAL DIAGNOSIS

- US can show microcephaly, ventriculomegaly, intracranial calcifications.
- Polymerase chain reaction (PCR) detects and quantifies viral DNA in amniotic fluid and fetal blood.

EXAM TIP

Most common cause of perinatal infections: CMV.

- microcephaly, ventriculomeg-
- periventricular calcification
- seizures
- sensorineural deafness
- hepatosplenomegaly + deafness
- blueberry muffin rash.

 WARD TIP

Previous CMV infection does **not** confer immunity.

viruses
- varcella: IgM/IgG Ab test (mum)
- parvo: IgM (mum)
- rubella: virul RNA (baby)
- cmv: PCR (baby); IgM/G for mum.

MANAGEMENT

- Routine maternal serologic screen is not recommended.
- Measurement of maternal serum IgM and IgG is used to confirm infection.
- If maternal primary infection confirmed, then invasive prenatal testing with US and amniocentesis.

TREATMENT

No maternal treatment. No fetal treatment or prophylaxis.

Group B Streptococcus (GBS)

A 27-year-old woman at 37 weeks presents with a 2-day history of fever of 101°F (38.3°C), loss of fluid from the vagina, and diffuse abdominal tenderness. What is the most likely diagnosis? What is the gold standard for diagnosis? What is the most common cause? How is it treated?
Answer: Chorioamnionitis (infection of the amniotic fluid, membranes, placenta or decidua—also known as intra-amniotic infection). Amniotic fluid culture is the gold standard for diagnosis. Most common cause is Group B streptococcus. It is treated with IV antibiotics: ampicillin + gentamicin +/− clindamycin.

Asymptomatic carrier state of GBS (*S. agalactiae*) in vagina and rectum is common.

COMPLICATIONS

- Preterm labor.
- Premature rupture of membranes (PROM).
- Chorioamnionitis.
- Fetal/neonatal infections.
- Pyelonephritis.
- Endometritis.
- Urinary tract infection.

NEONATAL SEPSIS

- Low-birth-weight and premature infants have worse outcome than term infants.
- **Early-onset disease:**
  - Neonatal infection <7 days after birth.
  - Can prevent with intrapartum prophylaxis.
  - Results from vertical transmission.
  - Sepsis, pneumonia, and meningitis are most common manifestations.
- **Late-onset disease:**
  - Infection 1 week to 3 months after birth.
  - Usually meningitis or bacteremia.
  - Not preventable with intrapartum prophylaxis.
  - Infection is community acquired or nosocomial.

PREVENTION

See Figure 9-1.
- Culture-based approach (recommended by CDC):
  - Culture all women for GBS at 35–37 weeks.
  - Intrapartum prophylaxis if GBS positive.

> Vaginal and rectal GBS screening cultures at 35–37 weeks' gestation for ALL pregnant women (unless patient had GBS bacteriuria during the current pregnancy or a previous infant with invasive GBS disease)

Intrapartum prophylaxis indicated

- Previous infant with invasive GBS disease
- GBS bacteriuria during current pregnancy
- Positive GBS screening culture during current pregnancy (unless a planned cesarean delivery, in the absence of labor or amniotic membrane rupture, is performed)
- Unknown GBS status (culture not done, incomplete, or results unknown) and any of the following:
    - Delivery at <37 weeks' gestation
    - Amniotic membrane rupture ≥18 hours
    - Intrapartum temperature ≥100.4°F (≥38.0°C)

Intrapartum prophylaxis not indicated

- Previous pregnancy with a positive GBS screening culture (unless a culture was also positive during the current pregnancy)
- Planned cesarean delivery performed in the absence of labor or membrane rupture (regardless of maternal GBS culture status)
- Negative vaginal and rectal GBS screening culture in late gestation during the current pregnancy, regardless of intrapartum risk factors

FIGURE 9-1. Intrapartum GBS prophylaxis. (Reproduced, with permission, from Cunningham FG, Leveno KJ, Bloom SL, et al. *Williams Obstetrics*, 22nd ed. New York, NY: McGraw-Hill, 2005: 1286.)

- Risk-based approach: For unknown GBS at the time of labor.
- **Penicillin:** First-line agent.
    - Penicillin allergy: Cefazolin if anaphylaxis risk low.
        - If anaphylaxis risk is high, perform sensitivities for erythromycin and clindamycin.
        - If resistant to above, give vancomycin.

> **WARD TIP**
>
> Penicillin: First line for GBS prophylaxis.

Toxoplasmosis

- *Toxoplasma gondii* transmitted by:
    - Eating infected raw or undercooked meat.
    - Infected cat feces.
- Maternal infections are usually asymptomatic.
- Infection confers immunity; pre-pregnancy infection almost eliminates vertical transmission.
- Infected fetus clears the infection from organs, but it may be localized to CNS.
- Severity of fetal infection depends on the GA at the time of the maternal primary infection.
- **Classic triad** of newborn complications:
    - Chorioretinitis
    - Intracranial calcifications.
    - Hydrocephalus.
- Can also cause intellectual disability and vision loss.

MANAGEMENT

- Routine screening not recommended.
- Confirm diagnosis:
    - By seroconversion of IgG and IgM or >4-fold rise in paired specimen.
    - Avidity IgG testing: If high-avidity IgG found, infection in the preceding 3–5 months is excluded.
    - PCR for *T. gondii* in amniotic fluid.

[handwritten notes:]
1.) previous pregnancy cx by GBS infection
2.) GBS Bacteriuria
3.) GBS+
4.) GBS status unknown.
- Do not need prophylaxis if GBS⊖ or C/S.

→ all neurological; sensorineural hearing loss also present.

mom: IgG/IgM.
Amniotic fluid: PCR for baby.

TREATMENT

- Prevents and reduces congenital infection. Does not eliminate the risk.
- Sulfadiazine + pyrimethamine: Presumptive treatment in late pregnancy. Higher potential toxicity.
- Spiramycin.

PREVENTION

- No vaccine available.
- Practice good hygiene when handling raw meat and contaminated utensils.
- Clean and peel fruits and vegetables.
- Wear gloves when cleaning cat litter or delegate the duty. Keep cats indoors.

Bacterial Vaginosis (BV)

A 32-year-old G2P1001 at 32 weeks' gestation presents with a 4-day history of vaginal discharge. She denies itching, burning, or pain. On physical exam, a homogenous white discharge is noted to coat the vaginal side walls. A wet mount of the discharge shows clue cells, and a fishy odor is noted when KOH is added to the discharge. What is the most likely diagnosis? What is the best treatment?

Answer: Symptoms and diagnosis based on Amsel's criteria is consistent with bacterial vaginosis. The treatment of choice in pregnancy is oral metronidazole.

Clinical syndrome that results from replacement of normal *Lactobacillus* in the vagina with anaerobic bacteria, *Gardnerella vaginalis*, *Mycoplasma hominis*.

DIAGNOSIS

- **Amsel clinical criteria:**
  - Homogenous, white discharge that coats vaginal walls.
  - Clue cells on microscopy.
  - Vaginal pH > 4.5.
  - Whiff test positive: Fishy odor when KOH added to vaginal discharge.
- Nugent criteria: Gram stain.
- Pap smears have low sensitivity for the diagnosis of BV—not used.
- Increased risk of antepartum complications:
  - Preterm birth.
  - PROM.
  - Preterm labor.
  - Chorioamnionitis.

TREATMENT

- Does not improve perinatal outcome.
- Oral metronidazole for symptoms.
- Treatment of partners not routinely recommended.

Candidiasis

Yeast infection on the vulva and in the vagina usually caused by *Candida albicans*.

DIAGNOSIS

Pseudohyphae seen on microscopy.

TREATMENT
- Topical treatment with antifungals preferred.
- Can give oral fluconazole.

Sexually Transmitted Infections (STIs)

See Chapter 31 for additional information on STIs.

SYPHILIS

- *Treponema pallidum* spirochetes cross the placenta and cause congenital infection.
  - Any stage of maternal syphilis may result in fetal infection.
- Newborns can have jaundice, hepatosplenomegaly, skin lesions, rhinitis, pneumonia, myocarditis, nephrosis.
- One screening test should be followed by one confirmatory test:
  - Screening tests:
    - Rapid plasma reagin (RPR)
    - Venereal Disease Research Laboratory (VDRL)
  - Confirmatory tests:
    - Fluorescent treponemal antibody absorption test (FTA-ABS)
    - Microhemagglutination assay (MHA-TP)
- US findings: Edema, ascites, hydrops, thickened placenta.
- **Penicillin** is the treatment of choice for all stages of syphilis (same as nonpregnant patients). If patient is penicillin allergic, then she must be desensitized and still treated with penicillin.
- **Jarisch-Herxheimer reaction** may occur with penicillin treatment. It involves uterine contractions and late decelerations in the fetal heart rate as the dead spirochetes occlude the placental circulation.

GONORRHEA

- The patient will often have concomitant *Chlamydia* infection.
- In pregnancy, usually limited to lower genital tract (cervix, urethra, periurethral glands, and vestibular glands). Acute salpingitis is rare in pregnancy.
- Prenatal screen should be done at the first prenatal visit. Repeat later in pregnancy if high risk or if required by state law.
- Diagnosed with nucleic acid PCR. (NAAT)
- **Complications:**
  - Septic abortion.
  - Preterm delivery.
  - PROM.
  - Chorioamnionitis.
  - Postpartum infections.
- Treat with ceftriaxone.
- Gonorrhea can cause conjunctivitis and vision loss in neonates. All newborns are given prophylaxis against conjunctivitis. + tx: azithromycin

CHLAMYDIA

- Most pregnant patients are asymptomatic.
- Can cause delayed postpartum uterine infection.
- Diagnosed with nucleic acid PCR. (NAAT) !

EXAM TIP

What are late manifestations of congenital syphilis?
Hearing loss with bone and teeth abnormalities
- Frontal bossing
- Short maxilla
- High palatal arch
- Saddle nose deformity
- Malformed teeth

EXAM TIP

Penicillin is the only syphilis therapy in pregnancy that prevents congenital syphilis.

WARD TIP

Infections associated with preterm delivery:
- Gonorrhea
- Chlamydia
- Bacterial vaginosis

- HIV, Syphilis, G/C
- Rubella — screen at the 1st visit
- HBV
- TB

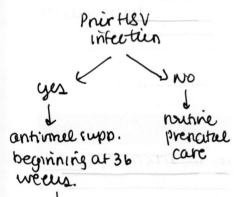

Prior HSV infection

yes → antiviral supp. beginning at 36 weeks.

no → routine prenatal care

lesions/prodromal sx occuring during labor?

no → NSVD

yes → C/S

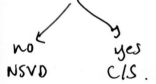

Avoid Breast feeding
- HIV
- HSV
- TB

- **Neonatal infections:**
  - Ophthalmia neonatorum: Conjunctivitis, blindness.
  - Pneumonia.
- Prenatal screen: Screen at the first prenatal visit. Repeat in T3 if at high risk or if required by state law.
- Treatment: Azithromycin or doxycycline.

HERPES SIMPLEX VIRUS

- **Signs and symptoms:** Numbness, tingling, pain (prodromal symptoms), vesicles with erythematous base that heal without scarring.
- **Treatment:** Acyclovir and valacyclovir can shorten the length of symptoms and amount of viral shedding. Shedding not completely eliminated.
  - Safe in pregnancy.
  - Suppression with acyclovir starting at 36 weeks is indicated for those with a history of herpes.
- Neonatal infections can occur via intrauterine (5%), peripartum (85%), and postnatal (10%).
- Newborn infection with three forms:
  - Skin, eye, mouth with localized involvement.
  - CNS disease with encephalitis.
  - Disseminated disease with multiple organ involvement.
- When patient presents in labor:
  - Ask about prodromal symptoms.
  - Examine perineum, vagina, cervix for lesions.
  - If prodromal symptoms or lesions are present, patient should be offered a cesarean delivery to ↓ the risk of vertical transmission.
- Can breast-feed, even when on antivirals. Avoid breast-feeding if herpes lesions on breast that can come in contact with infant.

HEPATITIS B VIRUS

A 30-year-old G1P0 at 39 weeks is admitted for active labor. Her prenatal course is complicated by an infection with chronic hepatitis B. How should the infant be treated once the delivery takes place?
Answer: The infant should receive the first dose of the hepatitis vaccine series and hepatitis immune globulin soon after birth.

- Chronic infection occurs in 70–90% of acutely infected infants leading to:
  - Cirrhosis.
  - Hepatocellular carcinoma.
- Screen at first prenatal visit and at delivery with hepatitis B surface antigen (HBsAg).
- Antiviral treatment not recommended during pregnancy.
- ↑ risk of preterm delivery.
- Small amount of transplacental passage.
- Most neonatal infection due to ingestion of infected fluid in the peripartum or with breast-feeding.
- ↑ risk of infectivity with ↑ levels of hepatitis B early antigen (HBeAg).
- Vaccine can be given during pregnancy.
- **Prevention** of neonatal infection: If mother with hepatitis B:
  - Give hepatitis B immunoglobulin (HBIG) to infant upon delivery.
  - Give first of three hepatitis B vaccines upon delivery.
  - Can breast-feed if infant given prophylaxis.

HUMAN IMMUNODEFICIENCY VIRUS (HIV)

- HIV screening recommended at first prenatal visit. Some states require a repeat test in T3. Opt-out approach used for HIV testing.
  - **Screening:** Enzyme-linked immunosorbent assay (ELISA).
  - **Confirmatory:** Western blot and/or PCR.
  - If available, currently the preferred algorithm uses a fourth-generation antigen/antibody combination HIV-1/2 immunoassay plus a confirmatory HIV-1/HIV-2 antibody differentiation immunoassay.
- The vast majority of cases of pediatric AIDS are secondary to vertical transmission from mother to fetus.
- Risk of perinatal transmission ~25%. If zidovudine (ZDV) is given during antepartum, intrapartum, and to neonate, risk of transmission is reduced to 8%.
- Combination antiretroviral therapy started in the antenatal period can reduce risk of vertical transmission to 2%.
- Reduce maternal viral load:
  - Antiretroviral therapy should be encouraged in **all** HIV-infected pregnant women regardless of CD4+ count and viral load in order to reduce vertical transmission.
  - In pregnancy, antiretroviral treatment usually consists of nucleoside reverse transcriptase inhibitor (NTRI) zidovudine-lamivudine because of its safety profile in pregnancy, combined with a protease inhibitor such as atazanavir-ritonavir.
  - CD4+ counts and viral loads should be monitored at regular intervals.
  - Blood counts and liver functions should be monitored monthly while patient is on antiretroviral therapy.
- Reduce vertical transmission:
  - Give maternal IV ZDV intrapartum.
  - Reduce duration of ruptured membranes.
  - Recommend cesarean delivery before labor or rupture of membranes if viral load >1000 copies.
  - Avoid breast-feeding.
  - Give infant post-exposure prophylaxis with ZDV for 6 weeks.

HUMAN PAPILLOMAVIRUS (HPV)

Chronic viral infection that can cause genital condyloma, cervical, vaginal, and vulvar cancer.

- Clearance of virus slower during pregnancy.
- Condyloma acuminata, external genital warts, ↑ in number and size in pregnancy.
- If size and location of lesions obstruct vaginal delivery, may need to perform a cesarean delivery.
- Lesions often regress spontaneously after delivery.
- Cesarean delivery not routinely recommended.

TREATMENT

- Trichloroacetic or bichloroacetic acid applied weekly for external warts.
- Cryotherapy.
- Laser.
- **Not** recommended for pregnancy:
  - Podophyllin resin.
  - Podofilox.
  - 5-fluorouracil.
  - Imiquimod.
  - Interferon.

EXAM TIP

HIV Testing
Opt-in approach: Patient must consent to receive the test.
Opt-out approach: Test is routinely done on all patients; patient must decline the test if she does not want it.

EXAM TIP

Two main strategies to ↓ vertical transmission of HIV:
- Antiretroviral therapy
- Cesarean delivery

EXAM TIP

With antiretrovirals and cesarean delivery, vertical transmission of HIV is reduced from 25% to 2%.

WARD TIP

HPV can cause laryngeal papillomatosis in fetus.

Handwritten notes:
intrapartum
- avoid artificial ROM, fetal scalp electrode, operative deliv.
- ≤1000: ART + NSVD
- ≥1000: ART + ZDV + C/S.

postpartum:
- mom: continue ART.
- infant: ≤1000: ZDV
- infant: ≥1000: multidrug ART.

Neonatal Infection

Juvenile-onset respiratory laryngeal papillomatosis: Rare benign neoplasm of the larynx.

- Hoarseness, respiratory distress.
- Due to HPV-6 and HPV-11.

TRICHOMONIASIS

- Diagnosis made when **flagellated organisms** seen on **wet prep**.
- Complications:
  - Preterm delivery.
  - Preterm premature ruptured membranes.
- Treat with oral metronidazole.

Vaccines during pregnancy

- recommended
- inactivated influenza
- Tdap
- Rh immunoglobin

- High risk pts
- Hep A/B.
- Hib, meningococcus pneumococcus
- VZV Ig

- contraindicated
- MMR
- Varicella
- HPV
- intranasal influenza.

Asymptomatic Bacteria

- Def'n: ≥ 100k CFU/mL bacteria
- RF
  - pregestation DM
  - hx of UTI
  - multiparity.
- Pathogens
  - E.coli
  - klebsiella
  - enterobacter
  - GBS.
- tx:
  - cephalexin
  - Amoxacillin-clavulenate
  - nitrofurantoin
  - fosfomycin

Twin Gestation

Twin pregnancy continues to ↑ in the United States secondary to assisted reproductive technologies and an advancing maternal age. Maternal and perinatal morbidity are ↑ in multiple gestations. Twin pregnancies have higher rates of almost every potential pregnancy complication, including preterm delivery, growth restriction, and congenital anomalies. Prenatal visits are more frequent with multiple gestations, since they are at increased risk for complications. Normal physiologic changes are increased, and there is an increase in cardiac output, iron requirements, plasma volume, blood volume, glomerular filtration rate, and caloric requirements.

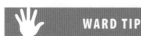

Maternal Adaptations

Maternal physiologic changes are more exaggerated compared to a singleton pregnancy.
- **Cardiac:**
    - ↑ heart rate, ↑ stroke volume, ↑ cardiac output is more secondary to the ↑ myometrial contractility and blood volume.
    - ↑ in uterine volume/weight.
- **Respiratory:** Further ↑ in tidal volume and oxygen consumption.
- **Renal:** ↑ GFR and ↑ in renal size.
- **Nutrition:**
    - Calories: Increase intake by 300 kcal/day above that for singleton pregnancy, or 600 kcal/day above that of a nonpregnant woman.
    - Weight gain: Avg/week is 1–1.75 pounds; total gain: 37–54 pounds for a normal weight woman.

Types of Twins

 A 22-year-old P2012 at 15 weeks presents for her first prenatal visit. She reports that fetal movement is present. On physical exam, her fundal height is 20 cm, at the level of the umbilicus. A bedside ultrasound reveals a twin gestation. Management of her prenatal care should include what important tests/procedures?
Answer: An ultrasound to determine chorionicity and serial ultrasounds to check for fetal growth restriction/discrepancy.

A **zygote** is the result of fertilization of an ovum with a spermatozoan.
- **Dizygotic twins** are the result of two ova fertilized by two different sperm. Risk factors include fertility drugs, race, advanced maternal age, and parity. These are fraternal twins.
- **Monozygotic twins** are the result of a single ovum fertilized by one sperm which subsequently divides. The frequency is 1 in 250 pregnancies (see Figure 10-1). These are identical twins.
- The timing of cell division within the monozygotic twin determines the amnionicity and chorionicity of twins.
    - Division of the ovum between days 0 and 3: Dichorionic, diamniotic monozygotic twins.
    - Division between 4 and 8 days: Monochorionic, diamniotic monozygotic twins.

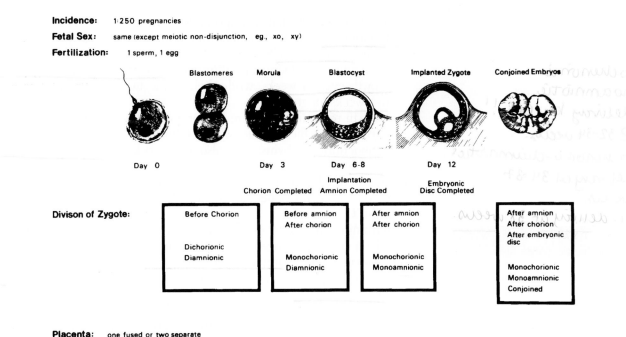

Incidence: 1:250 pregnancies

Fetal Sex: same (except meiotic non-disjunction, eg., xo, xy)

Fertilization: 1 sperm, 1 egg

FIGURE 10-1.   Mechanism of monozygous twinning. (Reproduced, with permission, from Cunningham FG, Leveno KJ, Bloom SL, et al. *Williams Obstetrics*, 22nd ed. New York: McGraw-Hill, 2005: 914.)

- Division between 9 and 12 days: Monochorionic, monoamniotic monozygotic twins.
- Division after 13 days: Conjoined twins.
- Monochorionic twins have more complications than dichorionic.
- Monoamniotic twins have more complications than diamniotic.

Prenatal Diagnosis

- Diagnosis and genetic counseling is important because of the ↑ risk of congenital anomalies.
- Both monozygotic and dizygotic twins are at ↑ for structural anomalies.
- Multiple gestation have an increased risk of aneuploidy.
  - First-trimester serum markers not as valid for multiple gestation.
  - Nuchal translucency is the preferred first-trimester marker.

Diagnosis and Management of Twins

- **Physical exam** may show a uterine size/gestational age (GA) difference with size greater than expected from GA.
- **Ultrasound** is used for the following in multiple gestations:
  - Confirm diagnosis.
  - Determine chorionicity.
  - Detect fetal anomalies.
  - Measure cervical length.
  - Evaluate for fetal growth.
  - Guide invasive procedures.
  - Confirm fetal well-being.

 WARD TIP

Vaginal delivery of twins can be performed but requires an obstetrician skilled in vaginal twin deliveries; otherwise, cesarean delivery is recommended.

 EXAM TIP

Differential diagnoses for a size/date discrepancy in pregnancy include:
- Twins
- Adnexal mass
- Distended bladder
- Fetal macrosomia
- Hydramnios
- Maternal obesity
- Uncertain LMP (wrong dates)
- Molar pregnancy

monochorionic
monoamniotic
– delivery by C/S !!
@ 32-34 weeks.
monochorionic-diamniotic
– delivery at 34-37
weeks
di-di: delivery at 38 weeks.

Multiple gestation pregnancies are at increased risk for complications such as diabetes mellitus, hypertension, congenital anomalies, and growth restriction.

Dizygotic twins are more common than monozygotic twins.

Monochorionic twins have higher complication rates than dichorionic twins, and require more frequent surveillance.

TWINS
Twin-twin transfusion: Serious complication in monochorionic twin gestations with high mortality.

- Determining chorionicity is important:
  - Chorionicity can best be determined in the first or early second trimester by ultrasound (US).
  - Monochorionic twins should undergo US examination to look for fetal growth every 4 weeks, while dichorionic twins can be scanned every 6–8 weeks for growth.
  - Growth restriction rates are higher among the monochorionic in comparison to the dichorionic twin gestation.
  - Monochorionic twins may also be at risk for twin-twin transfusion syndrome.
- Induction of labor of twins should be strongly considered when 38 weeks' gestation has been reached, as the rate of stillbirth and growth restriction ↑ after this GA.
- Determining the route of delivery (vaginal versus cesarean) should be based on the experience of the obstetrician, other obstetric indications (i.e., previa), and the presentation of both twins.
  - Trial of vaginal delivery is usually appropriate in situations where both twins are cephalic.
  - Cephalic presentation of Twin A and breech presentation of Twin B should be managed based on the experience of the provider. In some settings, vaginal delivery may be appropriate, with a plan for an internal podalic version of the second twin after delivery of the first versus vaginal breech delivery of the second twin.
  - Breech presentation of Twin A and cephalic presentation of Twin B may cause interlocking twins. Delivery should be cesarean.

monoamniotic twins at risk for cord entanglement.

Twin-Twin Transfusion

- A **serious complication** of monochorionic twin gestation in which blood/intravascular volume is shunted from one twin to another.
- The major risk is intrauterine fetal demise, in which one twin develops complications due to underperfusion (donor twin) and the other due to overperfusion (recipient twin).
- The theoretical cause is *unbalanced vascular anastomoses*.
- US is needed for diagnosis.
- Treatment is laser coagulation of the anastomoses.

– Lambda sign present in dichorionic pregnancies !
– T sign present in monochorionic pregnancies !

monochorionic/monoamniotic
– c/s at 32-34 weeks → risk of cord
entanglement!

CHAPTER 11

Abortions and Fetal Death

First-Trimester Bleeding

Bleeding in the first trimester can be from many causes that may or may not be related to the pregnancy.

DIFFERENTIAL DIAGNOSIS

■ Spontaneous abortion (including threatened abortion).
■ Ectopic pregnancy.
■ Hydatidiform mole.
■ Benign and malignant lesions (i.e., cervical polyp cervical cancer).
■ Trauma.
■ Infection.

WORKUP

■ History: Vaginal bleeding +/− abdominal pain.
■ Physical:
   ■ Vital signs (rule out shock/sepsis).
   ■ Pelvic exam (note the source of bleeding and cervical dilation).
■ Diagnostic tests:
   ■ Quantitative β-human chorionic gonadotropin (hCG) level.
   ■ Complete blood count (CBC).
   ■ Blood type and Rh. An anti-D immunoglobulin injection should be given to all D (Rh) antigen negative pregnant patients that have vaginal bleeding and a negative D (Rh) antibody screen.
      ■ Prevents maternal isoimmunization (generation of antibodies against fetal red blood cells in current or future pregnancies).
   ■ Ultrasound (US) assesses fetal viability and contents of the uterus.

Spontaneous Abortion

Spontaneous abortion (or miscarriage) is a clinically recognized pregnancy loss before 20 weeks' gestation. There are many risk factors, including advanced maternal age, maternal smoking, and history of previous spontaneous abortion.
■ **Abortion** = intentional or unintentional termination of a pregnancy <20 weeks' gestation or weight of <500 g.
■ Completed spontaneous abortion is the spontaneous expulsion of all fetal and placental tissue from the uterine cavity before 20 weeks' gestation.
■ Occurs in 8–20% of all recognized pregnancies.
■ Most miscarriages are clinically unrecognized because they occur before or at the time of the next expected menses (13–26%).

ETIOLOGIES

Chromosomal Abnormalities

■ Most common cause of spontaneous abortion, and accounts for 50% of all miscarriages. The majority of abnormal karyotypes are numeric abnormalities as a result of errors during gametogenesis, fertilization, or the first division of the fertilized ovum.
■ Frequency:
   ■ Aneuploidy (abnormal number of chromosomes): 85%.
   ■ Triploidy: 10%.
   ■ Tetraploidy: 4%.

Infections

Infectious agents in cervix, uterine cavity, or seminal fluid can cause abortions. These infections may be asymptomatic:

- *Toxoplasma gondii*
- Herpes simplex
- *Ureaplasma urealyticum*
- *Mycoplasma hominis*
- *Listeria monocytogenes*
- Chlamydia
- Gonorrhea

Structural Abnormalities

- Septate/bicornuate uterus: 25–30%.
- Cervical incompetence.
- Leiomyomas (especially submucosal).
- Intrauterine adhesions (i.e., from previous curettage).

*

Endocrine Abnormalities

- Progesterone deficiency.
- Polycystic ovarian syndrome (PCOS).
- Diabetes—uncontrolled.

Immunologic Factors

- Lupus anticoagulant.
- Anticardiolipin antibody (antiphospholipid syndrome).

antiphospholipid antibody
- ≥1 fetal death ≥10 weeks
- ≥3 spontaneous abortions < 10 weeks.
- preterm birth before 34 weeks

Environmental Factors

- Tobacco: ≥14 cigarettes/day ↑ abortion rates.
- Alcohol.
- Irradiation.
- Environmental toxin exposure.
- Caffeine: >5 cups/day.
- Trauma.

Types of Spontaneous Abortion

See Table 11-1.

THREATENED ABORTION

A 34-year-old G1P0 at 8 weeks presents to the ED with vaginal bleeding. She reports no cramping, trauma, or intercourse. She is afebrile and hemodynamically stable. Physical exam reveals a nontender abdomen. Sterile speculum shows 5 cc of dark blood in the vagina with no active bleeding. The cervix is closed and thick. US shows an 8-week intrauterine pregnancy with cardiac activity. What is the likely diagnosis? What is the best treatment for her condition? *→ threatened abortion*

Answer: Threatened abortion. The patient should be managed expectantly. Many patients have a normal pregnancy course; others may go on to miscarry.

TABLE 11-1.   **Types of Abortions**

	THREATENED	INEVITABLE	INCOMPLETE	COMPLETE	MISSED	SEPTIC
Clinical presentation	Vaginal bleeding	Cramping, bleeding	Cramping, bleeding (ongoing)	Cramping, bleeding (resolved)	Asymptomatic	Fever, abdominal/ pelvic pain, ruptured membranes
Passage of tissue	No	No	some but not all tissue passed	all tissue passed (done)	No	Variable
Cervical Os	Closed	Open	Open	Closed	Closed	Variable
Pregnancy viable	~50% will miscarry	100% will miscarry	No	No	No	Variable
Management	Transvaginal US hCG levels Expectant management	D&C vs. expectant management	D&C	Follow hCG levels to negative	D&C vs. expectant management	IV antibiotics, D&C

Threatened abortion is uterine bleeding from a gestation that is <20 weeks without cervical dilation or passage of tissue.

- Pregnancy may continue, but there is an increased risk of loss of pregnancy.
- It increases the risk of preterm labor and delivery and other adverse pregnancy outcomes.

DIAGNOSIS

- Speculum exam reveals blood coming from a **closed cervical os, without amniotic fluid or products of conception** (POC) in the endocervical canal.
- US will show an empty uterus if gestation very early, a gestational sac, or a fetus with cardiac activity. If uncertain of diagnosis, can follow serial hCGs; should ↑ by a minimum of 60% every 48 hr if normal pregnancy (peaks at ~10 weeks).

MANAGEMENT

Observation, pelvic rest.

INEVITABLE ABORTION

An 18-year-old G1P0 at 8 weeks presents to the ED complaining of cramping and vaginal spotting. She reports no passage of tissue. Physical exam shows bleeding from the cervical os, which is open. Ultrasound shows an intrauterine pregnancy with cardiac activity. What is the most likely diagnosis?

Answer: Vaginal bleeding before 20 weeks' gestation, open cervical os, and no expulsion of products of conception is an inevitable abortion.

Inevitable abortion is vaginal bleeding, cramps, and **cervical dilation at <20 weeks' gestation without expulsion of POC.** Expulsion of POC is imminent.

DIAGNOSIS

- Presence of menstrual-like cramps.
- Speculum exam reveals blood coming from an **open** cervical os.
- Fetal cardiac activity may or may not be present on US.

MANAGEMENT

- Surgical evacuation of the uterus with dilation and curettage.
- Medical uterine evacuation with misoprostol (prostaglandin E1).
- Expectant management.

INCOMPLETE ABORTION

Incomplete abortion is the **passage of some, but not all, POC** from the uterine cavity before 20 weeks' gestation.

Increased risk of:
- Ongoing bleeding requiring a blood transfusion.
- Ascending infection, septic abortion.

DIAGNOSIS

- Cramping and bleeding.
- Enlarged, boggy uterus; dilated internal os.
- POC present in the endocervical canal or vagina.
- POC retained in the uterus may be seen with US.

MANAGEMENT

- Assess hemodynamic status and stabilize (IV fluids, blood transfusion).
- Suction dilation and curettage (D&C) to remove the POC from the uterus.
- If stable, misoprostol medical evacuation may be appropriate.
- Karyotype POC if recurrent abortion.

EXAM TIP

Dilated cervix is seen with inevitable and incomplete abortions.

COMPLETE ABORTION

> A 24-year-old woman at 9 weeks presents to the ED with complaints of vaginal bleeding and cramping that is now decreased. She reports that she had an ultrasound 3 days prior showing a viable fetus. Vitals are normal. On physical exam there is no abdominal tenderness, there is 5 cc of dark blood in the vagina, and the cervix is closed. An ultrasound shows an empty uterus. What is the most likely diagnosis?
> **Answer:** Complete abortion.

Complete abortion is the **complete passage of POC**. The **cervical os is closed** after the abortion is completed.

DIAGNOSIS

- Pain has ceased.
- Uterus is well contracted. Cervical os may be closed.
- US shows empty uterus.

MANAGEMENT

- If possible, send POC to pathology to verify intrauterine pregnancy.
- Observe patient for further bleeding and signs of infection.
- Dilation and curettage usually reserved for patients with excessive bleeding or unstable vitals.

US criteria for Missed abortion:
- absence of fetal cardiac activity + CRL <7mm
- mean gestational sac diameter 20 mm w/no yolk sac or embryonal pole.

MISSED ABORTION

Missed abortion is **fetal demise** before 20 weeks of gestation **without expulsion of any POC.**

DIAGNOSIS

- The pregnant uterus fails to grow, and symptoms of pregnancy have disappeared.
- Intermittent vaginal bleeding/spotting/brown discharge and a closed cervix.
- Quantitative β-hCG may decline, plateau, or continue to ↑.
- US confirms absent fetal cardiac activity or empty gestational sac.

MANAGEMENT

- Expectant management.
  - Most women will spontaneously deliver a missed abortion within 2 weeks.
  - Risk of incomplete or septic abortion that may require a D&C.
  - Concern for coagulopathy if dead fetus is not evacuated, higher risk in T2 and T3.
- Suction D&C.
- Misoprostol (PG E$_1$) medical evacuation of the uterus.

WARD TIP

Low-normal range fibrinogen level: Early sign of consumption coagulopathy, especially:

- Low platelets
- Prolonged PT/PTT

SEPTIC ABORTION

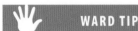 A 25-year-old G3P1011 presents to the ED with fever, lower abdominal pain, and foul-smelling discharge. She reported having a medical termination of pregnancy 6 days prior. Her temperature is 101.1°F (38.3°C), blood pressure 110/70, pulse 100, and respiratory rate 18. On physical exam, she appears lethargic and ill. She has lower abdominal tenderness, and sterile speculum exam shows a copious amount of foul-smelling discharge in the vagina. Bimanual exam reveals uterine tenderness and no adnexal masses. The cervix is dilated 1 cm and thick. Complete blood count (CBC) shows a white blood cell count (WBC) of 20K. US shows a large amount of heterogenous tissue in the uterus. What is the most likely diagnosis? What is the best treatment for her condition?

Answer: The patient has a septic abortion and should receive broad-spectrum IV antibiotics and a D&C.

- **Infected POC are present.**
- Less likely to occur with spontaneous abortion, and more likely to occur with induced abortion.
- The infection is usually polymicrobial.
- Infection can spread from endometrium, through myometrium, to parametrium and sometimes to peritoneum.
- Septic shock may occur.

DIAGNOSIS

- Fever, hypotension, tachycardia, generalized pelvic discomfort, uterine tenderness, signs of peritonitis.
- Speculum exam: Malodorous vaginal and cervical discharge.
- Leukocytosis.
- US shows retained POC.

MANAGEMENT

- Vaginal discharge culture, blood culture, check CBC, urinalysis (UA), serum electrolytes, liver function tests (LFTs), blood urea nitrogen (BUN), creatinine, and coagulation panel.
- Broad-spectrum IV antibiotics with excellent anaerobic bacteria coverage.

WARD TIP

If POC are not removed in a septic abortion, severe sepsis often occurs.

- D&C promptly after starting antibiotics and stabilizing patient.
- Hysterectomy if unable to evacuate the infected uterine contents.

RECURRENT ABORTION (RECURRENT PREGNANCY LOSS—RPL)

- Three or more successive clinically recognized pregnancy losses prior to 20 weeks gestation.
- Women with two successive spontaneous abortions have a recurrence risk of 25–30%.

ETIOLOGY

- Chromosome abnormalities: aneuploidy, parental chromosome rearrangements (balanced translocation is the most common).
- Anatomic uterine abnormalities: congential anomalies such as uterine didelphys, septate uterus, and bicornuate uterus. Septate uterus is the most common anomaly associated with RPL.
- Acquired uterine defects: Intrauterine synechiae (Asherman syndrome), submucous leiomyomas.
- Cervical incompetence: Painless cervical dilation leads to second-trimester pregnancy loss. Treat with cervical cerclage.
- Endocrine abnormalities: Diabetes mellitus, thyroid disorders, polycystic ovary syndrome (PCOS).
- Autoimmune conditions: Antiphospholipid syndrome (thrombosis results in fetal demise).
- Unexplained in a majority of cases.

MANAGEMENT

Investigate possible etiologies. Potentially useful tests include:
- Karyotype of abortus.
- Parental karyotypes: Balanced translocation in parents may result in unbalanced translocation in the fetus.
- Sonohysterogram, hysteroscopy: Evaluate uterine cavity.
- Immunologic workup: Anticardiolipin antibodies and lupus anticoagulant.
- Thyroid function tests.

Induced Abortion (Pregnancy Termination)

DEFINITIONS

- **Induced abortion:** Intentional termination of pregnancy before 20 weeks' gestation.
- **Elective termination of pregnancy:** Intentional termination performed based on the woman's desire.
- **Therapeutic abortion:** Intentional termination performed to maintain maternal health.

ASSESSMENT OF THE PATIENT

- **Confirm gestation age.**
  - US most reliable method and most commonly used.
  - Definitive LMP date and pelvic exam consistent with suspected dates is acceptable in T1.
  - Adequate dating helps determine legality of the procedure—states usually set gestational age limits.

EXAM TIP

Consumptive coagulopathy (DIC) is an uncommon but serious complication of septic abortion.

EXAM TIP

RPL is three or more pregnancy losses before 20 weeks.

EXAM TIP

After two miscarriages, women with a history of RPL have a 25–30% risk of recurrence.

Cervical incompetence- short cervix → dilates in 2nd trimester; tx w/ a cervical cerclage.

- **Blood type and Rh type:** If patient is Rh negative, anti-D immunoglobulins should be administered prophylactically.
- Careful patient counseling should be performed. Some states have mandatory requirements for waiting times and parental notification for minors.

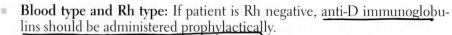

INDICATIONS FOR THERAPEUTIC ABORTION (NOT AN EXHAUSTIVE LIST)

Maternal

Severe maternal disease where continuation of pregnancy may be life-threatening: Severe cardiovascular disease, poorly controlled diabetes with end-organ damage, early severe preeclampsia (after 20 weeks), maternal malignancy requiring prompt chemotherapy.

Fetal

- Major malformation (e.g., anencephaly).
- Genetic (e.g., spinal muscular atrophy).

METHODS OF PREGNANCY TERMINATION

- Pharmacologic agents.
- Surgical methods.

Pharmacologic Agents

- Abortions in T1 and T2 can be performed with pharmacologic agents.
- **Prostaglandin E$_2$ E$_1$, F$_2\alpha$:**
  - Typically used for T2 pregnancy terminations.
  - Can be administered orally or vaginally, depending on the type of prostaglandin.
  - Given every 2–6 hr until uterus evacuated.
  - **Advantages:** Easy to use, can be safely used in women with prior cesarean delivery.
  - **Disadvantages:** Diarrhea, fever.
- **Mifepristone (RU 486) and misoprostol:**
  - Primarily used for T1 abortion.
  - Antiprogestin mifepristone 200 mg orally is followed by 800 μg buccal or oral misoprotol 24–48 hr later.
  - Ninety-two percent successful for pregnancy <49 days' gestation (7 weeks).
  - Seventy-seven percent successful for pregnancy 57–63 days' gestation (8–9 weeks).

Surgical Method

- May be used in T1 or T2.
- **Dilation and evacuation (D&E):**
- T1: Involves dilation of cervix and suction curettage of uterine contents. Sometimes referred to as **dilation and curettage (D&C).**
- T2: Involves dilation of cervix (osmotic, mechanical, pharmacologic) and extraction of fetal parts using various instruments.
  - **Advantages:** Less emotional stress for patient, avoid hospitalization, greater convenience.
  - **Disadvantages:** Need technical expertise, trauma to the cervix.
- Hysterotomy: Rarely performed unless contraindications to other methods.

WARD TIP

Differential diagnosis for T1 bleeding:

- Spontaneous abortion
- Ectopic pregnancy
- Molar pregnancy
- Vaginal/cervical lesions/lacerations

Pharm

1st Tri
- PGE1
- PGE2
- PGF2α

2nd tri
- mifepristone +
misoprostol.

WARD TIP

Differential diagnosis for T3 bleeding:

- Placental abruption
- Placenta previa
- Rupture of vasa previa
- Uterine rupture

EXAM TIP

Ninety percent of all pregnancy terminations are performed in the first trimester.

WARD TIP

Suction curettage:

- Most common procedure for pregnancy termination in T1.
- Safest surgical pregnancy termination method.

COMPLICATIONS OF SURGICAL PREGNANCY TERMINATIONS

- Infection: Most common complication.
- Incomplete removal of POC.
- Disseminated intravascular coagulation (DIC).
- Hemorrhage.
- Cervical laceration.
- Uterine perforation/rupture.
- Psychological sequelae.
- Risk of anesthesia.
- Death.

Fetal Death (Stillbirth)

Death of the fetus **>20 weeks'** gestation, **prior to complete expulsion** or extraction from the mother. Most states use 20 weeks as the cutoff distinguishing a fetal death from a miscarriage/abortion.

ETIOLOGY/RISK FACTORS

Three main classes are fetal, placental, and maternal causes.

Fetal

- Fetal growth restriction: Significant ↑ in the risk of stillbirth. It is associated with:
  - Fetal aneuploidies. ⎤ — 1st trimester **
  - Fetal infection. ⎦
  - Maternal smoking.
  - Hypertension.
  - Autoimmune disease.
  - Obesity.
  - Diabetes.
- Chromosomal and genetic abnormalities: Found in up to 8–13% of fetal deaths.
- Multiple gestation.

Placental

- Placental abruption is a common cause of fetal death (10–20% of all stillbirths).
  - Maternal cocaine and other illicit drug use.
  - Smoking.
  - Hypertension.
  - Preeclampsia.
- Placental infarction.
- Placental or membrane infection.
- Twin-twin transfusion syndrome.

Maternal

- Non-Hispanic black race.
- Nulliparity.
- Advanced maternal age.
- Obesity.
- Drugs, alcohol, smoking.
- Medical comorbidities:
  - Hypertension.
  - Diabetes.

WARD TIP

Complications are four times higher for T2 abortions than T1 abortions. Establishing GA is critical.

EXAM TIP

Death is a risk of pregnancy termination, but it is 10 times less than the risk of death from giving birth.

EXAM TIP

The most common method of induced pregnancy termination in the United States is D&C.

EXAM TIP

Medical methods of pregnancy termination are best used in the first 49 days.

EXAM TIP

PGF$_{2\alpha}$ is contraindicated for use in asthmatics, as it induces smooth muscle contraction.

PPH: methergine — HTN.

EXAM TIP

Most common reason for T2 abortions: Congenital anomalies.

CAUSES OF FETAL DEATH BASED ON TRIMESTER

T1 + infectus

- Chromosomal abnormalities.
- Environmental factors (i.e., medications, smoking, toxins).
- Maternal anatomic defects (i.e., müllerian defects).
- Endocrine factors (i.e., thyroid dysfunction, diabetes).
- Unknown.

T2

- Anticardiolipin antibodies.
- Antiphospholipid antibodies.
- Chromosomal abnormalities.
- Anatomic defects of uterus and cervix.
- Placental pathological conditions (e.g., circumvallate placentation, placenta previa). ↳ uteroplacental insufficiency

T3

- Anticardiolipin antibodies.
- Placental pathological conditions (e.g., circumvallate placentation, placenta previa, placental abruption).
- Infections (e.g., toxoplasmosis, CMV, parvovirus).

Time Nonspecific

- Trauma, including intimate partner violence.
- Cord accident.
- Maternal systemic disease (e.g., diabetes, hypertension).
- Maternal infection (e.g., chorioamnionitis).
- Substance abuse (e.g., cocaine).

DIAGNOSIS

- In late pregnancy, absent fetal movement detected by the mother is usually the first sign.
- Absent fetal heart tones by Doppler.
- **Real-time US** showing absent fetal cardiac activity is the **diagnostic method of choice**.

MANAGEMENT

- D&E may be used if fetal death occurs in T2. D&E has ↓ maternal mortality compared to PGE_2 labor induction, but also has the risk of uterine perforation.
- Labor induction if fetal death occurs in T3. Induction of labor with vaginal misoprostol is safe and effective even in patients with a prior cesarean delivery.
- Every attempt should be made to avoid a hysterotomy.
- The patient should be encouraged to seek counseling due to emotional stress caused by diagnosis of fetal death and length of time between diagnosis and delivery.

Intrauterine Adhesions (synechiae)
- RFs: infection (septic abortion, endometritis), surgery (D+C, myomectomy)
- AUB, infertility, amenorrhea, cyclic pelvic pain, recurrent pregnancy loss
- dx: hysteroscopy
- tx: lysis

Ectopic Pregnancy

Ectopic pregnancy is the leading cause of pregnancy-related maternal death during T1. Diagnose and treat *before* rupture occurs to ↓ the risk of death!

EXAM TIP

Most common site of ectopic pregnancy: Ampulla of fallopian tube.

[Handwritten notes in left margin:]

1st trimester bleeding:
- ectopic pregnancy
- hydatiform mole
- abortion
- trauma.

ampulla (FT) > AC > ovary > cervix
↓
cervical most dangerous as it has the highest risk of rupture.

Ectopic pregnancy is a pregnancy that is located <u>outside the uterine cavity</u>. The most common site is the **fallopian tubes** (97%), followed by the abdominal cavity, ovary, and cervix. Within the fallopian tubes, the **ampulla** is the most common site, followed by the isthmus and <u>fimbria</u>. <u>Cornual</u> pregnancies that occur in the intramural portion of the fallopian tube are the most dangerous due to ↑ <u>risk of uterine rupture</u> (see Figure 12-1). Rupture of the ectopic pregnancy can lead to rapid bleeding and death.

Epidemiology

- Incidence: 20/1000 reported pregnancies.
- Increased risk of recurrence.
- Three to four times more common in <u>women over age 35</u> compared to those in the 15- to 24-year-old age group.

Risk Factors

A 20-year-old G1P1001 presents to the ED with right lower quadrant (RLQ) pain and vaginal spotting. She reports that her menses have been regular, except that she is currently <u>3 weeks late</u> and her <u>last menstrual period (LMP)</u> was 7 weeks ago. She has a history of <u>pelvic inflammatory disease</u>, and she smokes one pack of cigarettes per day. Review of systems is positive for nausea and vomiting. Physical exam shows blood pressure 100/70, heart rate 90, and temperature 98.8°F (37.1°C). She has RLQ tenderness without rebound or guarding. Pelvic exam shows 5 cc of dark blood in the vault and right adnexal tenderness. Quantitative β-human chorionic gonadotropin (β-hCG) is <u>3000 mIU/mL</u>. Ultrasonography (US) shows an empty uterus. What is the most likely diagnosis?

Answer: Ectopic pregnancy. All reproductive-age women who present with abdominal pain and bleeding should have a β-hCG performed. The quantitative β-hCG is at a level where an intrauterine pregnancy should be visualized in the uterus. Since the uterus is empty, the pregnancy must be in an ectopic location.

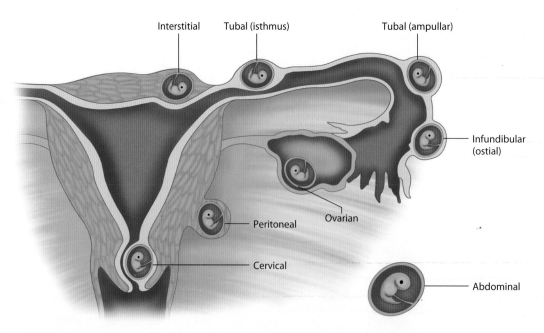

FIGURE 12-1. **Sites of ectopic pregnancy.** (Reproduced, with permission, from Ganti L. *Atlas of Emergency Medicine Procedures.* New York: Springer Nature; 2016.)

- Pelvic inflammatory disease (PID)/history of sexually transmitted infections (STIs) is a major risk factor. This can create scarring of the fallopian tubes.
- Previous ectopic pregnancy.
- Tubal scarring from prior surgery (tubal reanastamosis or sterilization).
- Current intrauterine device (IUD) use.
- Congenital malformations of the uterus: Septate uterus.
- Current smoking.
- Assisted reproductive technology: Ovulation-inducing drugs and in vitro fertilization.
- In utero diethylstilbestrol (DES) exposure.

EXAM TIP

Biggest risk factor for ectopic pregnancy: Prior ectopic pregnancy.

EXAM TIP

Ectopic pregnancy is the leading cause of pregnancy-related deaths (6%).

Exam

- Pelvic exam may reveal normal or slightly enlarged uterus.
- Vaginal bleeding.
- Pelvic pain.
- Palpable adnexal mass.
- Signs of ruptured ectopic:
  - Hypotension.
  - Tachycardia.
  - Abdominal exam with rebound and guarding.

EXAM TIP

Always check a pregnancy test on all reproductive age women with abdominal pain and/or vaginal bleeding.

Differential Diagnosis

Think of anything that can cause abdominal, adnexal pain, or bleeding in a premenopausal woman:
- Threatened abortion.
- Ovarian torsion.
- PID.
- Acute appendicitis.
- Ruptured ovarian cyst.
- Tubo-ovarian abscess.
- Degenerating uterine leiomyoma.

Diagnostic Studies

A 26-year-old G2P0010 at 6 weeks by LMP presents to the ED with left-sided abdominal pain and vaginal bleeding. She reports no chest pain, dizziness, or shortness of breath. She had a positive home pregnancy test 2 weeks ago, but has not received prenatal care yet. She was treated for pelvic inflammatory disease 1 year ago. The serum β-hCG is 2000 mIU/mL. What is the next step that will help to confirm or exclude the diagnosis of ectopic pregnancy?

Answer: Transvaginal ultrasound is the modality of choice and should be done next. The presence of an intrauterine pregnancy makes the risk of ectopic very low (not zero). The TVUS may show an empty uterus, an early intrauterine pregnancy, or findings consistent with an ectopic pregnancy.

- **Urine pregnancy test (UPT)** to confirm pregnancy: The UPT will be positive, with β-hCG levels >25 mIU/mL, approximately 1 week after conception.
- **Quantitative serum β-hCG:**
  - Should ↑ by at least 66% every 48 hr in the first 6–7 weeks of gestation after day 9.
  - Value of serial β-hCGs: Stable reliable patients can be followed with serial β-hCG levels. Inadequate rise in β-hCG is suggestive of ectopic or nonviable pregnancy.
- **Progesterone:** Not used routinely. Higher with viable IUP.
  - >25 ng/mL: Suggests normal intrauterine pregnancy (IUP).
  - <5 ng/mL: Suggests abnormal pregnancy (either ectopic or nonviable pregnancy).
  - 5–25 ng/mL: Unclear. Unfortunately, many results fall in this range and are not helpful.
- **US: Diagnostic modality of choice:**
  - Transvaginal sonography (TVUS) is more sensitive than transabdominal approach.
  - Ectopic pregnancy is suspected if a gestational sac is not seen within the uterine cavity with a serum pregnancy test at a threshold value. Threshold for detecting an IUP on TVUS is β-hCG = 1500–2000 mIU/mL. This is called the **discriminatory zone.**
    - The **discriminatory zone** is the serum β-hCG level above which a gestational sac should be visualized by TVUS if an IUP is present (see Figure 12-2).
  - US findings suggestive of ectopic pregnancy:
    - **Absence of intrauterine gestational sac.**
    - Ectopic gestational sac or cardiac activity.
    - Complex adnexal mass.
    - Fluid in the cul-de-sac: Fluid in the dependent portion of the pelvis can represent blood from the ruptured ectopic pregnancy.

Management

> A 30-year-old G2P1001 at 6 weeks presents to the ED with vaginal spotting and right lower quadrant pain. She reports no medical problems, prior surgeries, or substance abuse. She is afebrile with stable vital signs. She is tender in the right lower quadrant without rebound or guarding. Serum β-hCG is 4000 mIU/mL. TVUS shows an empty uterus with a 2.5-cm hyperechoic ring consistent with an ectopic in the right adnexa. There is a small amount of fluid in the cul-de-sac. What is the best treatment for this patient?
>
> **Answer:** Methotrexate. This hemodynamically stable patient has findings consistent with an ectopic pregnancy. With methotrexate, she avoids risks of surgery and can preserve the fallopian tube.

GENERAL

Determine if the patient is hemodynamically stable. Determine if the ectopic pregnancy is ruptured. Administer anti-D immunoglobulin if patient is D negative.

MEDICAL

Methotrexate (MTX) is an option for treatment of an unruptured early ectopic pregnancy.

[handwritten notes in margin:]
anti-D Ig indications:
- moth Rh⊖, baby Rh⊕
- abortion - spontaneous or septic
- vaginal bleeding
- ectopic pregnancy.

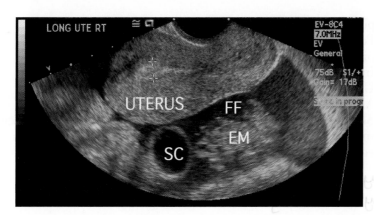

FIGURE 12-2. **Transvaginal ultrasound demonstrating an ectopic pregnancy.** Note the large amount of free fluid (FF) in the pelvis. No intrauterine pregnancy was seen. A large complex echogenic mass (EM) was seen in the left adnexa, consistent with an ectopic pregnancy. A simple cyst (SC) is also seen, in the right adnexa.

- Antimetabolite.
- Inhibits dihydrofolic acid reductase.
- Interferes with DNA synthesis.
- Treatment of certain neoplastic diseases, rheumatoid arthritis, psoriasis, and ectopic pregnancies.
- Indications:
  - Hemodynamically stable patient.
  - Ectopic pregnancy <3.5 cm.
  - Patient reliable for follow-up.
  - Intrauterine pregnancy ruled out.
  - β-hCG ≤5000 mIU/mL.
  - No fetal cardiac activity.
- Relative and/or absolute contraindications:
  - Fetal cardiac activity of ectopic pregnancy.
  - Quantitative β-hCG >15,000 mIU/mL.
  - Ectopic pregnancy >3.5 cm.
  - Hemodynamically unstable patient: MTX requires time to work.
  - Leukopenia: MTX can further suppress immune system.
  - Thrombocytopenia (<100K).
  - Active renal/hepatic disease (MTX is renally cleared and can be hepatotoxic).
  - Active peptic ulcer disease (MTX may worsen).
  - Possibility of concurrent viable intrauterine pregnancy.
  - Presence of ruptured ectopic pregnancy.
  - Breast-feeding.

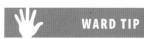

WARD TIP

Do not co-administer a nonsteroidal anti-inflammatory drug (NSAID) with MTX, as it can potentiate nephrotoxicity.

SURGICAL

- **Laparotomy** if patient is hemodynamically unstable:
  - Enter into the peritoneal cavity via a large incision on abdominal wall. Place two large-bore IVs to administer normal saline and type and cross for blood.
  - Most commonly used for hemodynamically unstable patient.
  - Fast access and minimal equipment needed.
- **Laparoscopy** if patient is hemodynamically stable:
  - Entry into peritoneal cavity via small incisions and visualization of abdominal and pelvic organs with a small camera.
  - Can be diagnostic (only visualize) or operative (perform surgical procedures).

EXAM TIP

Women who desire sterilization may have bilateral salpingectomies at the time of their surgery for ectopic pregnancy.

- **Salpingectomy:** Removal of the affected fallopian tube.
  - Performed to treat ruptured ectopic or severely damaged tube.
- **Salpingostomy:**
  - Incision on the antimesenteric portion of the tube.
  - Used for unruptured distal tubal ectopic pregnancy.
  - Allows pregnancy to be removed while sparing the tube.
  - Should follow the β-hCG down to zero as some pregnancy tissue may be left behind and continue to grow, which can cause a chronic ectopic.

Laparotomy – hemodynamically unstable
Laparoscopy – hemodynamically stable
salpingectomy - rupture or severely damage tube.
salping ostomy = unruptured, distal tubal.
        LD follow β-hCG to zero.

High-Yield Facts in Gynecology

CHAPTER 13

Contraception and Sterilization

Contraception

Contraception is a way to prevent pregnancy using medications, devices, or abstinence. Contraceptives can be used regularly prior to intercourse, at the time of intercourse, or after intercourse. A patient's choice of contraceptive method will be influenced by personal considerations, noncontraceptive benefits, efficacy, safety, cost, and contraceptive method (see Table 13-1).

TABLE 13-1. **Contraception Agents Compared Including Best-Suited Patients**

CATEGORY	AGENTS	MECHANISM	BEST SUITED FOR	DISADVANTAGES AND CONTRAINDICATIONS
Barrier	Diaphragm Cervical caps Condoms (male and female)	Mechanical obstruction	Breast-feeding Not desiring hormones **Decrease sexually transmitted infections (male condom provides the best protection against STI)**	Patient discomfort with placing devices on genitals **Lack of spontaneity** Allergies to material Diaphragm may be associated with more UTIs and risk of toxic shock syndrome
Combined hormonal (estrogen and progestin)	Combined oral contraceptives Contraception patch Vaginal ring	Inhibit ovulation Thickens cervical mucous to inhibit sperm penetration Alters motility of uterus and fallopian tubes Thins endometrium	Iron-deficiency anemia Dysmenorrhea Ovarian cysts Endometriosis **OCP**—take pill each day **PATCH—less to remember** **RING**–less to remember, vaginal irritation, and discharge	Known thrombogenic mutations Prior thromboembolic event Cerebrovascular or coronary artery disease (current or remote) Cigarette smoking (>15 cigarettes/day) at or over the age of 35 Uncontrolled hypertension Diabetic retinopathy, nephropathy, peripheral vascular disease Known or suspected breast or endometrial cancer Undiagnosed vaginal bleeding Migraines with aura Benign or malignant liver tumors, active liver disease, liver failure Known or suspected pregnancy
Progestin-only pill	Minipill	Thickens cervical mucus to inhibit sperm penetration Inhibit ovulation Alters motility of uterus and fallopian tubes Thins the endometrium	(Breast-feeding)	Very dependent on taking pill each day at same time Patient needs to remember to take pill
Injectables	Depot medroxy progesterone acetate	Inhibits ovulation Thins endometrium Alters cervical mucus to inhibit sperm penetration	Breast-feeding Iron-deficiency anemia **Sickle-cell disease** **Epilepsy** Dysmenorrhea Ovarian cysts Endometriosis	Depression Osteopenia/osteoporosis Weight gain

progestin only contraceptives for those who are breast feeding

TABLE 13-1.   Contraception Agents Compared Including Best-Suited Patients (*continued*)

CATEGORY	AGENTS	MECHANISM	BEST SUITED FOR	DISADVANTAGES AND CONTRAINDICATIONS
Implants (subdermal in arm)	Etonorgestrel Implant (Nexplanon)	Inhibits ovulation Thins endometrium Thickens cervical mucus to inhibit sperm penetration	Breast-feeding Desires long-term contraception (lasts for 3 years) Iron-deficiency anemia Dysmenorrhea Ovarian cysts Endometriosis	Hepatic tumors (benign or malignant), active liver disease Undiagnosed abnormal vaginal bleeding Known or suspected carcinoma of the breast or personal history of breast cancer Hypersensitivity to any of the components of etonogestrel implant **May lead to irregular vaginal bleeding**
IUD	Levonorgestrel intrauterine device	Thickens cervical mucus to inhibit sperm penetration Thins endometrium	Breast-feeding Desires long-term, reversible contraception Stable-mutually monogamous relationship Menorrhagia Dysmenorrhea (NOTE: decreased bleeding and dysmenorrhea)	Current STI or PID Unexplained vaginal bleeding Malignant gestational trophoblastic disease Untreated cervical or endometrial cancer Current breast cancer Anatomical abnormalities distorting the uterine cavity Uterine fibroids distorting endometrial cavity
IUD	Copper-T	Inhibits sperm migration and viability Changes transport speed of ovum Damages ovum	Desires long-term reversible con-traception (10 years) Stable, mutually monogamous relationship Contraindication to hormonal steroids	Current STI Current or PID within the past 3 months Unexplained vaginal bleeding Malignant gestational trophoblastic disease Untreated cervical or endometrial cancer Anatomical abnormalities distorting the uterine cavity Uterine fibroids distorting endometrial cavity **Wilson disease** **May cause more bleeding or dysmenorrhea**
Permanent sterilization	Bilateral tubal occlusion (can be postpartum, laparoscopic, or hysteroscopic)	Mechanical obstruction of tubes	Does not desire future fertility	Contraindications to surgery Risk of regret

(Reproduced, with permission, from Toy EC, Ross PJ, Baker B, Jennings JC. *Case Files: Obstetrics and Gynecology*. 5th ed. New York: McGraw-Hill Education, 2016. Table 44-2.)

General methods of preventing pregnancy include:

- Barrier.
- Hormonal (including oral, injectable, implants).
- Intrauterine device (IUD).
- Sterilization.
- Abstinence.

BARRIER METHODS

Female Condom

- Rarely used because of expense and inconvenience.
- It offers labial protection, unlike the male condom.
- Efficacy: 79%.

Male Condom

TYPES

- Latex: Most common, inexpensive, protects against sexually transmitted infections (STIs), some women have allergy/sensitivity.
- Synthetic (polyurethane): Expensive, protects against STIs, non-allergenic.
- Natural membrane (lamb skin): Least protection against STIs.

EFFICACY

86–97%, depending on proper and consistent use.

DRAWBACKS

- Must be placed properly before genital contact.
- ↓ sensation.
- May rupture.

Diaphragm

A flexible ring with a rubber dome that must be fitted by a gynecologist. It creates a barrier between the cervix and the lower portion of the vagina. It must be inserted with spermicide and left in place after intercourse for 6–8 hr. Does not protect against STIs.

EFFICACY

80–94%.

COMPLICATIONS

- If left in for too long, in rare cases may result in *Staphylococcus aureus* infection (which may cause **toxic shock syndrome**).
- May ↑ risk of urinary tract infection (UTI).

Cervical Cap

A smaller version of a diaphragm that fits directly over the cervix. Holds spermicide against the cervix to kill sperm. It is more popular in Europe than in the United States.

EFFICACY

- In women who have not given birth: 80–90%.
- In women who have given birth: 60–70%.

Spermicide

Foams, gels, creams placed in vagina up to 30 min before intercourse. Does not reduce the risk of STIs. Most effective when used in combination with barrier methods such as a condom or diaphragm.

TYPES

Nonoxynol-9 (most common) and octoxynol-3 are active ingredients of spermicide, which disrupt the sperm cell membrane; effective for only about 1 hr.

EXAM TIP

The only contraceptive method that protects against STIs is the male and female condom.

WARD TIP

Inconsistent condom use accounts for most failures.

EXAM TIP

Efficacy rates for spermicides are much higher when combined with other barriers (i.e., condoms, diaphragms).

EXAM TIP

P450 inducers will decrease the efficacy of oral contraceptives (OCPs) (e.g., phenytoin, rifampin, griseofulvin, carbamazepine, alcohol, barbiturates) due to increased clearance.

EFFICACY

74–94%.

Sponge

A polyurethane sponge containing nonoxynol-9 that is placed over the cervix. It can be inserted up to 24 hr before intercourse and should be left in place for 6 hours after intercourse. Available over-the-counter.

EFFICACY

84%.

RISK

Toxic shock syndrome.

HORMONAL AGENTS

A 37-year-old G2P2 woman desires a reversible form of contraception. Her history reveals that she smokes cigarettes, suffers from migraines with visual auras, has uncontrolled hypertension (HTN), and has a first-degree relative with a history of breast cancer. She requests combination oral contraceptives (COCs). How do you counsel this patient?

Answer: The patient should not be placed on COCs due to her risk factors for developing venous thromboembolism and strokes. Contraindications for OCP use include female smokers >35 years old, uncontrolled HTN, diabetes with vascular disease, migraines with visual aura, and benign or malignant liver tumors, liver disease, history of breast cancer, and pregnancy.

Combination Oral Contraceptives (COCs)

EFFICACY

- 92–99.9% (variability due to compliance).
- Contain estrogen and progestin; types include fixed dosing and phasic dosing:
  - **Fixed dosing:** Requires the same dose every day of cycle.
  - **Phasic dosing:** Gradual ↑ in amount of progestin as well as some changes in the level of estrogen.

MECHANISM OF ACTION

- **Estrogen** suppresses follicle-stimulating hormone (FSH) and therefore prevents follicular emergence. Maintains stability of endometrium.
- **Progesterone** prevents luteinizing hormone (LH) surge and therefore inhibits ovulation.
  - Thickens cervical mucus to pose as a barrier for sperm.
  - Alters motility of fallopian tube and uterus.
  - Causes endometrial atrophy.

SIDE EFFECTS

- Nausea.
- Headache.
- Bloating.

BENEFITS

- ↓ risk of ovarian cancer by 75%.
- ↓ risk of endometrial cancer by 50%.

EXAM TIP

Hormonal patch may be less effective in obese (≥200 lb) women.

WARD TIP

Types of estrogens:
  Estradiol: Reproductive life
  Estriol: Pregnancy
  Estrone: Menopause

EXAM TIP

Tension headaches are **not** a contraindication for oral contraceptive agents. Migraine headaches with visual aura can ↑ risk of stroke in patients who take combination hormonal contraception.

WARD TIP

The inactive pills in the COC simulate hormone withdrawal of the normal menstrual cycle, which results in menses.

EXAM TIP

COC: Estrogen and progesterone combined. Main mechanisms:
- Prevents ovulation
- Alters uterine and fallopian tube motility
- Thickens cervical mucus to prevent sperm penetration
- Causes endometrial atrophy

- ↓ bleeding and dysmenorrhea.
- Regulates menses.
- Reduces the risk of pelvic inflammatory disease (PID) (thicker mucus), fibrocystic breast change, ovarian cysts, ectopic pregnancy, osteoporosis, acne, and hirsutism.
- ↓ risk of anemia.

Risks

- ↑ risk of venous thromboembolism/stroke (3/10,000).
- ↑ risk of myocardial infarction (in smokers >35 years old).
- Mood changes.
- Migraines.

Contraindications

- Known thrombogenic mutations.
- Prior thromboembolic events.
- Cerebrovascular or coronary artery disease (current or remote).
- Cigarette smoking over age 35.
- Uncontrolled HTN.
- Diabetic retinopathy, nephropathy, peripheral vascular disease.
- Known or suspected breast or endometrial cancer.
- Undiagnosed vaginal bleeding.
- Migraines with visual aura.
- Benign or malignant liver tumors, active liver disease, liver failure.
- Known or suspected pregnancy.

Progestin-Only Oral Contraceptives

Efficacy

Slightly higher failure rate when compared to COCs (91–97% effective), but must be taken at same time each day (within 3 hr).

Mechanism of Action

- Thickens mucus to prevent sperm penetration.
- Alters motility of uterus and fallopian tubes.
- Causes thinning of endometrial glands.
- Contain only progestin: There is LH suppression and therefore no ovulation. The main differences from combination pills are:
  - A mature follicle is formed (but not released).
  - No placebo is used.
- Progestin-only pills are best for:
  - Lactating women (progestin, unlike estrogen, does *not* suppress breast milk).
  - Women for whom estrogen is contraindicated (e.g., estrogen-sensitive tumors).

Side Effects

- Breakthrough bleeding.
- Nausea (10–30% of women).

Transdermal (Ortho Evra)

- Efficacy similar to COCs (combined estrogen/progesterone).
- Apply and change patch once a week for 3 weeks. Remove for one patch-free week to have withdrawal bleed, then place new patch.
- May have reduced efficacy in obese women.
- May have better compliance.

- May come off and need replacement.
- Possible ↑ risk of thromboembolic events compared to COC users.

Vaginal Ring (NuvaRing)

- Efficacy similar to COCs (combined estrogen/progesterone).
- Insert and leave in place for 3 weeks. Remove for one ring-free week to have withdrawal bleed, then replace on same day of the week the old ring was removed.
- May have reduced efficacy in obese women.
- May have better compliance.

Injectable Hormonal Agents

(LARC)

A 20-year-old G0 desires long-acting reversible contraception. She has a history of grand mal seizures for which she takes an anticonvulsant. She still has seizures once about every 6 months. What is the best contraceptive method for her?

Answer: Medroxyprogesterone acetate injection can ↑ the seizure threshold and ↓ the number of seizures. It also ↓ the number of sickle cell crises in patients with sickle cell disease. It improves anemia, ↓ dysmenorrhea and ovarian cysts, and improves symptoms of endometriosis.

Medroxyprogesterone acetate (DMPA) IM injection given every 3 months.

EFFICACY

99.7%.

MECHANISM OF ACTION

Sustained high progesterone level to block LH surge (and hence ovulation). Thicker mucus and endometrial atrophy also contribute. There is no FSH suppression.

INDICATIONS

- Especially suitable for women who either cannot tolerate COCs or who are unable to take COCs as prescribed.
- DMPA can provide noncontraceptive benefits in:
  - Seizure disorder: ↓ the number of seizure episodes.
  - Sickle cell disease: ↓ the number of sickle cell crises.

SIDE EFFECTS

Epilepsy and Sickle cell dz

- Bleeding irregularity/spotting.
- Unknown when menstruation/fertility will resume after treatment cessation (can remain infertile for up to 9 months).
- ↑ hair shedding.
- Mood changes.
- ↓ high-density lipoprotein (HDL).
- ↓ libido.
- Weight gain.
- Osteopenia/osteoporosis. Reverse when stop using DMPA.

CONTRAINDICATIONS

- Known/suspected pregnancy.
- Undiagnosed vaginal bleeding.
- Breast cancer.

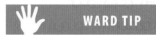

WARD TIP

There is no proven link between oral contraceptives and ↑ in breast cancer.

EXAM TIP

Side effects of estrogen:
- Breast tenderness
- Nausea
- Headache

EXAM TIP

Side effects of progestin:
- Depression
- Acne
- Weight gain
- Irregular bleeding

EXAM TIP

Why is estrogen a procoagulant? Estrogen ↑ factors VII and X and ↓ antithrombin III.

WARD TIP

Progestin-only pill requires strict compliance and requires taking the pill at the same time every day.

If contraindicated to COCs → consider nexplanen implant.

- Liver disease.
- Osteoporosis/osteopenia.

Implantable Hormonal Agents

Etonorgestrel (progestin) containing rod inserted in the subcutaneous tissue of the arm. It should be replaced every 3 years.

EFFICACY

99.8%.

MECHANISM OF ACTION

- Suppression of LH surge and inhibition of ovulation.
- Thickened mucus.
- Endometrial atrophy.

INDICATIONS

- Contraindication/intolerance to oral contraceptives.
- Smokers >35 years old.
- Women with diabetes mellitus, HTN, coronary artery disease (CAD).

SIDE EFFECTS

- Irregular bleeding.
- Acne.
- ↓ libido.
- Adnexal enlargement.
- Possible difficult removal.

CONTRAINDICATIONS

- Thrombophlebitis/embolism.
- Known/suspected pregnancy.
- Liver disease/cancer.
- Breast cancer.
- Concomitant anticonvulsant therapy.

INTRAUTERINE DEVICE

A 25-year-old G1P1, who delivered a full-term infant 6 months previously, reports a long-term, monogamous relationship. She denies a history of STIs or other medical conditions. She undergoes the insertion of an IUD without any apparent complications. The patient presents 4 days later with abdominal pain, nausea, vomiting, and fever. Speculum exam reveals malodorous discharge and IUD strings at the cervical os. What is the most likely cause for the patient's symptoms?

Answer: Endometritis due to contamination during insertion. Infections proximal to the time of IUD placement are due to contamination. Infections months to years after the IUD placement may be due to STIs.

WARD TIP

The IUD filament provides access for bacteria to the upper genital tract, so there is an ↑ risk for infection.

Insertion of a T-shaped device into the endometrial cavity with a nylon filament protruding through the cervix into the vagina to facilitate removal.

EFFICACY

97–99.1%.

MECHANISM OF ACTION

- Copper T:
    - Copper causes a sterile inflammatory reaction, creating a hostile environment.
    - Inhibits sperm migration and viability.
    - Damages ovum, changes ovum transport speed.
    - Used for 10 years.
- Levonorgestrel IUD:
    - Thickens cervical mucus.
    - Thins endometrium.
    - Used for 5 years.
    - Spermicidal.

INDICATIONS

- Oral contraceptives contraindicated/not tolerated.
- Smokers >35 years old.
- Levonorgestrel IUD can be used for menorrhagia.

CONTRAINDICATIONS

- Multiple sexual partners.
- Recent history of PID.
- Immunocompromised (e.g., HIV, sickle cell disease).
- Known/suspected pregnancy.
- Wilson disease. → *copper IUD*.
- Copper allergy.
- Absolute contraindications: Current or suspected pregnancy, undiagnosed abnormal vaginal bleeding, suspected gynecologic malignancy, acute infection (cervical, uterine, or salpingeal), history of PID, immunosuppressed patients, severe anatomical uterine distortion.

COMPLICATIONS

- PID.
- Uterine perforation.
- Ectopic pregnancy.
- Menorrhagia with Copper T.
- IUD expulsion.
- *Actinomyces* infection.

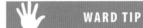

WARD TIP

Non-user-dependent methods like the IUD, subdermal implant, and injections have lower failure rates than OCPs.

WARD TIP

Contraindication for IUD placement: Women with multiple sex partners.

WARD TIP

Ectopic pregnancy is a dangerous complication of IUD use.

POSTCOITAL/EMERGENCY CONTRACEPTION

A 19-year-old G0P0 woman presents to the office concerned that she may have an undesired pregnancy after engaging in unprotected sex with her boyfriend 2 days ago. The patient does not remember the date of her last menstrual period. What therapy can you offer this patient?

Answer: Emergency contraception is effective when initiated within 72 hr of intercourse. It consists of high-dose progestin, high-dose OCPs, or insertion of a Copper T IUD.

WARD TIP

Copper and levonorgestrel IUD reduce the risk of ectopic pregnancy compared to no contraceptives, but not as much as OCPs.

Up to 3 Days After Intercourse

Levonorgestrel (Plan B): One 0.75-mg tablet taken within 72 hr of coitus. A second 0.75-mg tablet is taken 12 hr after the first dose. Efficacy: 89%.

Up to 5 Days After Intercourse

Copper T IUD: Can be left in the uterine cavity and provide contraception for up to 10 years. Efficacy: Nearly 100%.

Sterilization

Sterilization is an elective surgery that leaves a male or female unable to reproduce. With about 1 million procedures per year in the United States, sterilization is the most popular form of birth control. There are 1–4 pregnancies per 1000 sterilizations.

- Male type: Vasectomy.
- Female type: Tubal ligation or tubal occlusion.
- It is estimated that 10–12% of men who undergo vasectomies and 13–25% of women who undergo tubal ligations may experience regret after permanent sterilization. Higher regret rate is associated in women younger than age 25, women not married at the time of their tubal ligation or occlusion, or women whose tubal procedure was performed less than a year after delivery.

MALE STERILIZATION: VASECTOMY

- Excision of a small section of both vas deferens, followed by sealing of the proximal and distal cut ends (office procedure done under local anesthesia). Ejaculation still occurs.
- Sperm can still be found proximal to the surgical site, so to ensure sterility one must use contraception for 12 weeks or 20 ejaculations and then have two consecutive negative sperm counts.

FEMALE STERILIZATION

There are several methods of female sterilization.

Procedures can be performed (Figure 13-1) either postpartum (during cesarean section or immediately after vaginal delivery) or interval (remote from a pregnancy). An interval tubal occlusion should be performed in the follicular phase of the menstrual cycle in order to avoid the time of ovulation and possible pregnancy.

Laparoscopic Tubal Occlusion

Eighty to ninety percent of tubal occlusions are done laparoscopically. All methods occlude the fallopian tubes bilaterally.

Electrocautery

This involves the cauterization of a 3-cm zone of the isthmus. It is the most popular method (very effective but most difficult to reverse).

Clipping

The Hulka-Clemens clip (also Filshie clip), similar to a staple, is applied at a 90-degree angle on the isthmus. It is the most easily reversed method but also has the highest failure rate.

Banding

A length of isthmus is drawn up into the end of the trocar, and a silicone band, or Fallope ring, is placed around the base of the drawn-up portion of fallopian tube.

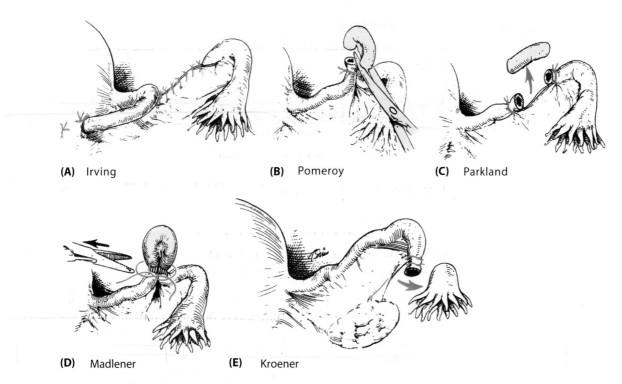

(A) Irving   (B) Pomeroy   (C) Parkland

(D) Madlener   (E) Kroener

FIGURE 13-1.   Various techniques for tubal sterility. (Reproduced, with permission, from Cunningham G, et al. *Williams Obstetrics*, 21st ed. New York: McGraw-Hill, 2001: 1556.)

Hysteroscopic Occlusion (Essure)

- Small polyester/nickel/titanium/steel coil implant is placed in the proximal fallopian tube, creating a mechanical blockage.
- Minimally invasive.
- Two-year data show 99.8% efficacy.
- Alternative contraception needed until tubal occlusion proved by hysterosalpingogram 3 months after implant placed.
- **Mechanism of action:** Scarring forms around implant over 3 months and prevents sperm to enter the fallopian tube.

Postpartum Tubal Occlusion

- **Pomeroy method:** A segment of isthmus is lifted and a suture is tied around the approximated base. The resulting loop is excised, leaving a gap between the proximal and distal ends. This is the most popular method.
- **Parkland method:** A window is made in the mesosalpinx and a segment of isthmus is tied proximally and distally and then excised.
- **Madlener method:** Similar to the Pomeroy but without the excision, a segment of isthmus is lifted and crushed and tied at the base.
- **Irving method:** The isthmus is cut, with the proximal end buried in the myometrium and the distal end buried in the mesosalpinx.
- **Kroener method:** Resection of the distal ampulla and fimbriae following ligation around the proximal ampulla.
- **Uchida method:** Epinephrine is injected beneath the serosa of the isthmus. The mesosalpinx is reflected off the tube, and the proximal end of the tube is ligated and excised. The distal end is not excised. The mesosalpinx is reattached to the excised proximal stump, while the long distal end is left to "dangle" outside of the mesosalpinx.

WARD TIP

Be sure to follow-up on pathology report after tubal ligation to ensure that tissue excised was fallopian tubes.

WARD TIP

Selection of patient for tubal ligation is important:

- Little to no history of pelvic adhesions
- Little to no history of significant PID
- Body habitus

Partial or Total Salpingectomy

Removal of part or all of the fallopian tube.

Luteal-Phase Pregnancy

A luteal-phase pregnancy is a *pregnancy diagnosed after tubal sterilization but conceived before*. Occurs around 2–3/1000 sterilizations. It is prevented by either performing sensitive pregnancy tests prior to the procedure or performing the procedure during the follicular phase.

Reversibility of Tubal Ligation

Around one-third of tubal ligations can be reversed such that pregnancy can result. **Pregnancies after tubal ligation reversal are ectopic until proven otherwise.**

Complications of Tubal Occlusion

- Failure of procedure (patient still fertile).
- **Poststerility syndrome:** Pelvic pain/dysmenorrhea, menorrhagia, ovarian cyst.
- **Fistula formation:** Uteroperitoneal fistulas can occur, especially if the procedure is performed on the fallopian tubes <2–3 cm from the uterus.
- Infection.
- Operative complications most commonly from anesthesia.

OTHER METHODS OF STERILIZATION

Colpotomy

Utilizes entry through the vaginal wall near the posterior cul-de-sac and occludes the fallopian tubes by employing methods similar to those performed in laparoscopy and laparotomy.

Hysterectomy

Removal of the uterus, either vaginally or abdominally; rarely performed for sterilization purposes. Failure rate is <1%. **Pregnancy after hysterectomy = ectopic pregnancy = emergency.**

Abstinence

CONTINUOUS ABSTINENCE

Abstaining from vaginal intercourse at any time. It is the only 100% effective way to prevent pregnancy.

NATURAL FAMILY PLANNING (NFP)

A form of birth control based on the timing of sex during a woman's menstrual cycle. It can be an effective, low-cost, and safe way to prevent an unwanted pregnancy. The success or failure of this methods will depend on the patient's ability to recognize the signs that ovulation is about to occur and abstain from having sex or use another form of contraception during the fertile period.

WARD TIP

NFP has a 75–99% success rate in preventing pregnancy, depending on patient compliance.

There are four methods of NFP:
1. Basal body temperature method.
2. Ovulation/cervical mucus method.
3. Symptothermal method.
4. Lactational amenorrhea.

Basal Body Temperature

The woman must take and record her basal body temperature every morning as soon as she wakes up. Her temperature should ↑ by 0.3–1°F for 3 consecutive days when she has a progesterone surge, indicating that she is ovulating. The couple can abstain if they do not desire pregnancy or have intercourse if they are trying to conceive.

Ovulation/Cervical Mucus Method (Billings Method)

The woman checks for the presence and change of cervical mucus at the opening of the vagina to determine if she is fertile. Most women will secrete mucus as they move closer to ovulation. At time of ovulation, a woman's mucus becomes more clear, profuse, wet, stretchy, and slippery, and is referred to as the "peak day" of fertility. After the peak day, the mucus will become thick again and go away. If couple does not desire pregnancy, they are advised to abstain from sex at the first signs of mucus until 4 days after the peak day.

Symptothermal Method

Combination of previous two methods. In addition to taking the temperature and checking for mucus changes every day, the woman checks for other signs of ovulation: Abdominal pain or cramps, spotting, and changes in the position and firmness of the cervix. This method requires that you abstain from sex from the day you first notice signs of fertility until the third day after the elevation in temperature. This method can be more effective than either of the other two methods because it uses a variety of signs.

Lactational Amenorrhea

The use of breast-feeding to space pregnancies through exclusive breast-feeding, which means no pacifiers, no bottles, and nursing on demand. This may be difficult for working mothers, so it may not be as reliable for child spacing.

ADVANTAGES OF NFP

- No side effects, allergies, breakthrough bleeding, bloating, or hormonal impact on libido.
- Low cost.
- Reversible.
- Improved knowledge and understanding of woman's fertility and normal cycle.
- Improve communication: The woman should communicate her fertility status to her partner.
- No impact on breast-feeding—no risk to baby.

DISADVANTAGES OF NFP

- Abstinence isn't always easy.
- Requires a committed and cooperative couple.
- No protection against STIs.
- Takes time to learn fertility awareness.

NOTES

COCs contraindications - explanation

E ↑ clotting factors
- x Thromboembolic dz
- x Thrombophilias

E ↑ RAAS activation → fluid retention
- x if pt has HTN

E ↑ risk of vascular events
- CAD, CVD, PAD x
- Diabetic nephropathy retinopathy x
- smokers ≥ 35 y/o x
- migraine w/ aura → ↑ stroke risk x

E ↑ risk of breast + endometrial cancer
- do not give if BC or EC.

E ↑ tumor growth in Liver
- x in benign or malignant liver dz

✗ Prevents preg
- contra in vaginal bleeding of unknown origin
- known or suspected pregnancy!

CHAPTER 14

Menstruation

Puberty

- Puberty is the transition from childhood to the final stage of maturation that allows for reproduction.
- Puberty is believed to begin with **disinhibition** of the pulsatile gonadotropin-releasing hormone (GnRH) secretion from the hypothalamus (mechanism is unknown).

SECONDARY SEX CHARACTERISTICS

Development of the secondary sexual characteristics proceeds in the following order:

1. **Thelarche** (breast budding). Average age 10 years. Due to increase in estradiol.
2. **Pubarche** (axillary and pubic hair growth). Average age 11 years. Due to increase in adrenal hormones.
3. **Menarche** (first menses). Average age 12 years. Due to increase in estradiol.

TANNER STAGES

The Tanner stages of development refer to the sequence of events of breast and pubic hair development.

- **Stage 1:** Prepubertal child. *
- **Stages 2–4:** Development stages.
- **Stage 5:** Adult. *

PRECOCIOUS PUBERTY

Appearance of the secondary sexual characteristics before 8 years of age is referred to as precocious puberty and requires investigation into the etiology. Cause may be central (gonadotropin-dependent) or peripheral (gonadotropin-independent).

ETIOLOGY (NOT AN EXHAUSTIVE LIST)

Central Causes

- Idiopathic: Most common (80–90%).
- Tumors of the hypothalamic-pituitary stalk: Prevent negative feedback.
- Inflammation of the hypothalamus: ↑ GnRH production.
- 21-hydroxylase deficiency.

Peripheral Causes

- Estrogen-secreting tumors (often ovarian tumors or cysts).
- Excess exogenous estrogen.
- Adrenal or thyroid abnormalities.
- McCune-Albright syndrome (triad of precocious puberty, café au lait spots, fibrous bone dysplasia).

Menstrual Cycle

The menstrual cycle is the cyclical changes that occur in the female reproductive system (see Figure 14-1 and Table 14-1). The hypothalamus, pituitary, ovaries, and uterus interact to allow ovulation approximately once per month (average 28 days [+/− 7 days]). The following description is based on a 28-day menstrual cycle.

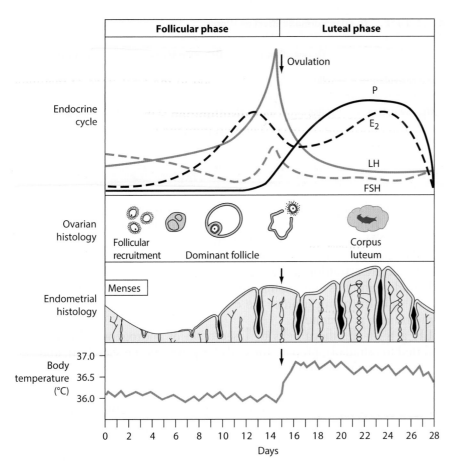

FIGURE 14-1. **The menstrual cycle.** (Modified, with permission, from Fauci AS, Braunwald E, Isselbacher KJ, et al. *Harrison's Principles of Internal Medicine*, 14th ed. New York: McGraw-Hill, 1998: 2101.)

TABLE 14-1. **Summary of Menstrual Cycle**

Menstruation: Withdrawal of progesterone causes endometrial sloughing.

Follicular phase:
- FSH causes follicle maturation and estrogen secretion.
- Estrogen causes endometrial proliferation.

Ovulation: LH surge causes oocyte to be released.

Luteal phase: Corpus luteum secretes progesterone, which causes:
- Endometrial maturation.
- ↓ FSH, ↓ LH.

- Many follicles are stimulated by follicle-stimulating hormone (FSH), but *the follicle that secretes more estrogen than androgen will be released.* This dominant follicle releases the most estradiol so that its positive feedback causes an LH surge.
- Average menses = 4 days. More than 7 days is abnormal.
- Blood loss in menstruation averages 30–50 mL and should not form clots; >80 mL is an abnormally high amount of blood loss.

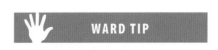

WARD TIP

Prostaglandins released from the endometrium cause dysmenorrhea.

TABLE 14-2.   Ovarian Hormone Effect on Uterus

	OVARIAN PHASE	**DOMINANT HORMONE**	**UTERINE PHASE**
Before ovulation	Follicular	Estrogen	Proliferative
After ovulation	Luteal	Progesterone	Secretory

DAYS 1–14: FOLLICULAR PHASE

- The follicular phase begins on the first day of menses. All hormone levels are low. Without any negative feedback, **GnRH** from the hypothalamus causes **FSH** release from the pituitary.
- **FSH** stimulates maturation of granulosa cells in the ovary. The granulosa cells secrete **estradiol** in response.
- **Estradiol** inhibits luteinizing hormone (**LH**) and **FSH** due to negative feedback. In the meantime, the **estradiol** secretion also causes the endometrium to proliferate.
- **LH** acts on the theca cells to ↑ secretion of **androgens** (which are converted to estradiol), prepare the cells for progesterone secretion, and cause further granulosa maturation.

DAY 14: OVULATION

- A critical level of estradiol triggers an LH surge.
- The **LH surge** causes the oocyte to be released from the follicle. The ruptured follicle then becomes the corpus luteum, which secretes progesterone.

DAYS 14–28: LUTEAL PHASE

- The corpus luteum secretes progesterone for only about 14 days in the absence of human chorionic gonadotropin (hCG).
- **Progesterone** causes the endometrium to mature in preparation for possible implantation. It becomes highly vascularized and ↑ glandular secretions (see Table 14-2).
- **Progesterone** also inhibits the release of **FSH** and **LH**.
- If fertilization does not occur, the corpus luteum involutes, **progesterone** and **estradiol** levels fall, with subsequent endometrial sloughing (menses). The hypothalamic-pituitary axis is released from inhibition, and the cycle begins again.

WARD TIP

Ovulation takes place 24–36 hr after LH surge and 12 hr after LH peak.

WARD TIP

The follicular phase is highly variable. The luteal phase is usually about 14 days due to the length of time the corpus luteum is able to secrete progesterone.

EXAM TIP

The corpus luteum is maintained after fertilization by hCG, which is released by the embryo.

CHAPTER 15

Premenstrual Syndrome/Premenstrual Dysphoric Disorder

Premenstrual syndrome (PMS) and premenstrual dysphoric disorder (PMDD) have many symptoms that overlap with anxiety and depression. A differentiation should be made because each has a different treatment. PMS and PMDD both have similar symptoms, but PMDD has markedly severe symptoms. The symptoms of PMS **do not impair** daily activities; however, the symptoms of PMDD **do affect** the activities of daily living. The symptoms occur in the luteal phase for both conditions.

Definition

- Refers to a group of behavioral and physical symptoms.
- Occur in luteal phase of the menstrual cycle and resolves shortly after menses begins.
- May interfere with work and personal relationships.
- Symptoms followed by a symptom-free period.
- Monitor for 3 months because symptoms can be variable month to month, and the diagnosis relies on symptoms for 3 consecutive months.

Premenstrual Syndrome Diagnostic Criteria

A 26-year-old woman complains of feeling sad and confused before her menses. She reports having headaches and breast pain. She feels better when she is alone, but she is able to work and take care of her two children. Once she begins menses, she no longer has these symptoms. What is the most likely diagnosis? What is the best way to make the diagnosis?

Answer: PMS. This patient has affective and somatic complaints that resolve with menses. She is able to continue her daily activities despite the symptoms. Best diagnostic method is keeping a prospective symptom diary for 3 months.

- At least one of the following affective and somatic symptoms during the luteal phase that leads to impaired functioning:
  - Affective symptoms:
    - Depression.
    - Angry outburst.
    - Irritability.
    - Anxiety.
    - Confusion.
    - Social withdrawal.
  - Somatic symptoms:
    - Breast tenderness.
    - Abdominal bloating.
    - Headache.
    - Extremity swelling.
- Relieved shortly after the onset of menses, providing a symptom-free interval.
- Symptoms occur in three prospectively monitored cycles.
- Exclude other diagnoses—depression and anxiety may present all throughout the cycle.

Premenstrual Dysphoric Disorder Diagnostic Criteria (diagnosis made using DSM-V Criteria)

A 17-year-old G0 complains of being sad 4 days right before she starts menstruating. She reports low energy, fatigue, hopelessness, anxiety, mood swings, bloating, breast tenderness, headache, and sleep disturbances during these days. These symptoms disappear 2 days after the start of menses. They occur on a monthly basis. She reports that she misses school on a monthly basis because she cannot get out of bed for 3 days. What is the most likely diagnosis? What is the best objective test to confirm the diagnosis?

Answer: PMDD. This patient has symptoms consistent with PMS, but with markedly severe symptoms that affect daily activities. She should monitor her symptoms in relation to her menses and record them prospectively.

- Physical and behavioral symptoms with prospectively monitored cycles for most of the preceding year.
- Symptoms must cause significant stress or interference with normal daily activities.

DSM-V DIAGNOSTIC CRITERIA

- One or more of the following symptoms:
  - Feeling sad, hopeless, or having self-deprecating thoughts.
  - Anxiety or tension.
  - Mood lability and crying.
  - Persistent irritability, anger, ↑ interpersonal conflicts.
- In addition, one or more of the following symptoms must be present to reach a total of five symptoms overall:
  - Problems concentrating.
  - Changes in appetite.
  - Anhedonia.
  - Decreased energy.
  - Feeling overwhelmed.
  - Physical symptoms, i.e., breast tenderness, bloating.
  - Sleep disturbances.

SIGECAPS + Moods sx.

— sad/depressed
— anxieus
— mood liability
— anger
+ SIGECAPS
+ Physical sx.

EXAM TIP

Diagnosis of PMS should be made from recording symptoms on a prospective calendar.

Tests

- Prospective calendar of symptoms in relation to menses.
- Validated prospective self-administered questionnaire: Daily Record of Severity of Problems (DRSP) form.

Treatment

No drugs are currently FDA approved for the treatment of PMS or PMDD, but several drugs are helpful when used off label. There are also some dietary and lifestyle modifications that have been helpful. Treatment can be recommended based on severity of symptoms.

EXAM TIP

The therapy with most evidence for effectiveness for PMS/PMDD: SSRIs and ovulation blocking agents.

- **Supportive therapy:**
  - Reassurance and information counseling.
  - Relaxation therapy for severe symptoms has been shown to help.
  - Stress reduction. + *exercise*
- **Aerobic exercise** reduces affective symptoms, especially depression.
- **Dietary supplementation:** ⟨Vitamin E ↓ mastalgia⟩
- **Selective serotonin reuptake inhibitors (SSRIs):**
  - Fluoxetine and sertraline have been well studied and shown to help. Other SSRIs may have similar efficacy.
  - Can be administered throughout the menstrual cycle or just with symptoms during the luteal phase of the cycle.
- **Oral contraceptives:**
  - Cyclic combined oral contraceptives (COCs) with 4- rather than 7-day placebo may be more effective.
  - If symptoms do not improve with cyclic COCs, consider continuous COCs.
  - Monophasic COCs are best.
- **Other therapies:**
  - Nonsteroidal anti-inflammatory drugs (NSAIDs).
  - Gonadotropin-releasing hormone (GnRH) agonists: Severe symptoms that do not respond to SSRIs or COCs.
  - Bilateral salpingo-oophorectomy (+/− hysterectomy): Reserved as a last resort for severe cases of PMDD. Patients must have improvement with GnRH agonists, and have completed childbearing.

stress red + exercise

SSRIs + COCs

NSAIDs, GnRH agonists

Bilateral Salpingo oophorectomy.

PMS (depression, anxiety, irritability larger, confusion + physical sx
→ breast tenderness, HA, abd. bloating, extremity swelling)
→ NO social/occupational impairment

PMDD – Dep, anxiety, mood lability, anger + SIG ECAPS + physical sx
– significant social/occ impairment

CHAPTER 16

Infertility

The monthly conception rate is 20% in a group of normal fertile couples. Infertility ↑ with increasing age of the female partner.

- Female factors account for 50–60% of infertile couples.
- Male factors account for 26% of infertile couples.
- In 40% of infertile couples, there are multiple causes.

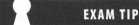

EXAM TIP

Infertility is defined as a failure to conceive after 1 year of unprotected intercourse in a woman under age 35.

Definition: Infertility

- The inability to conceive **after 12 months** of unprotected sexual intercourse in a woman under age 35, and after **6 months** of regular intercourse in a woman ~~under~~ over age 35.
- Affects 15% of couples.

Types

- **Primary infertility:** Infertility in the absence of previous pregnancy.
- **Secondary infertility:** Infertility after previous pregnancy.

Female Factors Affecting Infertility

- Multifactorial: 40%.
- Unexplained: 28%.
- Ovulatory dysfunction: 21%.
- Tubal disease: 14%.
- Endometriosis: 6%.

Male Factors Affecting Infertility

- Abnormal sperm function.
- Abnormal sperm production.
- Obstruction of ductal system (seminiferous tubules to urethral orifice).

Infertility Workup

The workup should include a complete history and physical examination. Both partners should be evaluated concurrently.

See Table 16-1.

MALE FACTOR

EXAM TIP

Calcium channel blockers and furantoins can impair sperm number and function.

Semen Analysis

Performed after at least 48 hr of abstinence, with examination of the sperm within a maximum of 2 hr from time of ejaculation (for those who prefer to collect at home). Two properly performed semen analyses should be obtained at least 1–2 weeks apart. The analysis reflects sperm production that occurred 3 months ago.

TABLE 16-1. Evaluation of Infertile Couple

Male factor: Semen analysis.

Ovulation factor: Serum progesterone, day 3 FSH, prolactin.

Uterine factor: Ultrasonography, hysterosonogram, hysterosalpingogram, hysteroscopy.

Tubal factor: Hysterosalpingogram, laparoscopy.

Endometriosis: Laparoscopy.

[handwritten margin note: ovarian → chemical: β-hCG, progesterone, prolactin. uterine → mechanical: US, hysterosalpingogram, sono hysterogram, hysteroscopy. fallopian → mechanical: hysterosalpingogram, lap.]

CHARACTERISTICS

- Volume: Normal >2 mL.
- Semen count: Normal >20 million/mL.
- Motility: Normal >50% with forward movement.
- Morphology: Normal >40%.

TREATMENT FOR ABNORMAL SEMEN ANALYSIS

- Depends on the cause.
- Refer to urologist.
- Smoking and alcohol cessation.
- Avoid lubricants with intercourse.
- Clomiphene citrate or aromatase inhibitors (for the male partner) to block negative feedback of estrogens and increase LH, FSH, and testosterone production.
- Assisted Reproductive Technologies (with partner or donor sperm):
  - Intrauterine insemination: Sperm injected through cervix.
  - Intracytoplasmic sperm injection (ICSI).
  - In vitro fertilization.
- If semen analysis is normal, continue workup of other factors.

WARD TIP

Most male infertility is idiopathic.

[handwritten: - ↓EtOH/Tob - clomiphene citrate or aromatase inhibitors. - IVF, IUI, intracytoplasmic sperm injection]

OVARIAN FACTOR

A 28-year-old G0 has been unable to conceive with her husband over one year. Her periods are irregular. She has a BMI of 30, displays coarse facial hair, and a dark velvety pigmentation on the back of her neck. What is the likely diagnosis in this patient? What is the reason she is unable to conceive?

Answer: Polycystic ovarian syndrome (PCOS) affects approximately 5% of all women, and is a leading cause of infertility. Her exam shows evidence of hyperandrogenism and insulin resistance. She is anovulatory and will need an ovulation induction agent to conceive.

WARD TIP

Initial workup for infertility:
- Assess ovulatory function and ovarian reserve
- Semen analysis
- Hysterosalpingogram

METHODS OF ASSESSING OVULATION

- **History of regular monthly menses** is a strong indicator of normal ovulation, especially if accompanied by symptoms of breast tenderness, bloating, etc.
- **Basal body temperature (BBT):** Body temperature rises about 0.5–1°F during the luteal phase due to the ↑ level of progesterone. Elevation of BBT is a good indicator that ovulation is taking place, but it can be hard to interpret and therefore is not used widely.
- **Day 21 (mid-luteal) serum progesterone:** May be low <3 ng/mL if anovulatory. If >3 ng/mL, the patient is likely to be ovulatory.
- **Ovulation predictor kit:** Available over the counter and tests for LH surge, which is highly predictive of ovulation.

[handwritten: - <3 ng/mL prog → anovulatory - >3 ng/mL prog → ovulatory]

PCOS
— ovulation induction
 1.) Clomiphene citrate
 2.) Gonadotropins
 3.) Aromatase inhibitors
— metformin + weight loss.

↑ FSH, LH } POF
↓ Estrogen

ovulating fx
— regularity of menstrual cycle
— luteal prog
— LH sing kit
— Basal Body Temp.

Ovarian Reserve.
— Day 3 FSH → N ↓
— Clomiphene citrate challenge.
— Antral Follicle count w/ TVUS
— AMH: ∝ to primordial pool.

semen
↓
ovaries
↓
uterus
↓
fallopian tubes
} infertility evaluation

HSG = fluoroscopy w/ dye.
Hysteroscopy = camera
Sonohysterogram = saline fluid + US.
Laparoscopy = mullerian defects or endometriosis

POSSIBLE CAUSES AND TREATMENTS OF ANOVULATION

- **Hypogonadotropic Hypogonadism:** i.e., hypothalamic amenorrhea from stress or starvation. Treat with lifestyle modification +/− ovulation induction.
- **Hyperprolactinemia:** Administer bromocriptine, a dopamine agonist, which suppresses prolactin. May also require ovulation induction.
- **Normogonadotropic Normoestrogenic:** i.e., PCOS: Treat with ovulation induction agent +/− metformin, weight loss. Ovulation induction agents include clomiphene citrate, gonadotropins, and aromatase inhibitors.
- **Hypergonadotropic Hypoestrogenic:** i.e., premature ovarian failure. Treat with IVF with donor eggs.

METHODS OF ASSESSING OVARIAN RESERVE

- **Day 3 FSH:** Early low levels of FSH indicate adequate production of ovarian hormones.
- **Clomiphene Citrate Challenge Test (CCCT):** 100-mg clomiphene citrate days 5–9 with measurement of FSH on days 3 and 10, and estradiol on day 3.
- **Antral Follicle Count (AFC):** TVUS in early follicular phase to count antral follicles; a low count indicates poor reserve.
- **Anti-Müllerian Hormone (AMH):** Biochemical marker of ovarian function; serum levels decline as the primordial follicle pool declines with age.

UTERINE FACTORS

A 30-year-old G0 is undergoing an evaluation of her uterus as part of the workup for infertility. What procedure to evaluate the uterus would be both diagnostic and therapeutic?

Answer: Hysteroscopy allows diagnosis of a uterine anomaly and treatment at the same time.

If ovulation analysis and semen analysis are normal, analysis of the internal architecture of the uterus and fallopian tubes is performed to determine if there is an anatomic obstruction causing infertility. In most cases, an internal architecture study is part of the initial workup.

- **Hysterosalpingogram (HSG):**
  - First-line test for evaluation of tubal patency and also allows visualization of the uterine cavity.
  - Radiopaque dye is injected into the cervix and uterus. Dye passes through the fallopian tubes to the peritoneal cavity. It should outline the inner uterine contour and both fallopian tubes when imaged with fluoroscopy.
  - Performed during follicular phase (avoid possibility of pregnancy).
  - Subfertile women who undergo HSG have higher pregnancy rates than subfertile women who do not undergo HSG. Appears to be both diagnostic and therapeutic.
- **Hysteroscopy:**
  - A hysteroscope is a telescope that is connected to a video unit with a fiber-optic light source.
  - It is introduced through the cervix and allows visualization of the uterine cavity.
  - It can be diagnostic and therapeutic. It can view the abnormality and treat it at the same time (i.e., resection of a uterine septum).

- Operative hysteroscopy is useful in:
  - Asherman syndrome (lyse intrauterine adhesions).
  - Endometrial polyps (polypectomy).
  - Congenital uterine malformations (i.e., uterine septum).
  - Submucosal fibroids (resect).
- **Sonohysterogram:**
  - Fluid is instilled in the endometrial cavity concurrently with a pelvic ultrasound.
  - Outlines intrauterine pathology (i.e., polyps, submucosal fibroids).
  - Can be done with an ultrasound in an office setting.
- **Ultrasound:**
  - In office study. Can allow diagnosis of fibroids.
- **Laparoscopy:**
  - A telescope is placed through the skin of the abdominal wall into the peritoneal cavity.
  - Can visualize outside of the uterus to assist in diagnosis of some müllerian malformations (and also for evaluation of endometriosis). Often performed in conjunction with hysteroscopy in the OR.

CAUSES AND TREATMENTS FOR UTERINE FACTOR INFERTILITY

- Submucosal fibroid: Resection, myomectomy.
- Intrauterine septum: Hysteroscopic resection of septum.
- Uterine didelphys: Metroplasty—a procedure to unify the two endometrial cavities.
- Asherman syndrome: Hysteroscopic lysis of intrauterine adhesions.

TUBAL FACTOR

A 30-year-old G0 has been having unprotected intercourse for 18 months without getting pregnant. She reports regular menstrual cycles. She had two episodes of pelvic inflammatory disease (PID) in the past. What is the best diagnostic modality to evaluate this patient? What will be the best treatment for her infertility?

Answer: Hysterosalpingogram will help determine if there is tubal blockage due to PID. If tubal blockage is present, the most effective treatment is in vitro fertilization.

EVALUATION

- Hysterosalpingogram (HSG)
- Laparoscopy

CAUSES AND TREATMENTS FOR TUBAL FACTOR INFERTILITY

- Adhesions:
  - Lysis of adhesions via laparoscopy.
  - Microsurgical tuboplasty.
  - Neosalpingostomy (blocked tubes are opened).
  - In vitro fertilization (IVF). Preferred in most cases.
- If the evaluation up to this point is within normal limits, then a diagnostic laparoscopy should be performed.

PERITONEAL FACTORS

Laparoscopy is diagnostic and therapeutic.

CAUSES AND TREATMENTS FOR PERITONEAL FACTOR INFERTILITY

- **Adhesions:** Lysis of adhesions via laparoscopy.
- **Endometriosis: Excision or ablation of implants.**

WARD TIP

Damage from tubal surgery can result in ectopic pregnancy. Most reproductive endocrinologists recommend in vitro fertilization if tubal factor is present. If the obstruction is distal and the patient is young, surgery may be an option.

Assisted Reproductive Technologies

Assisted reproductive technologies (ARTs) include clinical and laboratory techniques that are used to achieve pregnancy in infertile couples. ARTs are employed when correction of the underlying cause of infertility is not feasible.

DEFINITION

Directly retrieving eggs from the ovary followed by manipulation and replacement. The following are examples. Aside from intrauterine insemination, ARTs can utilize patient or donor egg and/or sperm.

WARD TIP

IVF ↑ the chances of multiple gestation.

INTRAUTERINE INSEMINATION

- Washed sperm is injected into the uterus.
- Must have a normal fallopian tube for fertilization to take place.

IN VITRO FERTILIZATION (IVF) AND EMBRYO TRANSFER

- Egg cells are fertilized by sperm outside the uterus.
- Consists of ovarian stimulation, egg retrieval, fertilization, selection, and embryo transfer into uterus.
- Success rate of IVF is about 20%.
- Expensive.

INTRACYTOPLASMIC SPERM INJECTION (ICSI)

- Subtype of IVF.
- Injection of spermatozoan into oocyte cytoplasm.
- Revolutionized treatment of infertility in men with severe oligospermia (low number), azoospermia (absence of live sperm), asthenospermia (low motility), teratospermia (abnormal morphology).
- Pregnancy rate: 25–30% per cycle.
- Increased risk of multifetal gestation.
- Not influenced by cause of abnormal sperm.
- Can use spermatozoa from testicular biopsies.
- Expensive.

GAMETE INTRAFALLOPIAN TRANSFER (GIFT)

- Egg and sperm are placed in a normal fallopian tube for fertilization.
- Success rate is about 25%.

ZYGOTE INTRAFALLOPIAN TRANSFER (ZIFT)

- Zygote created via fertilization in vitro and placed in fallopian tube, where it proceeds to uterus for natural implantation.
- Success rate is about 30%.

ARTIFICIAL INSEMINATION WITH DONOR SPERM

- Success rate is 75% in six cycles.
- Donor sperm is used for ARTs.

Amenorrhea

Infertility Simplified:

1.) Assess male first
- sperm count → anabolic steroids can ↓
- Scrotal temp → hyperthermia in varicocele.
- testicular damage?
- psychogenic? (↓ libido, erectile dysfx)
- assess for possible Kallmann

2.) assess female - ovulatory fx
- Basal body temp rise during luteal phase
- Hormones
    - mid luteal progesterone.
    - FSH, TSH, prolactin, B-hCG, androgens.

3.) Assess patency of uterus/fallopian tubes.
- hysterosalpingogram (1)
- sonohistogram (2)
    ↳ if either abn → hysteroscopy, or laparoscopy.

4.) examine cervix for abn.

The causes of <u>amenorrhea</u> are quite varied. The hypothalamic-pituitary-ovarian (HPO) <u>axis</u> is involved in the regulation of the menstrual cycle, the uterus responds to the HPO axis, and a normal cervix and vagina allow the outflow of menstrual blood. An abnormality in any one of these components will result in amenorrhea.

- **Primary amenorrhea:** <u>Absence of menses by age 16</u> with normal growth and secondary sexual characteristics, or absence of menses <u>by age 13 with no secondary sexual characteristics.</u> Usually caused by a genetic or anatomic abnormality.
- **Secondary amenorrhea:** Absence of menses for (≥6 months) in a woman who previously had normal menses. Usually caused by an underlying medical condition.

Primary Amenorrhea

The causes of primary amenorrhea have been traditionally classified based on where the abnormality takes place along the HPO axis. It is more clinically useful to group the causes of primary amenorrhea on the basis of whether secondary sexual characteristics (breasts) and female internal genitalia (uterus) are present or absent. The external female genitalia are normal for these patients, but noting breast and uterus development on physical exam can indicate the diagnostic tests that will be most helpful.

BREASTS ABSENT, UTERUS PRESENT

Patients <u>without breasts</u> and with a uterus have <u>no ovarian estrogen</u>. It is important to distinguish the disease processes because it can have an impact on fertility.

- **Gonadal dysgenesis (hypergonadotropic hypogonadism):** The most common cause of primary amenorrhea, and is usually due to a chromosomal deletion or disorder. The ovaries are replaced by a <u>band of fibrous tissue</u> called *gonadal streak*. Due to the absence of ovarian follicles, there is no synthesis of ovarian steroids. Due to low levels of estrogen, breast development does not occur. Follicle-stimulating hormone (FSH) and luteinizing <u>hormone (LH) levels</u> are markedly elevated because the ↓ levels of estrogen do not provide negative feedback. Estrogen is not necessary for müllerian duct development or wolffian duct regression, so the internal and external genitalia are phenotypically female.
- **Turner syndrome (45,X):** In addition to primary amenorrhea and absent breasts, these patients have other phenotypic abnormalities such as <u>short stature (most prevalent)</u>, <u>webbing of the neck</u>, <u>short fourth metacarpal</u>, and <u>cubitus valgus</u>. Also may have cardiac abnormalities (coarctation of the aorta), renal abnormalities, and hypothyroidism. At puberty, the patient is given estrogen and progesterone to allow secondary sexual characteristics to develop. These patients also receive <u>growth hormone</u>.
- **Structurally abnormal X chromosome:** May have the same abnormalities as Turner syndrome patients.
- **17α-hydroxylase deficiency:** Can occur in 46,XX or 46, XY. Patients have ↓ cortisol and adrenal/gonadal sex steroid secretion. They have hypertension, hypernatremia, and hypokalemia due to excess <u>mineralocorticoid</u>. These patients need replacement with <u>sex steroids</u> and <u>cortisol</u>. Despite low levels of sex steroids, pregnancies have been achieved with IVF. Those with karyotype <u>46,XY</u> and 17α-hydroxylase deficiency will have no breasts or female internal <u>genitalia.</u>

- **Hypothalamic-pituitary disorders:** Low levels of estrogen are due to low gonadotropin release.
    - **Anatomic lesions:** Anatomic lesions of the hypothalamus or pituitary can result in low gonadotropin production.
        - Congenital: Stenosis of aqueduct, absence of sellar floor.
        - Acquired: Prolactinoma, chromophobe adenoma, craniopharyngiomas.
    - **Inadequate gonadotropin-releasing hormone (GnRH) release (hypogonadotropic hypogonadism):** Will have normal levels of gonadotropins if stimulated with GnRH. These patients should receive estrogen-progesterone supplementation to induce breast development and allow for epiphyseal closure. Human menopausal gonadotropins or pulsatile GnRH is administered for fertility. Clomiphene does not work due to low levels of endogenous estrogen.
        - **Kallmann syndrome:** Anosmia associated with low gonadotropins.
    - **Isolated gonadotropin deficiency (pituitary disease):** Associated with:
        - Prepubertal hypothyroidism.
        - Kernicterus.
        - Mumps encephalitis.
        - Thalassemia major: Iron deposits in the pituitary.
        - Retinitis pigmentosa.

BREASTS PRESENT, UTERUS ABSENT

> An 18-year-old G0 presents with primary amenorrhea. Her sister experienced menarche at age 12. She reports no use of drugs, heavy exercise, or significant weight loss. She is 5'5" and 130 lb. Her blood pressure is 110/60. She has Tanner stage IV breasts, but no axillary or pubic hair. She has a blind vaginal pouch. What is the most likely diagnosis?
>
> **Answer:** Androgen insensitivity. Breasts are present; uterus and axillary/pubic hair is absent in androgen insensitivity.

- **Androgen insensitivity (testicular feminization):** This condition results from the absence of androgen receptors or lack of responsiveness to androgen stimulus. These patients have an XY karyotype and normally functioning male gonads that produce normal male levels of testosterone and dihydrotestosterone. The müllerian ducts regress due to the presence of antimüllerian hormone, and the wolffian ducts do not develop because they are not stimulated by testosterone. Patients with this condition have no male or female internal genitalia, have normal female external genitalia, and have either a short or absent vagina. These patients have normal breasts and scant or absent axillary and pubic hair. Testes may be located intra-abdominally or in the inguinal canal, and have an ↑ risk of developing a malignancy (gonadoblastoma or dysgerminoma), usually after age 20. The gonads should be removed after puberty to allow for breast development and adequate bone growth. Estrogen is then given. These patients are raised as females.
- **Müllerian agenesis (Mayer-Rokitansky-Kuster-Hauser syndrome):** In this condition, the patients have no uterus and have a shortened vagina, but have normally ovulating ovaries, normal breast development, and normal axillary and pubic hair. These patients have associated renal and skeletal abnormalities and should be screened with an ultrasound or MRI. They have normal endocrine function and do not need supplemental hormones. They may undergo surgical reconstruction of the vagina or use vaginal dilators to make the vagina functional (see Table 17-1).

WARD TIP

17α hydroxylase deficiency:
  46,XX: Breast absent, uterus present
  46,XY: Breast absent, uterus absent

EXAM TIP

Androgen insensitivity: Patients look female externally. No pubic hair. Remove gonads after puberty to avoid risk of malignancy (gonadoblastoma or dysgerminoma).

[handwritten margin notes:]

males (XY)
- AMH → müllerian duct regression
- testosterone = internal male genitalia → seminal vesicles, epididymus, ejaculatory duct.

Androgen insens.
XY
↓
testes

Breasts?
uterus?
axillary hair?

TABLE 17-1. Comparison of Androgen Insensitivity and Müllerian Agenesis

	ANDROGEN RESISTANCE	MÜLLERIAN AGENESIS
Karyotype	XY	XX
Breast	Present	Present
Uterus	Absent	Absent
Pubic/axillary hair	Absent	Normal
Testosterone	Normal male levels	Female levels
Further evaluation	Need gonadectomy	Renal/skeletal abnormalities

testicular cancer. (handwritten annotation)

BREASTS ABSENT, UTERUS ABSENT

17α-hydroxylase deficiency: These patients are XY, have testes, but lack the enzyme needed to synthesize sex steroids. They have female external genitalia. Antimüllerian hormone causes the regression of the müllerian ducts. Low testosterone levels do not allow the development of internal male genitalia. There is insufficient estrogen to allow breast development. Those with karyotype 46, XX, will have no breasts, but a uterus will be present.

BREASTS PRESENT, UTERUS PRESENT

- This is the second largest category of individuals with primary amenorrhea (chromosomal/gonadal dysgenesis #1). These women should be evaluated similar to those with secondary amenorrhea.
- **Imperforate hymen; transverse vaginal septum.** These patients present with cyclic pelvic pain due to menstrual blood not having an egress. A hematocolpos (accumulation of menstrual blood in the vagina from an imperforate hymen) can be palpated as a perirectal mass on physical exam. The treatment is to excise the obstruction.

Evaluation of Primary Amenorrhea

HISTORY

- Other stages of puberty reached? Lack of any pubertal development suggests ovarian/pituitary cause.
- Family history.
- Height compared to other family members.
- Neonatal/childhood health problems.
- Symptoms of virilization.
- Recent stress, weight change, exercise.
- Drugs: Heroin/methadone can affect hypothalamus.
- Galactorrhea: Antipsychotics, Reglan (metoclopramide) can cause hyperprolactinemia.
- Headaches, vision problems, fatigue, polyuria, polydipsia: Hypothalamic/pituitary disorders.

PHYSICAL EXAM

- Height, weight, growth chart, arm span.
- Blood pressure:
  - Turner syndrome with coarctation of aorta.
  - Adrenal disorders.
- Breast development (Tanner staging): Marker of ovary function and estrogen action.
- Genital exam:
  - Clitoral size.
  - Tanner staging of pubic hair.
  - Hymen.
  - Vaginal depth.
  - Vaginal or rectal exam to evaluate internal organs.
- Skin: Hirsutism, acne, striae, acanthosis nigricans, vitiligo.
- Turner stigmata: Low hairline, web neck, shield chest, widely spaced nipples.

STUDIES

- Confirm presence of uterus: [Ultrasound, rarely MRI.]
- Uterus absent: Karyotype, serum testosterone: Müllerian anomalies have 46,XX with normal female levels of testosterone. Androgen insensitivity has 46,XY with male levels of testosterone.
- Uterus present. No other anatomic findings:
  - β-hCG to rule out pregnancy.
  - FSH
    - High: Indicative of primary ovarian failure. Karyotype: Turner syndrome (46,X); 17α-hydroxylase deficiency—(46, XX) electrolytes, ↑ progesterone, ↑ deoxycorticosterone, ↓ 17α-hydroxyprogesterone. Remove testes if Y chromosome present.
    - Low/normal: Functional hypothalamic amenorrhea, GnRH deficiency, hypothalamic/pituitary disorders. Head CT or MRI to evaluate for infiltrative disease or adenoma. Prolactin, thyroid-stimulating hormone (TSH). Testosterone and dehydroepiandrosterone sulfate (DHEA-S) if signs of hyperandrogenism.
    - Normal: With normal breast and uterus. Focus workup on secondary amenorrhea.

Secondary Amenorrhea

> 🧍 A 30-year-old G2P2002, with last menstrual period (LMP) 8 weeks ago, complains of no menses for 2 months. She usually has menses every 28 days lasting for 5 days. She reports no medical or surgical history. She has had two-term spontaneous vaginal deliveries. She uses combination oral contraceptive pills (OCPs), and has not missed any pills recently. What is the next step in management of this patient?
>
> **Answer:** The most common cause of amenorrhea in a reproductive-age woman is pregnancy, so a urine or serum β-hCG should be checked. Contraception use does not prevent pregnancy 100% of the time.

CAUSES

- Pregnancy.
- Hypothalamus (35%).

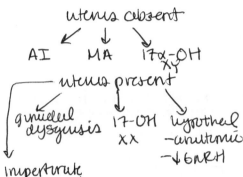

[Handwritten annotation:]

uterus absent

AI   MA   17α-OH
                  XY

uterus present

müllel dysgensis   17-OH   hypothal
          XX   —anutmia
                          —↓GnRH

imperforate hymen/
vaginal sept.

[Handwritten annotation:]

2° amenorrhea

BhCG ⊕→ pregnancy
↓ ⊖
other labs
(TSH, prolactin, FSH, ---)

- Pituitary (19%).
- Ovary (40%).
- Uterus (5%).
- Other (1%): Cervical, endocrine.

Hypothalamic

Low levels of gonadotropins, estrogen, absent withdrawal bleed with progesterone.
- **Lesions:** Craniopharyngiomas, granulomatous disease, encephalitis sequelae.
- **Drugs:** OCPs act at the level of the hypothalamus and pituitary. Postpill amenorrhea can occur up to 6 months after stopping the pill.
- Stress and exercise
- **Weight loss/anorexia nervosa:** Those who are malnourished have a ↓ reproductive ability. Weight gain will allow menses to resume. (↓ Leptin)
- **Functional hypothalamic amenorrhea:** ↓ GnRH secretion, without other causes (very rare).

Pituitary (Hypoestrogenic Amenorrhea)

- **Neoplasms:** Chromophobe adenomas are the most common non-prolactin-secreting pituitary tumors. Prolactinomas will be discussed in a later section. Treatment may involve suppression with medication (prolactinomas) or excision.
- **Lesions:** The pituitary gland can be damaged from anoxia, thrombosis, or hemorrhage. May be associated with ↓ secretion of other pituitary hormones like adrenocorticotropic hormone (ACTH), TSH, LH, and FSH. The patients may have hypothyroidism and adrenal insufficiency.
  - **Sheehan syndrome:** Pituitary cell destruction occurs due to hypotensive episode during pregnancy (usually due to catastrophic hemorrhage). Treatment includes replacement of pituitary hormones.
  - **Simmonds disease:** Pituitary damage unrelated to pregnancy.

ischemic necrosis

Ovarian (Hypergonadotropic Hypogonadism)

A 35-year-old G3P3003 complains of absence of menses for 8 months. She reports menarche at age 12 with menses every 40–50 days until recently. She reports a 20 lb weight gain over the last year. She used clomiphene to become pregnant with her last two pregnancies. Vitals show height 5'4", weight 220 lb, BP 120/80. She has hair on her upper lip and chin, acne, and oily skin on her face. What is the most likely diagnosis? If left untreated, what is this patient at ↑ risk for?
  Answer: Polycystic ovarian syndrome (PCOS). Diagnosis of PCOS is established with two out of three of the following: a history of oligomenorrhea/amenorrhea, features of hyperandrogenism (acne, hirsutism), and multiple ovarian cysts seen on ultrasound. This patient is at ↑ risk for endometrial hyperplasia or cancer if left untreated.

A 35-year-old G2P2002 with LMP 1 year ago presents with hot flashes and vaginal dryness. Her serum FSH is very high. What is the most likely diagnosis?
  Answer: Premature ovarian failure. Symptoms are similar to those in menopause and diagnosis is confirmed with elevated FSH.

- **Premature ovarian failure (POF):** Depletion of oocytes resulting in amenorrhea before the age of 40. The cause is often unknown, but could be due to:
  - Radiation or systemic chemotherapy.
  - Autoimmune conditions can be present.

clomiphene citrate inhibits hypothalamic Estrogen receptors, preventing ⊖ feedback. given to ↑FSH/LH →↑ ovulation

- Fragile X premutation. (FX POI)
- Turner syndrome.
- Treatment may include hormone replacement. Need strategies for bone protection.
- **Surgical:** Bilateral salpingo-oophorectomy.
- **Polycystic ovaries:** Hyperandrogenism.
  - **Diagnosis:** Established if two out of three of the following are present:
    - Polycystic ovaries on ultrasound.
    - Signs of androgen excess (hirsutism, acne).
    - Oligomenorrhea/amenorrhea.
  - **Signs:**
    - Hirsutism.
    - Acne.
    - Oligomenorrhea/amenorrhea.
    - Obesity.
    - Acanthosis nigricans (gray, brown velvety skin discoloration present most commonly on neck and axilla).
    - Premature pubarche and/or precocious puberty.
  - **Treatment**
    - Manage hirsutism, i.e., cosmetic methods, spironolactone.
    - Treat infertility (ovulation induction). – clomiphene
    - Protect the endometrium from endometrial hyperplasia or cancer: start cyclic or continuous OCPs/hormone therapy.
    - Evaluate and treat metabolic issues, i.e., insulin resistance, obesity, dyslipidemia.

Handwritten margin note:
- ↑Androgens – hirsutism, acne
- ↑ovarian cysts seen on US.
- oligo/amenorrhea.
- insulin resistance → acanthosis nigricans.

Uterine

- **Asherman syndrome:** Intrauterine adhesions can obliterate the endometrial cavity and cause amenorrhea.
  - Most frequent cause is endometrial curettage associated with pregnancy.
  - Adhesions may form after myomectomy, metroplasty, or cesarean delivery.
  - Confirm the diagnosis with hysterosalpingogram (HSG) or hysteroscopy.
  - Treat via hysteroscopic resection of adhesions. Estrogens administered to stimulate regrowth of endometrium.
- **Endometrial ablation:** This procedure may have been performed for menorrhagia.
- **Infection:** Endometritis or tuberculosis.

Handwritten margin note: Intrauterine or D&C.

Cervical

Stenosis due to loop electrosurgical excision procedure (LEEP) or cold-knife cone. Treat with cervical dilation.

Endocrine

Can cause secondary amenorrhea.
- Hyper/hypothyroidism.
- Diabetes mellitus.
- Hyperandrogenism (neoplasm, exogenous androgens).

WARD TIP

Progestin challenge test: Give oral progestin for 10 days. If the endometrium has been primed with estrogen from ovaries or peripheral fat, the withdrawal of progestin after 10 days will cause endometrial sloughing with resultant menses. No menses indicates absence of ovaries, estrogen deficiency, or outflow obstruction.

EXAM TIP

Asherman syndrome is intrauterine adhesions secondary to uterine curettage with resultant scarring. It can cause secondary amenorrhea.

EXAM TIP

The most common cause of Asherman syndrome is curettage performed during pregnancy or shortly thereafter.

Handwritten margin note:
Asherman's: – cyclic pelvic pain
– 2° amenorrhea
– infertility.
– AUB
– recurrent pregnancy loss

EVALUATION

HISTORY

- Recent stress, weight change, new diet or exercise habits, illness.
- Acne, hirsutism, deepening of voice.

- Symptoms of hypothalamic-pituitary disease:
  - Headaches.
  - Galactorrhea.
  - Visual field defects.
  - Fatigue.
  - Polyuria, polydipsia.
- Symptoms of estrogen deficiency:
  - Hot flashes.
  - Vaginal dryness.
  - Poor sleep.
  - ↓ libido.
- Obstetric emergency with hemorrhage (Sheehan syndrome).
- Medications:
  - Initiation or discontinuation of OCPs.
  - Androgenic drugs.
  - High-dose progestins.
  - Metoclopramide, antipsychotics: Cause ↑ prolactin leading to amenorrhea.

PHYSICAL EXAM

- Body mass index (BMI): >30 kg/m² in women with PCOS.
- Signs of systemic illness/cachexia, anorexia.
- Genital tissue with signs of estrogen deficiency: POF.
- Breast exam for galactorrhea.
- Neurologic exam for visual fields: Pituitary adenoma.
- Skin:
  - Hirsutism, acne, acanthosis nigricans: PCOS.
  - Thin/dry skin, thickened skin: Thyroid disorders.

STUDIES

- Serum prolactin, TSH, FSH. FSH is high in POF. Consider karyotype.
- DHEA-S and testosterone if signs of hyperandrogenism.
- Estrogen status:
  - Serum estradiol.
  - Progestin withdrawal test with Provera (medroxyprogesterone) 10 mg for 10 days. If bleeding occurs, then adequate estrogen is present in the body.

TREATMENT

Treatment is individualized based on the etiology of amenorrhea.

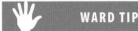

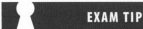

WARD TIP

Absence of vaginal bleeding after progesterone challenge is due to very low levels of estrogen.

EXAM TIP

Premature ovarian failure is often idiopathic.

Handwritten notes:

⊕ prog withdrawal.
– estrogen present
⊖ prog withdrawal.
– estrogen absent.

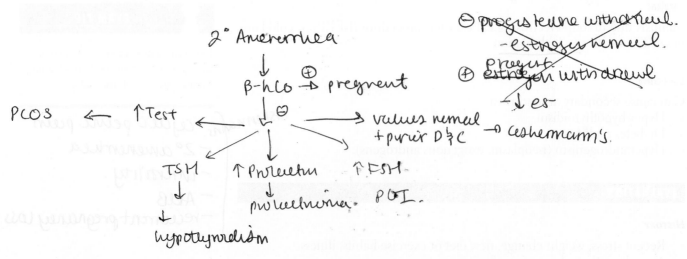

Hyperandrogenism

Definitions

- **Hirsutism:** Presence of hair in locations where it is not normally found in a woman, specifically in the midline of the body (upper lip, chin, back, intermammary region). Also known as male-pattern hair growth.
- **Virilization:** Signs of masculinization in a woman (temporal balding, deepening voice, clitoromegaly, ↑ muscle mass).
- **Hypertrichosis:** Generalized ↑ in the amount of body hair in its normal location.
- **Vellus hairs:** Fine, short hairs found on most parts of the body. They are barely visible.
- **Terminal hairs:** Coarse, darker hairs found, for example, in the axilla and pubic region. Androgens facilitate the conversion of vellus to terminal hairs.

Sources of Androgens

Androgens are produced in the ovary and the adrenal gland. The ovary primarily makes testosterone. It also secretes androstenedione and dehydroepiandrosterone (DHEA) to a smaller degree, and these are converted to testosterone in peripheral tissue. The adrenal gland makes dehydroepiandrosterone sulfate (DHEA-S) and DHEA. To produce a biologic effect, the enzyme 5α-reductase in the peripheral tissue converts testosterone to more potent 5α-dihydrotestosterone (DHT).

ADRENAL PRODUCTION OF ANDROGENS

- The **zona fasciculata** and the **zona reticularis** of the adrenal cortex produce androgens, as well as cortisol. ACTH regulates production.
- A third layer of the adrenal cortex, the **zona glomerulosa**, produces aldosterone and is regulated by the renin-angiotensin system.
- All three hormones—cortisol, androgens, and aldosterone—are derived from cholesterol. Androgen products from the adrenal are found mostly in the form of DHEA and DHEA-S. Elevation in these products represents ↑ adrenal androgen production.

OVARIAN PRODUCTION OF ANDROGENS

Luteinizing hormone (LH) stimulates the ovarian theca cells to produce androgens (androstenedione and testosterone). Next, follicle-stimulating hormone (FSH) stimulates ovarian granulosa cells to convert these androgens to estrone and estradiol. When LH levels become disproportionately greater than FSH levels, androgens become elevated.

Idiopathic Hirsutism (Peripheral Disorder of Androgen Metabolism)

A 35-year-old G3P3003 complains of increasing facial hair that began 2 years ago. She reports menses every 30 days lasting for 4 days. She reports her sister has similar symptoms. On physical exam, she is normotensive and has normal female genitalia.

(continued)

She has moderately dark hair on her upper lip and chin. Serum levels of testosterone and DHEA-S are normal. What is the most likely diagnosis?

Answer: Idiopathic hirsutism. Gradual onset of hirsutism with normal menses, testosterone, and DHEA-S indicates idiopathic hirsutism.

Handwritten margin note:
Idiopathic hirsutism
– normal menses
– ↑ hair / hirsutism
– Testosterone / DHEA-S normal.
↑ 5α-reductase activity in the periphery!

This condition manifests with signs of hirsutism, regular menses, and normal levels of testosterone and DHEA-S. This disorder is due to ↑ activity of 5α-reductase activity in the periphery. Antiandrogens that block the peripheral activity of testosterone or inhibit the enzyme 5α-reductase can be used to treat the hirsutism.

Adrenal Etiologies

CUSHING SYNDROME AND CUSHING DISEASE

- **Cushing syndrome:** An adrenal tumor produces ↑ levels of cortisol with clinical findings—hirsutism, menstrual irregularity, central obesity, moon face, buffalo hump, abdominal striae, weakness, and muscle wasting. Exogenous or endogenous cortisol can be the cause. Confirm diagnosis with dexamethasone suppression test.
- **Cushing disease** (pituitary disease) is a subset of Cushing syndrome. A benign pituitary adenoma causes an ↑ in the secretion of adrenocorticotropic hormone (ACTH) which results in ↑ cortisol levels. It accounts for 70% of Cushing syndromes. Virilization and hirsutism are associated with this condition because the ACTH stimulates androgen production as well.
- **Paraneoplastic syndromes,** in which tumors (usually small cell lung cancer) produce ectopic ACTH, also cause ↑ cortisol. These account for 15% of Cushing syndromes.
- **Adrenal tumors** (adenoma or carcinoma) account for the remaining 15% of Cushing syndromes. In general, adenomas produce only cortisol, so no hirsutism or virilization is present. Carcinomas, by contrast, often produce androgens as well as cortisol, so they may present with signs of hirsutism and virilization. DHEA-S is markedly elevated, and hirsutism and virilization have a rapid onset. Computed tomography (CT) or magnetic resonance imaging (MRI) can confirm the diagnosis.

Handwritten margin note:
start w/ 24 hr low dose dexamethasone → suppression test, 24 hr urinary cortisol, or evening salivary cortisol ↓ if ↑ in pt ↓ ACTH ↙ ↘ ↓Adrenal dz   ↑pituitary vs ectopic – high dose Dex or CRH suppression

CONGENITAL ADRENAL HYPERPLASIA (CAH)

- Caused by a congenital defect in an enzyme that produces cortisol.
  - **21-hydroxylase deficiency:** The most common form of congenital adrenal hyperplasia. The condition has various levels of severity. Affected individuals lack an enzyme crucial to cortisol and mineralocorticoid production. Therefore, the ↑ precursors of cortisol are shunted to androgen production. Elevated serum 17-hydroxyprogesterone is used as a marker for establishing the diagnosis of 21-hydroxylase deficiency. In the severe form, affected females have ambiguous genitalia at birth, along with severe salt wasting and cortisol insufficiency. Late-onset 21-hydroxylase deficiency presents with varying degrees of virilization and hirsutism in females after puberty.
  - **11β-hydroxylase deficiency:** Associated with ↓ cortisol, but ↑ mineral corticoids and androgens. A typical patient with this enzyme deficiency

Nonclassical CAH
- 17-OHprogesterone is normal.
- acne, hirsutism, menstrual irregularity in postpubertal girls indistinguishable from PCOS
- basal morning 17-OHprog levels ≥ 200 in the follicular phase are suggestive
- if > 200 → ↑ dose ACTH stim test; if 17-OHprog ≥ 1500 → dx.

PCOS
* ↑ ovarian + endometrial cancer risk!

TABLE 18-1. Clinical Findings in Congenital Adrenal Hyperplasia

	21-HYDROXYLASE DEFICIENCY	11β-HYDROXYLASE DEFICIENCY
Androgens	High	High
Cortisol	Low	Low
Mineralacorticoids	Low → hypotension	High → hypertension
Marker	↑ 17-hydroxyprogesterone	↑ 11-deoxycortisol

has severe hypertension with virilization/hirsutism (which results in pseudohermaphroditism of female babies). 11-deoxycortisol levels are high in 11β-hydroxylase deficiency (see Table 18-1).

Ovarian Etiologies

POLYCYSTIC OVARIAN SYNDROME (PCOS)

- PCOS is a common condition (affecting 5% of reproductive-age women) and is diagnosed by the presence of two out of three clinical findings: hyperandrogenism (i.e., acne, hirsutism), oligomenorrhea/amenorrhea, and multiple ovarian cysts on ultrasound.
- An abnormal release of gonadotropin-releasing hormone (GnRH) causes a persistently elevated LH. The LH:FSH ratio is often >3:1. There are ↑ levels of androgens produced from the adrenal gland and the ovary. Serum testosterone is elevated. These women also have higher levels of estradiol that is not bound to sex hormone–binding globulin (SHBG), although the total estradiol level is not elevated. There is ↑ estrone due to adipose conversion of androgens.
- These patients also may have acanthosis nigricans, obesity, insulin resistance, dyslipidemia, and infertility. In the future, they are at ↑ risk for diabetes mellitus, hypertension, cardiovascular disease, endometrial cancer, and ovarian cancer. The risk of endometrial and ovarian cancer is reduced with the use of oral contraceptive pills (OCPs).

STROMAL HYPERTHECOSIS

- LH stimulates theca cells in the ovary resulting in stromal hyperplasia. Theca cells produce large amounts of testosterone.
- Presents with gradual onset of anovulation, amenorrhea, and hirsutism.
- Testosterone secretion is progressively ↑ as a woman ages, resulting in virilization and bilaterally enlarged ovaries up to 5–7 cm in diameter.

THECA LUTEIN CYSTS

- Theca cells produce androgens, and granulosa cells transform the androgens to estrogens.
- Theca lutein cysts produce abnormally high levels of androgens, in excess of the amount that can be converted to estrogens.
- Diagnosis is made by ovarian biopsy.

cystic bilateral ovarian masses

WARD TIP

The most common cause of hirsutism and irregular menses is PCOS.

WARD TIP

A 24-year-old obese woman with facial hair complains of amenorrhea. Serum testosterone is elevated. *Think: PCOS.*

WARD TIP

A baby with ambiguous genitalia is born to a mother who complains of ↑ facial hair growth over last few months. *Think: Luteoma of pregnancy.*

LUTEOMA OF PREGNANCY

- A benign tumor that grows in response to human chorionic gonadotropin (hCG).
- Virilization may occur in both the mother and the female fetus.
- The tumor usually disappears postpartum, as do maternal clinical features.

keep feature: regression after delivery

ANDROGEN-SECRETING OVARIAN NEOPLASMS

> A 25-year-old G0 complains of a 2-month history of increasing dark hair on her upper lip and chin, thinning hair on her head, and deepening of her voice. On exam, she is normotensive, has hair growth as stated above, and has temporal balding. Her pelvic exam demonstrates clitoromegaly. What is the most likely diagnosis? What is the next step in management?
> **Answer:** Due to the rapid presentation of virilization, this is most likely an adrenal or ovarian tumor. Drawing serum total testosterone and DHEA-S will help differentiate the source. Pelvic US will confirm the presence of an ovarian mass. A CT or MRI will confirm the presence of an adrenal mass.

- **Sertoli-Leydig cell tumors** and **hilar (Leydig) cell tumors** are rare conditions in which the neoplasms secrete androgens.
- Sertoli-Leydig cell tumors are distinguished from hilar cell tumors in that Sertoli-Leydig tumors usually present in young women with palpable masses and hilar cell tumors are found in postmenopausal women with nonpalpable masses.
- Neoplasms present with rapid signs of virilization.

—can present several trimester; ↑ maternal and fetal virilization; tx: surgical removal, in 2nd trimester or postpartum.

History

- Pregnancy: Theca lutein cysts, luteoma of pregnancy.
- Timing of hirsutism, virilization: Rapid onset suggestive of ovarian or adrenal tumors. Gradual onset suggestive of idiopathic etiology.

Physical Exam

- Note distribution of terminal hair.
- Note signs of virilization.
- Bimanual exam: Pelvic mass.
- Hirsutism, menstrual irregularity, central obesity, moon face, buffalo hump, abdominal striae, weakness, and muscle wasting: Cushing syndrome.

Studies

- Serum total testosterone (ovarian), DHEA-S (adrenal): Distinguish ovarian versus adrenal source. *x*
- Ultrasound: Confirm ovarian mass.
- CT/MRI: Confirm adrenal mass.
- Dexamethasone suppression test: Distinguish the etiology of the ACTH stimulation.

- Serum 17-hydroxyprogesterone: Elevated in 21-hydroxylase deficiency.
- Serum 11-deoxycortisol: Elevated in 11β-hydroxylase deficiency.

Treatment

- Ovarian and adrenal tumors:
  - Sertoli-Leydig cell tumors: Unilateral salpingo-oophorectomy if not completed childbearing. / or 2nd trimester.
  - Hilar cell tumors: Usually in postmenopausal women. Total abdominal hysterectomy (TAH), bilateral salpingo-oophorectomy (BSO).
  - Adrenal adenoma or carcinoma: Surgical removal.
  - Stromal hyperthecosis: TAH, BSO.
- Late-onset 21-hydroxylase deficiency:
  - Androgen excess and menstrual irregularities can be treated as PCOS.
  - Infertility: Supplement with glucocorticoids to suppress androgens and allow ovulation.
- PCOS:
  - Weight loss.
  - OCPs for acne and menstrual irregularity. Estrogen component in the OCP ↑ SHBG; SHBG binds androgens; free androgen levels are then ↓. Progestins in the OCP inhibits 5α-reductase activity in the skin.
  - Cyclic progesterone for menstrual irregularity.
  - Infertility: Ovulation induction with clomiphene and metformin.
- Skin disorders:
  - Peripheral antiandrogens: Spironolactone, finasteride, cyproterone acetate.
  - Androgenic acne responds quickly to treatment. Hirsutism moderately responsive; alopecia least responsive to treatment.
- Idiopathic hirsutism:
  - Peripheral androgen activity inhibitor. May take 3 months to work (length of hair life cycle).
  - Electrolysis, laser, or intense pulsed light therapy.
  - OCPs, medroxyprogesterone acetate.
  - Vaniqa (eflornithine hydrochloride cream) topical treatment for unwanted facial hair.
  - Spironolactone: Blocks androgen receptors, ↓ ovarian testosterone production, inhibits 5α-reductase.
  - Finasteride (5α-reductase inhibitor), flutamide (nonsteroidal antiandrogen): Similar effectiveness to spironolactone.

idiopathic hirsutism → tx w/ spironolactone!

or can do finesteride to treat overactive 5α-reductase!

Hyperprolactinemia and Galactorrhea

WARD TIP

Physiologic stimuli for PRL release:
- Breast and nipple palpation
- Exercise
- Stress
- Sleep
- Noonday meal

WARD TIP

Stress is the most common cause of mildly elevated prolactin.

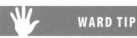
WARD TIP

Confirm galactorrhea by visualizing fat droplets with microscope.

EXAM TIP

Medications are the most common cause of galactorrhea and hyperprolactinemia.

metoclopramide, antipsych.

EXAM TIP

The most common pituitary adenoma associated with hyperprolactinemia is prolactinoma.

WARD TIP

Fifty percent of women with hyperprolactinemia will have a prolactinoma. If PRL is >200 ng/mL, nearly 100% will have prolactinoma.

Definitions

- **Hyperprolactinemia:** Elevated levels of the hormone prolactin (PRL).
- **Galactorrhea:** Watery or milky fluid secreted from the breast that is not in relation to pregnancy.
- **Prolactinoma:** Prolactin-secreting pituitary tumor.

Etiology

A 35-year-old G2P2002 complains of milky discharge from her breasts for 6 months. She also reports no menses for 6 months. She used to have menses every 28 days, lasting for 4 days. She has started to have hot flashes in the last 4 months. She denies the use of any medications. She is normotensive. No masses are palpated on the breast exam, but a milky discharge is expressed from both breasts. Her vagina is dry. Her serum β-human chorionic gonadotropin (β-hCG) is negative. What is the most likely diagnosis? What studies should be ordered next?

Answer: This patient has galactorrhea, amenorrhea, and low estrogen most likely due to hyperprolactinemia. Serum prolactin and thyrotropin-stimulating hormone (TSH) should be drawn to initiate the evaluation.

- Prolactin (PRL) is a peptide hormone produced by the anterior pituitary gland and is important for lactation. The main function of PRL is to stimulate growth of mammary tissue as well as produce and secrete milk into the alveoli. ↑ secretion of prolactin, hyperprolactinemia, may lead to galactorrhea. PRL secretion is stimulated by thyrotropin-releasing hormone (TRH) and serotonin; it is inhibited by dopamine.
- Hyperprolactinemia inhibits the pulsatile release of gonadotropin-releasing hormone (GnRH), resulting in amenorrhea/oligomenorrhea, anovulation, inappropriate lactation, and galactorrhea.
- **Causes** of hyperprolactinemia:
  - Drugs: Tranquilizers, tricyclic antidepressants (TCAs), antipsychotics, antihypertensives, narcotics, oral contraceptive pills (OCPs).
  - Hypothyroidism: ↓ negative feedback of thyroxine (T4) on the hypothalamic-pituitary axis causing a ↓ in TRH. TRH stimulates PRL secretion.
  - Hypothalamic: Craniopharyngioma, sarcoidosis, histiocytosis, leukemia. Interferes with portal circulation of dopamine.
  - Pituitary: Prolactinoma. Microadenoma (<1 cm), macroadenoma (>1 cm). See the following section on prolactinoma.
  - Hyperplasia of lactotrophs: Present very similarly to those having microadenomas.
  - Empty sella syndrome: Intrasellar extension of subarachnoid space which causes compression of the pituitary gland and an enlarged sella turcica.
  - Acromegaly: Pituitary gland secretes growth hormone as well as PRL.
  - Acute/chronic renal disease: ↓ metabolic clearance of PRL.
  - Chest surgery or trauma: Breast implants, herpes zoster at breast dermatome.

• Renal Failure can ↑ prolactin in serum obtain a creatinine level.

Prolactinoma

- One-tenth of people in the general population have an incidental prolactinoma.
- Fifty percent of women with hyperprolactinemia have a prolactinoma.
- Most prolactinomas are microadenomas.
- Majority of microadenomas do not enlarge.
- Hyperprolactinemia with or without a microadenoma follows a benign clinical course and treatment is not necessary unless estrogen levels are low or pregnancy is desired.
- Microadenoma growth is **not** stimulated by:
  - Pregnancy.
  - OCPs.
  - Hormone replacement.

HISTORY

- Amenorrhea/oligomenorrhea.
- Galactorrhea.
- Headaches.
- Bitemporal visual field deficit.

PHYSICAL EXAM

- Visual field testing if macroadenoma is present. Macroadenomas can exert pressure on the optic chiasm.
- Breast exam.

STUDIES

[handwritten: mere mild elevation in drug inelleed or hypothyroid]

- PRL level. *(≥ 200 ng/mL if prolactinoma)*
- TSH, triiodothyronine (T_3), T_4: Evaluate for hypothyroidism if PRL is elevated.
- Magnetic resonance imaging (MRI): Most sensitive for diagnosis of pituitary masses and empty sella syndrome due to greater soft tissue contrast.

TREATMENT

- **Drugs:** Stop the suspected drug, and repeat PRL after 1 month. If medication cannot be stopped and PRL level above 100 ng/mL, image the sella turcica to determine the presence of macroadenoma.
- Patient with galactorrhea and normal menses: **No further therapy** if normal PRL, normal TSH.
- **Bromocriptine:** Dopamine receptor agonist.
  - For patients with macroadenoma: Can reduce tumor mass.
  - For those that desire to conceive, are anovulatory, with hyperprolactinemia: Discontinued after conception as it crosses the placenta. Not known to be teratogenic.
  - For those with galactorrhea only: Inhibits secretion of PRL.
  - Side effects: Severe orthostatic hypotension (fainting, dizziness), nausea, vomiting.
  - Administered orally or vaginally (reduced side effect of nausea and vomiting).
  - Long-term treatment is required.

WARD TIP

Most macroadenomas enlarge with time. Most microadenomas do not.

EXAM TIP

The most common symptoms of hyperprolactinemia are galactorrhea and amenorrhea.

WARD TIP

Sixty percent of women with galactorrhea have hyperprolactinemia. Ninety percent of women with galactorrhea, amenorrhea, and low estrogen have hyperprolactinemia.

EXAM TIP

MRI: Modality of choice to diagnose pituitary adenomas or empty sella syndrome.

EXAM TIP

Bromocriptine is the drug of choice for women with PRL-secreting microadenoma who want to conceive.

EXAM TIP

Cabergoline is the drug of choice for reducing PRL levels and shrinking tumors.

EXAM TIP

Pregnancy ↑ the likelihood that PRL levels will ↓ or become normal overtime.

EXAM TIP

Bromocriptine induction of pregnancy is not associated with ↑ congenital abnormalities, spontaneous abortion, or multiple gestation.

WARD TIP

Cabergoline is more effective and better tolerated than bromocriptine.

- **Cabergoline:** Long-acting dopamine receptor agonist. Less frequent and less severe side effects.
- **Transsphenoidal microsurgical resection:**
  - Recommended only if macroadenoma and fail medical therapy.
  - Risk of diabetes insipidus, iatrogenic hypopituitarism.
  - Fifty percent cure for microadenomas, 25% cure for macroadenoma.
- **Radiation:** Adjunctive treatment following incomplete removal of large tumors.
- **Osteoporosis treatment/prophylaxis:** Low levels of estrogen resulting from hyperprolactinemia can result in bone loss.

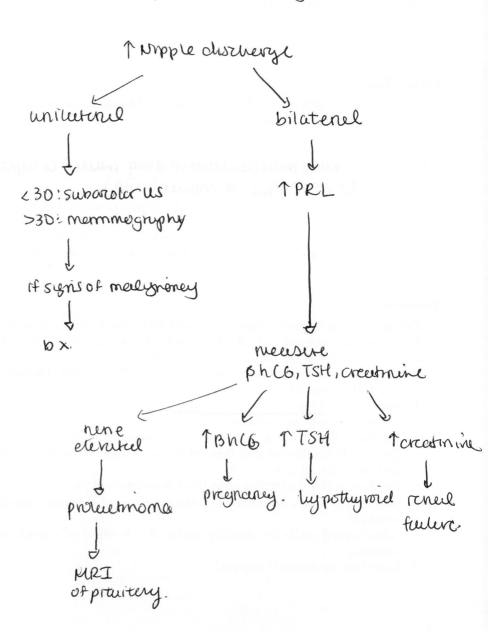

Abnormal Uterine Bleeding

Definitions

Menstrual abnormalities include:

- **Polymenorrhea:** Uterine bleeding that occurs more often than every 21 days.
- **Menorrhagia:** Prolonged (>7 days) or excessive (>80 mL) uterine bleeding occurring at regular intervals.
- **Oligomenorrhea:** Uterine bleeding that occurs less frequently than every 35 days.
- **Metrorrhagia:** Bleeding that occurs in between periods or at irregular intervals.
- **Menometrorrhagia:** Combination of both menorrhagia and metrorrhagia; uterine bleeding that is prolonged or excessive, frequent, and irregular.
- **Dysfunctional uterine bleeding:** Bleeding that occurs after organic, systemic, and iatrogenic causes have been ruled out. May be anovulatory or ovulatory.

These terms are falling out of favor (but you may still hear them a lot) in an effort to be more descriptive about the nature of uterine bleeding. The PALM-COEIN system provides terminology to describe uterine bleeding by bleeding pattern and etiology. The term Abnormal Uterine Bleeding (AUB) is paired with descriptive terms Heavy Menstrual Bleeding (HMB) instead of menorrhagia, and Intermenstrual Bleeding (IMB) instead of metrorrhagia. AUB is further classified by one of the following letters that describes the etiology:

PALM: Refers to structural causes of AUB.
P—Polyp (AUB-P)
A—Adenomyosis (AUB-A)
L—Leiomyoma (AUB-L)
M—Malignancy & hyperplasia (AUB-M)

COEIN: Refers to nonstructural causes of AUB.
C—Coagulopathy (AUB-C)
O—Ovulatory dysfunction (AUB-O)
E—Endometrial (AUB-E)
I—Iatrogenic (AUB-I)
N—Not yet classified (AUB-N)

Abnormal Uterine Bleeding: Reproductive Age

 A 24-year-old G0P0 presents with irregular menses occurring every 3–4 months. Her periods are heavy and last 7–9 days. She complains of severe acne since puberty. Her body mass index (BMI) is 40, and her exam is otherwise normal. She was recently diagnosed with type 2 diabetes. What initial lab tests should be ordered in the evaluation of this patient?

Answer: β-hCG, follicle-stimulating hormone (FSH), thyrotropin-stimulating hormone (TSH), prolactin (PRL). These tests cover the top differential diagnosis of pregnancy, premature ovarian failure, thyroid dysfunction, and hyperprolactinemia as the cause of abnormal uterine bleeding (AUB). If all of the results are normal, further workup can be done.

A normal menstrual cycle occurs every 21–35 days (28 ± 7 days) with menstruation for 2–7 days. The normal blood loss is less than 80 mL total (average 35 cc),

EXAM TIP

Characteristics of normal menstrual bleeding: every 21–35 days, fairly regular, <80 mL, 5 days.

EXAM TIP

Questions to quantify blood loss: # of tampons/pad used? How often change protection? Change protection at night? Clots? History of anemia? Bleeding onto clothes or bedding?

WARD TIP

Two main mechanisms for hemostasis during menstruation are hemostatic plug formation and vasoconstriction.

EXAM TIP

Metrorrhagia: The metro never comes according to schedule (bleeding at frequent, irregular intervals).

which represents <u>8 or fewer soaked pads</u> per day with usually <u>no more than 2 heavy days</u>. AUB is any disturbance of the above. It can occur at any age and has many causes.

Most cases of reproductive age bleeding are related to pregnancy, structural uterine pathology, anovulation, coagulopathy, or neoplasia. Less common causes include trauma and infection.

ETIOLOGY

- **Organic:**
  - Reproductive tract disease.
  - Accidents of pregnancy (threatened, incomplete, missed abortion; ectopic pregnancy; trophoblastic disease).
  - Malignancy: Most commonly <u>endometrial</u> and <u>cervical cancers</u>. Estrogen-producing ovarian tumors (i.e., <u>granulosa-theca cell tumors</u>) may present with excessive uterine bleeding.
  - Infection: Endometritis presents with episodic intermenstrual spotting. Cervicitis and severe vaginal infections can present with bleeding.
  - Structural causes (fibroids, polyps, adenomyosis).
  - Foreign bodies: Tampons retained in the vagina or intrauterine devices for contraception can cause bleeding.
  - Traumatic vaginal lesions.
- **Systemic:**
  - von Willebrand disease can cause ↑ bleeding due to coagulopathy.
  - Prothrombin deficiency.
  - Leukemia.
  - Sepsis.
  - Idiopathic thrombocytopenic purpura.
  - Hypersplenism.
  - Thyroid dysfunction: Hypothyroidism causes anovulation and is frequently associated with <u>menorrhagia</u> and <u>intermenstrual bleeding</u>.
  - <u>Cirrhosis</u>: Excessive bleeding secondary to the <u>reduced capacity of the liver to metabolize estrogens</u>.
- **Iatrogenic:**
  - Anticoagulation medications.
  - Oral or injectable steroids used for contraception.
  - Hormone replacement therapy (HRT).
  - Psychotropic drugs: Interfere with neurotransmitters responsible for inhibition and release of hypothalamic hormones, leading to anovulation and AUB.
  - **Ovulatory:** After adolescence and before perimenopausal years. Usually presents as menorrhagia and/or intermenstrual bleeding. Due to abnormal endometrial hemostasis for any reason.
  - **Anovulatory:** <u>There is continuous estradiol production without corpus luteum formation</u> or progesterone production. This steady state of estrogen stimulation results in <u>constant endometrial proliferation</u> without progesterone-mediated maturation and shedding. Fragments of overgrown endometrium sheds sporadically. Anovulation can manifest in:
    - Polycystic ovarian syndrome (PCOS). ✗
    - Obesity.
    - Adolescents (perimenarchal). ✗ *Rx w/ OCPs. to normalize cycle.*
    - Perimenopause.

HISTORY

- Bleeding history: frequency, interval, duration, and amount of bleeding.
- Assess changes in menstrual pattern.
- Ask about the presence of clots.

WARD TIP

A patient with postcoital bleeding should be evaluated for cervical cancer and cervicitis.

WARD TIP

Most common cause of hospital admission for <u>menorrhagia in adolescents</u> = <u>von Willebrand disease</u>.

WARD TIP

Ovarian tumors (benign and malignant) may present with menorrhagia or metrorrhagia.

WARD TIP

Anovulation → ↑ estradiol → endometrial proliferation → disorganized shedding.

WARD TIP

Signs of PCOS
- Oligomenorrhea
- Hyperandrogenism (i.e., hirsutism, acne)
- Obesity
- Cystic ovaries

WARD TIP

Irregular bleeding is often associated with anovulation.

- Instruct the patient to keep a bleeding calendar to record duration and flow.
- Ask how many sanitary pads or tampons she uses per day, and whether she has to change protection at night. (This is very subjective, but gives you an indication of the inconvenience the bleeding causes).
- Menorrhagia present since menarche or new?
- Family history of bleeding?
- History of epistaxis, gum bleeding, postpartum bleeding, surgical bleeding?
- Cold intolerance, skin or hair changes.

PHYSICAL EXAM

- Bimanual may reveal bulky uterus/discrete fibroids.
- Obesity, hirsutism, acanthosis nigricans (PCO).
- Exophthalmos, goiter, delayed DTRs, dry skin/hair (thyroid disorder).
- Visual field deficits, galactorrhea (hyperprolactinemia).
- Petechia (coagulopathy).

DIAGNOSTIC TESTS

- Pap smear.
- Pregnancy test.
- Hemoglobin, serum Fe, serum ferritin.
- TSH.
- FSH.
- Prolactin.
- Coagulation panel: von Willebrand factor for adolescents with menorrhagia.
- EMB for women ≥35 years of age or with history of unopposed estrogen or morbid obesity.
- Pelvic ultrasound.
- Sonohysterogram (pelvic US combined with intrauterine saline infusion to outline the uterine cavity).
- Hysteroscopy.

EXAM TIP

Hysteroscopy can be used to diagnose and treat the uterine abnormality at the same time.

TREATMENT

> A 28-year-old G2P2002 presents to the ED complaining of heavy vaginal bleeding for one week that has worsened over the past 24 hr. She also reports shortness of breath and dizziness. On exam, she appears pale and diaphoretic; HR 110, BP 85/60. Sterile speculum exam shows active bright-red bleeding and a normal cervix. What is the best treatment for this patient?
> **Answer:** Dilation and curettage (D&C) is the treatment of choice for a patient with heavy bleeding and hemodynamic instability. Its effect is immediate.

- Address organic, systemic, iatrogenic causes as indicated.
- Medical management: First-line treatment. Used for women who desire future fertility or those who will reach menopause within a short period of time.
    - Nonsteroidal anti-inflammatory drugs (NSAIDs) (tranexamic acid/mefenamic acid).
    - Iron supplements.
    - Hormones: OCP is the mainstay for anovulatory bleeding. Combination pill or estrogens are used in the management of acute bleeding. Progestin intrauterine device (IUD) can also be used for AUB.
- D&C: Indicated mainly for women with heavy bleeding leading to hemodynamic instability. Once the acute episode of bleeding is controlled, the patient can be started on medical management.

- Endometrial ablation: Used as a minimally invasive alternative to hysterectomy when medical management fails, or when there are contraindications to their use. It should **not** be used in women who wish to maintain their reproductive capacity.
- Myomectomy: Reserved largely for women who wish to maintain reproductive capacity.
- Hysterectomy: Reserved for women with other indications for hysterectomy, such as leiomyomas or uterine prolapse, or in whom medical and/or minimally invasive options have failed.

Postmenopausal Bleeding (PMB)

 A 55-year-old with LMP 5 years ago presents with a chief complaint of vaginal spotting. She also reports painful intercourse and burning in the vagina. Her spotting is not related to sexual activity. She has no medical problems, and is not on any medications. Pelvic exam reveals a dry vagina with ↓ rugae and no blood in the vagina. What is the most likely diagnosis?

Answer: Bleeding due to atrophy is the most common cause for postmenopausal bleeding.

Postmenopausal bleeding is defined as bleeding that occurs after 1 year of menopausal amenorrhea. All vaginal bleeding in postmenopausal women must be evaluated. Postmenopausal bleeding can be due to atrophy or endometrial carcinoma, along with various other causes.

ETIOLOGY

- Vaginal/endometrial atrophy (most common): Hypoestrogenism causes atrophy of the endometrium and vagina. In the uterus, the collapsed, atrophic endometrial surfaces contain little or no fluid to prevent intracavitary friction. This results in microerosions of the surface epithelium which is prone to light bleeding or spotting.
- Postmenopausal HRT: Many postmenopausal women who take HRT develop vaginal bleeding; the frequency depends upon the regimen used.
- Endometrial hyperplasia:
  - Endogenous estrogen production from ovarian or adrenal tumors or exogenous estrogen therapy is the possible cause.
  - Obese women have high levels of endogenous estrogen due to the conversion of androstenedione to estrone and the aromatization of androgens to estradiol, both of which occur in peripheral adipose tissue.
- Adenomyosis:
  - Confirmed by pathologic examination following hysterectomy.
  - Symptomatic adenomyosis occurs after menopause only in the presence of postmenopausal HRT.
- Post-radiation therapy:
  - A late effect of radiation therapy.
  - Radiation devascularizes tissue, causes sloughing, and bleeding.
  - Vaginal vault necrosis causes uncontrolled bleeding and pain.
- Iatrogenic anticoagulant effect.
- Neoplasia:
  - Endometrial cancer.
  - Cervical cancer. Vaginal bleeding occurs because the cancer outgrows its blood supply. The necrotic and denuded tissue bleeds easily and causes a malodorous discharge.

EXAM TIP

Most common cause of postmenopausal bleeding: atrophy of genital tract. Most common lethal cause: endometrial cancer.

WARD TIP

HRT for menopausal woman with a uterus must contain progestin with estrogen to prevent endometrial hyperplasia/carcinoma.

WARD TIP

Postmenopausal bleeding = endometrial cancer until proven otherwise by tissue biopsy.

- Vulvar cancer.
- Estrogen-secreting ovarian tumor.
- Leiomyomata uteri.
- The diagnosis of a **uterine sarcoma** should be considered in postmenopausal women with rapidly growing leiomyomata.
- Polyps: Endometrial growths of unknown etiology. Growth of polyps can be stimulated by estrogen therapy or tamoxifen. They may be benign, premalignant, or malignant.
- Infection: Uncommon cause of postmenopausal bleeding.
- Trauma.

HISTORY

- Onset, frequency, duration, and amount of bleeding.
- Associated signs/symptoms, i.e., weight loss, fever.
- History of trauma or bleeding in relation to sexual activity.
- Medication—hormones, anticoagulants, tamoxifen, over the counter herbal supplements.
- Past medical and surgical history.
- Family history of bleeding, gynecologic cancer, breast cancer.

PHYSICAL EXAM

- Note any suspicious lesions, lacerations, discharge, or foreign bodies.
- Classic signs of atrophy include pale, dry vaginal epithelium that has lost its rugae.
- Assess the size, contour, and tenderness of the uterus.

STUDIES

- Vaginal probes and wet mount for infections.
- Pap smear for cervical dysplasia, neoplasia.
- Endometrial biopsy for endometrial hyperplasia or cancer.
- Transvaginal ultrasound to assess endometrial stripe. If endometrial stripe is <4 mm, endometrial sampling may be deferred unless the patient has persistent bleeding. Rationale is thin lining due to atrophy.
- Diagnostic hysteroscopy with D&C.

TREATMENT

A 65-year-old presents with vaginal bleeding. Her last period was 15 years ago. She reports 3 days of dark-red spotting that has now resolved. An office endometrial biopsy shows complex endometrial hyperplasia with atypia. What is the next best step in management?

Answer: The next step is hysteroscopy with D&C. Approximately 30% of women with this diagnosis on biopsy will have a concurrent endometrial cancer. Once cancer is diagnosed or excluded, the patient should undergo hysterectomy with possible staging.

Treatment of postmenopausal bleeding is dependent on the cause:
- Local estrogen cream is used to treat vaginal atrophy and post-radiation effect limited to the vaginal region.
- Hysteroscopy with D&C and polypectomy or hysterectomy can be offered if symptoms are due to benign lesions like polyps and fibroids.

- Endometrial hyperplasia without atypia can be managed with progestin and ongoing monitoring.
- Endometrial hyperplasia with atypia should be treated as if there is underlying cancer. Approximately 30% will have underlying cancer. Hysteroscopy D&C can rule this out prior to performing hysterectomy as the treatment of choice.
- If endometrial carcinoma, consult gynecologic oncology to determine the best treatment (chemotherapy, radiation, or surgery). Endometrial carcinoma associated with complex endometrial hyperplasia is usually low grade, and can be managed with hysterectomy.

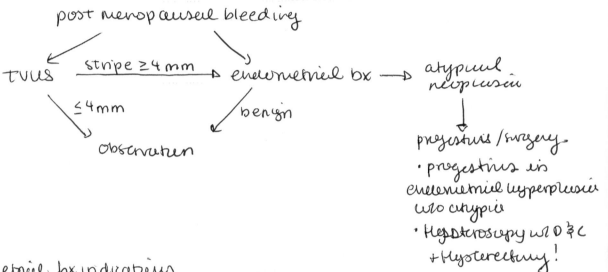

Endometrial bx indications

age ≥ 45 : AUB or PMB

age < 45 : AUB + unopposed estrogen, failed medical mgmt, Lynch syndrome.

age ≥ 35 : abnormal glandular cells on pap test.

NOTES

CHAPTER 21

Pelvic Pain

Chronic Pelvic Pain

A 35-year-old G2P2, with a history of uterine fibroids, presents with a 1-year history of pelvic pain lasting 20 min, three to four times a week. The pain is not relieved by Tylenol. Pelvic exam reveals a 16-week size uterus with tenderness directly over the fundus. Her cervix and adnexa are nontender. Her pregnancy test is negative. What is her most likely diagnosis? What diagnostic test should be ordered? What is the next best step in management?

Answer: The most likely diagnosis is a fibroid uterus with degeneration. It can be diagnosed with a pelvic ultrasound. Medical therapy is instituted first, typically with NSAIDs. If the pain persists despite conservative therapy, a surgical intervention may be considered.

Sometimes chronic pelvic pain may be attributed to a pathophysiological process that can be identified in an end organ, such as inflamed endometriosis lesions found on the ovaries; other times, no obvious pathology is found, such as in fibromyalgia.

Chronic pelvic pain (CPP) is one of several chronic pain conditions, which afflict more than 100 million Americans. More than 50% of them have more than one chronic pain condition, many of which affect either solely or predominantly women. The co-existence of one or more chronic pain conditions (Figure 12-1) is termed *chronic overlapping pain condition* (COPC). Patients with a COPC demonstrate common abnormalities in neural, immune, and endocrine functions, which may explain the overlapping nature of some of these conditions as well as increased risk for developing an additional COPC if a patient has an existing COPC.

CPP and COPCs are associated with higher levels of physical and mental disability, poorer sexual function, higher rates of drug addiction, and suicide when compared to controls without chronic pain. They are also more stigmatized by society and the health care system.

DEFINITION AND CRITERIA

- Pelvic pain that lasts at least 6 months.
- Symptoms cause significant distress or impairment in social, occupational, or other important areas of functioning (i.e., missed work, depression, sexual dysfunction).
- Pain that is located below the umbilicus but between the hips.

WORKUP

- **Detailed history** (focusing on above etiologies):
  - Temporal pattern: Timing and duration of symptoms.
  - Pain characteristics: Pain may be constant, intermittent, or with monthly menses (cyclic).
  - Associated symptoms/relieving factors: Pain may be associated with positional changes, fever, or nausea/vomiting.
  - Past surgeries: Adhesions may form after previous surgeries. Adhesions are fibrous tissue that forms between two internal organs and may be a source of pain.
  - Last menstrual period (LMP) and menstrual history.
  - Gastrointestinal (GI) complaints such as nausea, vomiting, diarrhea, dyschezia, or constipation associated with the pain.

WARD TIP

Pelvic pain accounts for 20% of hysterectomies, 40% of diagnostic laparoscopies, and 10% of referrals to a gynecologist.

WARD TIP

Mittelschmerz is pelvic pain associated with ovulation. It occurs at the time an egg is released from the ovary.

WARD TIP

Chronic pelvic pain etiologies—Think of "**LEAP²ING**" pain

Leiomyoma
Endometriosis/Endometritis
Adhesions/Adenomyosis
Psychological/Psychiatric (i.e., abuse history, depression).
Pelvic floor myalgia, myofascial pain
Infections (i.e., urinary tract infection, pelvic inflammatory disease)
Neoplasia
Gastrointestinal tract (i.e., inflammatory bowel disease, diverticulosis, or irritable bowel syndrome [IBS])

- Sexual history: Dyspareunia (deep versus insertional).
- Social history (marital discord, depression, stress, history of physical or sexual abuse): Pelvic pain may be associated with psychiatric factors and childhood sexual abuse.
- **Physical exam:** Look for:
  - Masses on abdominal and pelvic exam: May suggest an enlarged ovary or a uterine fibroid.
  - Cervical motion tenderness: If present may indicate an infection, such as PID or endometritis. In some cases, may reveal endometriosis.
  - Vulvar tenderness: May suggest vulvodynia.
  - Anal tenderness: May suggest hemorrhoids, abscesses, or a fistula. The rectovaginal exam may demonstrate uterosacral nodularity or a fixed, tender, retroverted uterus consistent with endometriosis.
  - Bladder tenderness (palpate anterior vagina): May suggest interstitial cystitis.
  - Pelvic floor: Assess muscles for tone and tenderness.
- **Labs**
  - Complete blood count (CBC) with differential: An elevated white blood cell count (WBC) may indicate an infection.
  - Pregnancy test.
  - Testing for gonorrhea and chlamydia.
  - Urinalysis (UA) and urine culture.
  - Fecal occult blood.
- **Imaging studies**
  - Pelvic ultrasound: Best to evaluate for ovarian cysts or uterine fibroids. May be suggestive of adenomyosis.
  - Computed tomography (CT)/magnetic resonance imaging (MRI)— best to evaluate for abdominopelvic masses or malignancies. May also better define masses seen on ultrasound, and MRI can help diagnose adenomyosis.
- **Referrals**
  - Gastroenterology referral for colonoscopy to evaluate for diverticulosis, irritable bowel syndrome, or inflammatory bowel disease.
  - Urology referral for cystoscopy to evaluate for interstitial cystitis.
  - Psychiatry referral to evaluate for psychosomatic pain and for depression.

Acute Pelvic Pain

A 22-year-old G0 presents with a 2-day history of severe, sharp right lower quadrant pain. Her LMP was 13 days ago, and she has no significant medical or surgical history. Her pain is not relieved with ibuprofen. Her vitals show T = 98.2, P = 100, BP 85/60. A pregnancy test is negative. Her hematocrit dropped from 38% to 30%. On exam, her abdomen is soft and tender with rebound and guarding. An ultrasound reveals a normal left ovary and a 4-cm right ovary, with a moderate amount of fluid in the cul-de-sac (pouch of Douglas). What is her diagnosis? What is the best next step in management?

Answer: The most likely diagnosis is a ruptured corpus luteal cyst. She recently ovulated, since her period was 2 weeks ago. She has vitals and an exam consistent with an acute abdomen. Given her drop in hematocrit, the fluid in the cul-de-sac is likely blood from the ruptured cyst. She needs surgical treatment with a diagnostic laparoscopy to diagnose and treat.

Acute pelvic pain is any pain in the pelvic cavity that lasts <6 months.

WARD TIP

PID is the most common cause of chronic pelvic pain in women less than 30 years old. Endometriosis is the most common cause in women greater than 30 years old.

WARD TIP

Laparoscopy is the final, conclusive step in diagnosing pelvic pain, but it should only be done once psychogenic and gastrointestinal etiologies have been evaluated.

WARD TIP

Differential for acute pelvic pain—
A ROPE

Appendicitis/**A**bscess/**A**bortion
Ruptured ovarian cyst
Ovarian torsion
PID (or tubo-ovarian abscess)
Ectopic pregnancy

WARD TIP

An elevated WBC may be due to infection (PID or appendicitis), inflammation/necrosis related to adnexal torsion, or a degenerating leiomyoma.

ETIOLOGIES

- Gynecologic—may require surgery if pain is severe:
  - Ruptured ovarian cyst.
  - Adnexal torsion.
  - Tubo-ovarian abscess, PID.
  - Endometriosis.
  - Dysmenorrhea.
- Obstetric:
  - Ectopic pregnancy.
  - Abortion.
- GI/genitourinary (GU):
  - Diverticulitis or diverticulosis.
  - Appendicitis.
  - Inflammatory bowel disease (IBD), or irritable bowel syndrome (IBS).
  - UTI.
  - Nephrolithiasis.

WORKUP

- **History:** Include temporal characteristics (cyclic, intermittent, or noncyclic), location, and severity of pain.
- **Physical exam:** Look for localized/point tenderness, cervical motion tenderness, adnexal tenderness, and abdominal tenderness. The latter three may be signs of PID. Look for signs of an acute abdomen such as guarding, rebound, or severe tenderness.
- **Labs:**
  - Pregnancy test.
  - CBC with differential.
  - UA and culture, if indicated.
  - Culture (nucleic acid DNA amplification) tests for chlamydia and gonorrhea.
- Pelvic ultrasound: Look for ovarian cysts/neoplasm, ovarian torsion (check Dopplers), an intrauterine/ectopic pregnancy, uterine fibroids, or a tubo-ovarian abscess.

TREATMENT

- Depends on the etiology of the pain.
- Start with conservative management, i.e., NSAIDs or other pain management.
- Surgical therapy: Consider if signs of an acute abdomen, if the diagnosis is unclear, or if the differential diagnosis includes potentially life-threatening or organ-threatening conditions, such as appendicitis, or ovarian torsion.
- Surgery: May consist of a diagnostic laparoscopy (if hemodynamically stable) or an exploratory laparotomy (if hemodynamically unstable).

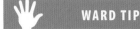

WARD TIP

All women of reproductive age, regardless of reported sexual history or contraception, should undergo a pregnancy test during evaluation of abdominal or pelvic pain.

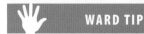

WARD TIP

A ruptured ovarian cyst is a common cause of acute pelvic pain.

EXAM TIP

A woman with new-onset pelvic pain and a positive pregnancy test has a complex adnexal mass and an empty uterus on ultrasound. What is the most likely diagnosis? An ectopic pregnancy.

CHAPTER 22

Endometriosis and Adenomyosis

Endometriosis

A 32-year-old G0P0 presents with a 3-year history of infertility. She reports menarche at age 13, with regular menses every 28 days. She complains of severe pain 2–3 days before her period, pain during her period, and pain with intercourse. She reports no history of STDs. Her husband has one child from a previous marriage. On exam, she has uterosacral nodularity and a fixed, retroflexed uterus. What diagnostic test would be the most appropriate at this point to make the diagnosis? What findings would you see on a tissue biopsy?

Answer: The patient has classic symptoms of endometriosis: dysmenorrhea and dyspareunia. Endometriosis is often associated with infertility. Although history and exam may suggest endometriosis, diagnostic laparoscopy is required to make a definitive diagnosis. The tissue biopsy would show endometrial glands, stroma, and hemosiderin-laden macrophages. The most common sites of involvement are the ovaries and pouch of Douglas.

DEFINITION

Endometrial glands and stroma growing outside of the uterus, often causing pain and/or infertility.

INCIDENCE

- 10–15% of reproductive-aged women.
- Occurs primarily in women in their 20s and 30s.
- Accounts for 20% of chronic pelvic pain.
- One-third to one-half of women with infertility have endometriosis.

PATHOPHYSIOLOGY

- The ectopic endometrial tissue is physiologically functional. It responds to ovarian hormones (especially estrogen).
- The result of this ectopic tissue is "ectopic menses," which cause bleeding, peritoneal inflammation, pain, fibrosis, and, eventually, adhesions.

SITES OF ENDOMETRIOSIS

Common

- Ovary (bilateral): 60%.
- Peritoneum over uterus.
- Anterior and posterior cul-de-sacs.
- Broad ligaments/fallopian tubes/round ligaments.
- Uterosacral ligaments.
- Bowel.
- Appendix.

Less Common

- Rectosigmoid: 10–15%.
- Cervix.
- Vagina.
- Bladder.

Rare

- Nasopharynx.
- Lungs. } → hemoptysis w/ menses.
- Central nervous system (CNS).
- Abdominal wall.
- Abdominal surgical scars or episiotomy scar.

EXAM TIP

Endometriosis is the most likely cause of infertility in a menstruating woman over the age of 30, without a history of pelvic inflammatory disease.

WARD TIP

A 37-year-old woman complains of hemoptysis during her period.
Think: Endometriosis of the nasopharynx or lung.

WARD TIP

Severity of symptoms does not necessarily correlate with quantity of ectopic endometrial tissue, but may correlate with the depth of penetration of the ectopic tissue.

THEORIES OF ETIOLOGY

Though the mechanisms and etiology are unknown, there are four theories commonly cited. It is likely that multiple theories may explain the diverse nature of this disorder:

- **Retrograde menstruation:** Endometrial tissue is transported in a retrograde fashion through the fallopian tubes, and implants in the pelvis with a predilection for the ovaries and pelvic peritoneum.
- **Coelomic (peritoneal) metaplasia:** Under certain conditions, peritoneal tissue develops into functional endometrial tissue, thus responding to hormones.
- **Vascular/lymphatic transport:** Endometrial tissue is transported via blood vessels and lymphatics. This can explain endometriosis in locations outside of the pelvis (i.e., lymph nodes, pleural cavity, kidneys).
- **Altered immunity:** There may be deficient or inadequate natural killer (NK) or cell-mediated response. This can explain why some women develop endometriosis, whereas others with similar characteristics do not.
- **Iatrogenic dissemination:** Endometrial glands and stroma can be implanted during a procedure (i.e., cesarean delivery), and result in endometriosis in surgical scars.

GENETIC PREDISPOSITION

- A woman with a first-degree relative with endometriosis has a 7% chance of being similarly affected, as compared with 1% in unrelated persons.
- Patients with a positive family history may develop endometriosis at an earlier age.

CLINICAL PRESENTATION

- Pelvic pain (may be dysmenorrhea or chronic pelvic pain):
  - Secondary dysmenorrhea (pain usually begins 2–3 days before menses, lasts throughout menses, and may persist several days after menses).
  - Dyspareunia (typically with deep penetration rather than insertion) results due to endometriotic implants in the pouch of Douglas and rectovaginal septum.
  - Dyschezia (pain with defecation): Also due to deep implants in the pouch of Douglas and rectovaginal septum.
- Infertility.
- Cyclic bowel or bladder symptoms (i.e., hematuria).
- Up to one-third of women may be asymptomatic.

SIGNS

- Fixed, tender, retroflexed uterus, with scarring posterior to uterus.
- "Nodular" uterosacral ligaments or thickening and induration of uterosacral ligaments.
- Ovarian endometriomas: Tender, palpable, and freely mobile adnexal masses that arise from implanted endometrial tissue within the ovary. This creates a small blood-filled cavity in the ovary, classically known as a "chocolate cyst." ✖✖
- Blue/brown vaginal implants (rare).

DIAGNOSIS

- **Laparoscopy or laparotomy:** The gold standard for definitive diagnosis is laparoscopy with biopsy, but visual inspection is considered satisfactory for diagnosis. If surgery is planned for diagnostic purposes, typically consent would be obtained to treat the endometriosis at the same time with ablation or excision.

WARD TIP

Long-term complications of endometriosis:
- Prolonged bleeding of ectopic tissue causes scarring (adhesions).
- Adhesions may contribute to infertility, small bowel obstruction, pelvic pain, and difficult surgeries.

WARD TIP

Congenital anomalies that promote retrograde menstruation may be found in adolescents with endometriosis.

WARD TIP

Chronic pelvic pain may result from endometriosis with associated adhesive disease.

EXAM TIP

Classic findings of endometriosis: Dysmenorrhea, dyspareunia, and dyschezia.

EXAM TIP

The classic findings on physical exam are nodularities on the uterosacral ligament and a fixed retroverted uterus.

- The colors of endometrial implants vary widely:
  - Red implants—new.
  - Brown implants—older.
  - White implants—oldest (scar tissue).
  - The cardinal features of a tissue biopsy include endometrial glands, stroma, and hemosiderin-laden macrophages.

CLINICAL COURSE

- Thirty-five percent are asymptomatic.
- Symptomatic patients may have increasing pain and possible bowel pain and possible bowel complications.
- Often, there is improvement with pregnancy secondary to temporary cessation of menses.
- May be associated with infertility.

TREATMENT

Medical

The primary goal is to induce amenorrhea and cause regression of the endometriotic implants. Many of these options suppress estrogen.
- First line treatment is NSAIDs and oral contraceptive pills (OCPs).
  - Oral contraceptives (OCPs): May use cyclic or continuous regimen.
  - Nonsteroidal anti-inflammatory drugs (NSAIDs): Treats dysmenorrhea.
  - Gonadotropin-releasing hormone (GnRH) agonists (i.e., leuprolide): Suppresses FSH and induces a pseudomenopause.
  - Progestins: Medroxyprogesterone acetate (Depo-Provera), oral progestins (i.e., norethindrone acetate), etonogestrel implant (Nexplanon®), levonorgestrel IUD (Mirena®).
  - Danazol: An androgen derivative that suppresses FSH/LH, causing pseudomenopause. Not often used due to androgenic side effects.

EXAM TIP

The pulsatile release of endogenous GnRH stimulates FSH secretion. GnRH agonists cause down regulation of pituitary receptors and suppress FSH secretion. This creates a pseudomenopause state.

Surgical

- Conservative (retain reproductive potential): Laparoscopic lysis, ablation, and/or excision of adhesions and endometriotic implants.
- Definitive: Hysterectomy +/− bilateral salpingo-oophorectomy. Reserved for refractory cases when childbearing is complete).

Adenomyosis

WARD TIP

The only way to definitively diagnose adenomyosis is with microscopic examination of the uterus after hysterectomy.

A 39-year-old G4P4 presents with worsening menorrhagia and dysmenorrhea. On physical exam, the uterus is 14 weeks' size, globular, boggy, slightly tender, and mobile. What is the next best step in management?

Answer: There is no proven medical therapy for adenomyosis, and hysterectomy is the only guaranteed treatment. However, conservative management with hormonal therapy is a reasonable next step. NSAIDs and OCPs can improve dysmenorrhea and regulate the heavy menses.

WARD TIP

When an enlarged uterus is found on exam, ultrasound can help differentiate between adenomyosis and uterine fibroids.

DEFINITION

Ectopic endometrial glands and stroma are found *within the myometrium*, resulting in a symmetrically enlarged and globular uterus.

INCIDENCE

- Occurs in 30% of women.
- Usually in parous women in their 30s to 50s. Rare in nulliparous women.
- May coexists with other processes that cause heavy menses and dysmenorrhea, such as uterine fibroids, endometrial polyps, and endometriosis.

SIGNS AND SYMPTOMS

Common:
- **Chronic** pelvic pain.
- Symmetrical uterine enlargement.
- Dysmenorrhea (25%).
- Menorrhagia (60%).

DIAGNOSIS

Either ultrasound or MRI can be used to differentiate between adenomyosis and uterine fibroids.

TREATMENT

- **No proven medical therapy for treatment.**
- GnRH agonist, NSAIDs, and OCPs may be used for pain and bleeding.
- Hysterectomy: Definitive therapy if childbearing is complete. The diagnosis is usually confirmed after histologic examination of the hysterectomy specimen.
- Endometrial ablation and uterine artery embolization have both been shown to be helpful for some women.

Adenomyosis Vs. Endometriosis

- **Adenomyosis:**
  - Typically found in older, multiparous women.
  - Tissue is not as responsive to hormonal stimulation.
  - Noncyclic pain.
- **Endometriosis:**
  - Typically found in young, nulliparous women.
  - Tissue is responsive to hormonal stimulation.
  - Cyclic pain.

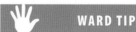

WARD TIP

The diagnosis of adenomyosis is suggested by characteristic clinical findings (i.e., menorrhagia, dysmenorrhea, enlarged uterus) after endometriosis and leiomyomas have been ruled out.

EXAM TIP

Adenomyosis is described as an enlarged, globular, "boggy" uterus on physical exam.

NOTES

CHAPTER 23

Differential Diagnoses of Pelvic Masses

Masses in the pelvis may be cystic or solid and can occur at any age. They can originate from the cervix, uterus, or adnexa, or from other organ systems.

DIFFERENTIAL DIAGNOSES

- Physiologic/functional cyst (follicular, corpus luteal, or theca lutein).
- Pregnancy (ectopic pregnancy).
- Infection/inflammation (tubo-ovarian abscess [TOA], diverticular abscess, appendicitis).
- Benign: Fibroid, ovarian neoplasms (most common—cystic teratoma), endometriomas.
- Malignant: Ovaries, fallopian tubes, colon, cervix, metastatic.

Diagnostic Tests for Various Causes of Pelvic Masses

The primary diagnostic tests are physical exam, pelvic ultrasound (US), and a pregnancy test.

- **Pregnancy:** Pregnancy test.
- **Functional/Physiologic ovarian cysts:** Physical exam + ultrasound to confirm.
- **Leiomyoma:** Physical exam + US to confirm.
- **Malignant ovarian neoplasm:** US, computed tomography (CT) scan to look for metastatic disease, CA-125, surgical exploration if malignancy suspected due to imaging studies, age, family history.
- **Benign ovarian neoplasm:** Physical exam, US, CA-125.
- **TOA:** Physical exam, US or CT, history of pelvic inflammatory disease (PID) with a palpable adnexal mass on exam (Figure 23-1).

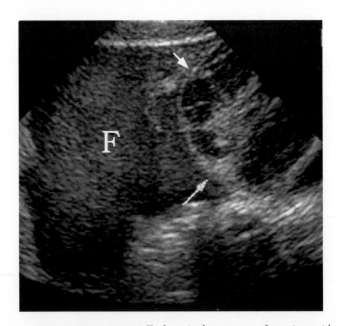

FIGURE 23-1. **Tubo-ovarian abscess.** Endovaginal sonogram of a patient with pelvic pain, vaginal discharge, and fever. The sonogram demonstrates echogenic fluid (F) in the cul-de-sac and a large cystic mass with internal echoes (arrows) in the left adnexa. This patient was known to have pelvic inflammatory disease and was successfully treated with antibiotics. (Reproduced, with permission, from Callen PW. *Ultrasonography in Obstetrics and Gynecology*, 5th ed. Philadelphia, PA: Saunders; 2007.)

Functional Ovarian Cysts

A 24-year-old G0 with a LMP 1 week ago presents with sudden severe right-sided pelvic pain. She also reports dizziness and feeling "weak." A urine pregnancy test is negative. What should be your next step in management?

Answer: Ultrasound. This patient presents with symptoms common for a ruptured ovarian cyst, which may require surgical intervention.

Functional ovarian cysts include follicular cysts and corpus luteum cysts.

FOLLICULAR CYSTS

Follicular cysts are the most common functional ovarian cysts.

PHYSIOLOGY

Failure of rupture or incomplete resorption of the ovarian follicle results in a cyst. Just like the original follicle, the ovarian cyst is granulosa cell lined and contains a clear to yellow estrogen-rich fluid.

SIGNS AND SYMPTOMS

- Usually asymptomatic when small (<5 cm). The larger the size, the more pain they cause and the higher the risk of ovarian torsion.
- Abnormal uterine bleeding.
- Unilateral abdominal and pelvic pain.
- Acute pelvic pain with findings of rebound and guarding on exam often signify rupture of the ovarian cyst. → provoked by sex or vigorous exercise

DIAGNOSIS

- Physical exam: Pelvic and abdominal exams.
- US confirms the diagnosis and is also helpful to see whether the cyst is ruptured. May show a simple (fluid-filled) ovarian cyst or fluid in the cul-de-sac, which is consistent with a ruptured cyst.

TREATMENT

- No treatment is necessary for most cysts, since they usually resolve spontaneously within 2 months. US may be repeated in 4–6 weeks to confirm resolution of the cyst. *no tx necessary.
- Oral contraceptive pills (OCPs) may help prevent formation of future cysts, especially in patients with recurrent cysts.
- If the cyst is unresolved after 2 months, it is more likely to be a neoplasm rather than follicular cyst, and laparoscopy with ovarian cystectomy or oophorectomy may be indicated to diagnose and treat the cyst. surgery for cyst if present for >2 months or >5 cm.
- Laparoscopic cystectomy or oophorectomy can also be considered for symptomatic or asymptomatic cysts >5 cm, which are at an increased risk for ovarian torsion.

LUTEIN CYSTS

There are two types of lutein cysts: **corpus luteum cysts** and **theca lutein cysts.**

Corpus Luteum Cyst

- The corpus luteum fails to involute and continues to enlarge. It can produce progesterone for weeks longer than normal, and may delay menses.
- **Corpus hemorrhagicum** is formed when there is hemorrhage into a corpus luteum cyst.
- If this ruptures, the patient can present with acute lower-quadrant pain and vaginal bleeding, and may develop signs of shock and hemoperitoneum.
- These cysts rarely grow >5 cm.

SIGNS AND SYMPTOMS

- Unilateral adnexal tenderness and pain.
- Abnormal uterine bleeding.

DIAGNOSIS

History and pelvic exam, US.

TREATMENT

- Observe for 2 months. Can start OCPs.
- If symptomatic: Analgesics, OCPs, laparotomy/laparoscopy if exam shows an acute abdomen and torsion or rupture is suspected.

Theca Lutein Cyst

↑ levels of human chorionic gonadotropin (hCG) can cause **follicular overstimulation** and lead to theca lutein cysts, which are often multiple and bilateral.

Tubo-Ovarian Abscess (TOA)

An abscess involving the ovary and fallopian tube that most often arises as a consequence of pelvic inflammatory disease (PID).

PHYSIOLOGY

- Primary TOA may arise as a complication of an ascending infection of the reproductive tract.
- Secondary TOA may develop as a result of bowel perforation (appendicitis, diverticulitis) from intraperitoneal spread of infection.
- TOA can also develop in association with pelvic surgery or malignancy.

SIGNS AND SYMPTOMS

- Pelvic and/or abdominal pain.
- Leukocytosis.
- Fever.
- Vaginal discharge.
- Palpable mass.

DIAGNOSIS

- Physical exam: Pelvic and abdominal.
- US or CT confirms the diagnosis and allows the opportunity to assess for other abscesses.

TREATMENT

- Antimicrobial therapy.
- Laparoscopic or US-guided drainage if no response to antibiotics.

Endometriomas

Endometriomas arise as a result of ectopic endometrial tissue in the ovary. They are commonly referred to as "chocolate cysts" due to the thick, brown, tarlike fluid that they contain.

PHYSIOLOGY

Endometriomas arise in women who have endometriosis. Endometriosis is a condition in which endometrial glands and stroma occur outside the uterine cavity.

SIGNS AND SYMPTOMS

- Pelvic pain.
- Dysmenorrhea.
- Dyspareunia.

DIAGNOSIS

- Clinical diagnosis can be made in women with a history of endometriosis, pelvic pain, and an ovarian cyst. As many as 50% of women with endometriosis will develop an endometrioma.
- Definitive diagnosis is made by laparoscopy and a biopsy containing hemosiderin-laden macrophages. However, it can be strongly suspected based on history, physical exam, and ultrasound.

TREATMENT

- **Only surgical; medical therapy is not effective treatment for an endometrioma.**
- Conservative surgery (ovarian cystectomy): Entire cyst (endometrioma) can be excised by laparoscopy of laparotomy. Aspiration has proven to be ineffective.
- Definitive surgery (oophorectomy): Alternative to cystectomy. Endometriomas are less likely to recur after oophorectomy, and it is a good option for women who have completed childbearing.

WARD TIP

An endometrioma = chocolate cyst.

Cystectomy > oophorectomy.

Benign Cystic Teratomas

A 25-year-old G1P1 presents for an annual well-woman exam. She reports a 3-month history of left-sided intermittent dull pain. She is afebrile. Pelvic exam demonstrates left adnexal enlargement and tenderness. The right adnexa is nontender without palpable masses. An ultrasound reveals a 5-cm, left hypoechoic unilocular cyst containing calcifications and internal debris. What is the most likely diagnosis? What is the best treatment for this patient?

Answer: Diagnosis—benign cystic teratoma. Treatment—laparoscopy with an ovarian cystectomy.

- Benign mature cystic teratomas (dermoid cysts) are the most common ovarian germ cell tumor.
- Germ cell tumors arise primarily in young women age 12–30 and account for 70% of tumors in this age group.

*[handwritten margin note: cx: * struma ovarii * ovarian tissue]*

PHYSIOLOGY

- Cystic teratomas contain tissue of ectodermal, mesodermal, and endodermal origin. The tissue is mature (benign) and may include skin, bone, teeth, and hair.
- The diverse tissue found within a teratoma is believed to develop from the genetic material in a single oocyte.
- Oocytes that are able to develop into teratomas undergo an arrest in development after meiosis I.
- Almost all mature cystic teratomas have a 46,XX karyotype.
- Malignant transformation develops in only 1–3% of cases.

DIAGNOSIS

US is the primary imaging tool used for diagnosis. Teratomas have a characteristic appearance, which usually includes cystic and solid components along with calcifications.

TREATMENT

- Excision of the teratoma by laparotomy or laparoscopy.
- An ovarian cystectomy is preferred in women who have not completed childbearing.
- If there is no viable ovarian tissue, if the patient is >40, or if the patient has completed childbearing, then an oophorectomy is preferred.
- Evaluate other ovary carefully—teratomas are bilateral in 15% of cases.

EXAM TIP

A young woman with a dermoid cyst can be treated with an ovarian cystectomy rather than an oophorectomy—the ovary can be preserved.

[handwritten margin note:]
- no viable ovarian tissue
- >40 y/o
- completed childbearing
→ oophorectomy

Malignancies

Malignant ovarian tumors are the leading cause of death from reproductive tract cancer. The lifetime risk of developing ovarian cancer is 1.6%. This risk is ↑ to 5% with one affected first-degree relative.

PATHOLOGY

Origins of the three main types of ovarian tumors:
- Epithelial: Repeated stimulation (i.e., ovulation) of the ovarian surface epithelium is hypothesized to result in malignant transformation. These tumors include serous, mucinous, endometrioid, clear cell, and transitional cell. Ninety-five percent of ovarian cancers are epithelial.
- Sex-cord stromal: These include granulosa cell, Sertoli cell, Sertoli-Leydig, and fibromas/fibrothecomas.
- Germ cell: These include teratoma, dysgerminoma, yolk-sac, and embryonal choriocarcinoma.

RISK FACTORS

- Family history in first-degree relative.
- Age (>50).
- Nulliparity.
- History of breast cancer.

SIGNS AND SYMPTOMS

- GI symptoms: Abdominal pressure, fullness, swelling, or bloating.
- Urinary urgency.
- Pelvic discomfort or pain.
- Often ovarian neoplasms are **asymptomatic.**

TABLE 23-1. **Pelvic Sonographic Findings Suggestive of Malignancy**

Solid component of mass, not hyperechoic, presence of nodularity
Multiloculated (fluid trapped in different compartments)
Thick septations (thick walls between compartments)
Presence of ascites
Peritoneal masses, **matted bowels, enlarged nodes**

DIAGNOSIS

- An elevated serum CA-125 (>35 units) indicates an ↑ likelihood that an ovarian tumor is malignant. Note that CA-125 is typically only elevated in epithelial ovarian cancers.
- Ultrasound is helpful in distinguishing between masses that are likely to be malignant and benign (see Table 23-1).
- Definitive diagnosis is tissue biopsy (which typically occurs at time of surgical staging).

TREATMENT

- Complete surgical staging must be conducted for all women with ovarian cancer.
- In a woman with early-stage ovarian cancer, an abdominal hysterectomy with bilateral salpingo-oophorectomy, omentectomy, lymphadenectomy, appendectomy, and peritoneal washings would be performed.
- With more advanced disease, aggressive removal of all visible disease improves survival ("optimal cytoreduction" is residual disease <1 cm in diameter).
- Ovarian cancer is one of the few cancers in which "surgical debulking" even in the presence of distant metastasis is helpful.
- Postoperative chemotherapy with a platinum and a taxane agent is indicated for women with advanced epithelial ovarian cancer.

PROGNOSIS

- Seventy-five percent of women are diagnosed with advanced disease after regional or distant metastases have occurred.
  - Overall 5-year survival.
  - 17% with distant metastases.
  - 36% with local spread.
  - 89% with early disease.

Leiomyomas (Fibroids)

 A 40-year-old woman presents with heavy, painful menses. She also reports occasional bleeding in between her periods, along with pelvic pain and pressure. On exam, the uterus is 16 weeks in size and irregular. The adnexae are not palpable. What is your next step in management?

Answer: This patient likely has uterine fibroids. A pelvic exam and imaging with US will help to confirm the diagnosis.

EXAM TIP

Ovarian cancers present with vague GI symptoms (fullness, early satiety, bloating) at a more advanced cancer stage.

WARD TIP

CA-125 is elevated in 80% of women with epithelial ovarian cancer overall but in only 50% of women with early disease.

WARD TIP

Leiomyomas typically present with heavy/prolonged menses and/or pelvic pain/pressure.

Leiomyomas are localized, benign, **smooth muscle tumors** of the uterus, which are hormonally responsive.

EPIDEMIOLOGY

- Clinically found in 25–33% of reproductive-age women and in up to 50% of black women. ↑ association w/ AA's.
- They are almost always multiple.
- The most common indication for hysterectomy.

SEQUELAE

Changes in uterine fibroids over time include:
- Hyaline degeneration.
- Calcification.
- Red degeneration (painful interstitial hemorrhage, often with pregnancy).
- Cystic degeneration—may rupture into adjacent cavities.

UTERINE LOCATIONS OF LEIOMYOMAS

- **Submucous:** Just below endometrium, protruding into the uterine cavity; more likely to cause abnormal bleeding.
- **Intramural:** Within the uterine wall. May enlarge enough to distort the uterine cavity.
- **Subserous:** Just below the serosa/peritoneum. May have a broad or pedunculated stalk.
- **Cervical:** Located in the cervix.
- **Parasitic:** The fibroid obtains blood supply from another organ (i.e., omentum).
- **Interligamentous:** The fibroid grows laterally into the broad ligament (likely started out subserosal).

SYMPTOMS

- **Asymptomatic** in >50% of cases.
- **Bleeding +/– anemia:** One-third of cases present with heavy or prolonged menstrual bleeding. Bleeding may be caused by:
  - Abnormal blood supply.
  - Pressure ulceration.
  - Abnormal endometrial covering.
- **Pain:** Secondary dysmenorrhea.
- **Pelvic pressure:** May be due to enlarging fibroids ("bulk symptoms").
- **Infertility:** May distort uterine cavity and lead to difficulty conceiving (i.e., tubal obstruction) or increased risk of miscarriage.

DIAGNOSIS

- **Physical exam** (bimanual pelvic and abdominal exams): Fibroids are usually midline, enlarged, irregularly shaped, and mobile.
- **Ultrasound** (may also be visualized by x-ray, magnetic resonance imaging [MRI], CT, hysterosalpingogram [HSG], hysteroscopy).
- Depending on patient characteristics, abnormal bleeding may be evaluated with Pap smear, ECC, endometrial biopsy, hysteroscopy with D&C.

TREATMENT

- **No treatment** is indicated for asymptomatic women, as this hormonally sensitive tumor will likely shrink with menopause.
- Pregnancy is usually **uncomplicated.** Some fibroids may grow in size during pregnancy. Bed rest and narcotics are indicated for pain with red degeneration.

EXAM TIP

Leiomyomas are the most common pelvic tumor found in women.

EXAM TIP

A rapidly enlarging myoma = think leiomyosarcoma.

WARD TIP

Submucosal and intramural types of fibroids usually present with heavy menses. Subserosal fibroids may become pedunculated and present with acute pain and torsion.

EXAM TIP

Pregnancy with fibroids carries ↑ risk of:
- Placental abruption
- First-trimester bleeding
- Dysfunctional labor
- Malpresentation
- Cesarean delivery

WARD TIP

The most common location for a uterine fibroid = subserosal.

- Treatment is usually initiated when:
  - Bleeding is not able to be managed with medications.
  - Hematocrit falls.
  - Fibroids compress adjacent structures (i.e., bladder or bowel symptoms, hydronephrosis).
  - Symptoms limit lifestyle.
- Medical management:
  - OCPs or progestins (implants, injections, pills) may be used to manage bleeding, but are inconsistently effective.
  - Levonorgestrel-containing IUD (Mirena®) may be used to manage bleeding if the uterus is not significantly enlarged and if the uterine cavity is not distorted.
  - Gonadotropin-releasing hormone (GnRH) agonists can be given for up to 6 months to shrink tumors (i.e., before surgery) and control bleeding (i.e., allow improvement of anemia).
- Surgical management:
  - **Endometrial ablation:** Women who have completed childbearing and have small fibroids (<4 cm) may be candidates.
  - **Uterine artery embolization:** Minimally invasive option for women who want to preserve their uterus but not their fertility.
  - **Myomectomy:** Surgical removal of the fibroid by hysteroscopy, laparoscopy, or laparotomy. A myomectomy is reserved for women who desire to retain their uterus for childbearing.
  - **Hysterectomy:** Indicated for symptomatic women who have failed conservative management and completed childbearing.

EXAM TIP

About one-third of fibroids recur following myomectomy.

WARD TIP

The treatment for *asymptomatic* fibroids is observation.

WARD TIP

Definitive treatment for fibroids = hysterectomy.

Bleeding
pelvic pain/pressure } → uterine leiomyoma.
infertility

NOTES

CHAPTER 24

Cervical Dysplasia

Cervical Dysplasia

Cervical dysplasia describes abnormal cells of the cervix that can be precursors to cancer. Papanicolaou (Pap) smears are performed regularly to assess for cervical dysplasia. Further workup and treatments include colposcopy, cone biopsy, and the loop electrosurgical excision procedure (LEEP) as well as cryotherapy or laser therapy. Approximately 80% of cervical dysplasia is related to human papillomavirus (HPV) infection. A vaccine against high-risk strains of this virus can be offered to young women (and men).

Cervical dysplasia and cervical cancer lie on a continuum of conditions. Cervical dysplasia can take one of three paths:
1. Progress to cancer.
2. Remain the same and not progress.
3. Regress to normal.

WARD TIP

Vaccines against high-risk strains of HPV are currently FDA approved for girls and boys between the ages of 9 and 26 years.

Risk Factors for Cervical Dysplasia and Cervical Cancer

- Human papillomavirus (HPV) infection:
    - Eighty percent of cases.
    - Risk highest if infected >6 months.
    - Types 16, 18, 31, 33, 45—high oncogenic potential.
- ↑ sexual activity (↑ risk of viral/bacterial infections):
    - Multiple sexual partners.
    - Intercourse at early age (<18 years).
- Low socioeconomic status.
- Genetic predisposition.
- Cigarette smoking (increases risk for squamous cell cancers but not adenocarcinomas).
- Alcohol, 2–4 drinks/wk, can ↑ sexual behavior which leads to HPV infection.
- Oral contraceptive pills (OCPs), particularly with use >5 years (condoms ↓ risk in these women).
- Immunosuppression.

EXAM TIP

HPV typical associations:
- Types 6 and 11: Anogenital warts
- Types 16 and 18: Cervical cancer

Human Papillomavirus (HPV)

- HPV is a sexually transmitted infection. Infection can occur through sexual contact–infected intact skin, mucous membranes, or bodily fluids from an infected partner.
- Abstinence, condoms, and decreasing the number of sexual partners can lower the risk of contracting HPV.
- There is a high prevalence of HPV in sexually active women, but most infections are subclinical (asymptomatic).
- Most young women will clear the virus within 24 months.
- There are more than 100 genotypes of HPV.
- HPV types 16 and 18 cause 70% of cervical cancers and 50% of cervical cancer precursors.

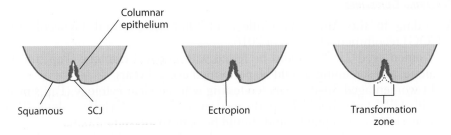

Columnar epithelium

Squamous | SCJ

Ectropion

Transformation zone

FIGURE 24-1. Sites of cervical cancers.

Squamocolumnar Junction (SCJ)

- Located on the cervix, this is the border between the squamous lining of the vagina and the columnar cells of the uterus.
- Most cervical cancers arise at this site.
- Position is variable (see Figure 24-1).
- In nulliparous women, it is usually located at the external cervical os.
- In pregnancy, it migrates out and is visible to the naked eye.
- The area near the ectocervix where columnar cells undergo metaplasia and become squamous cells, is referred to as the **transformation zone (TZ).**
- The TZ is the area between the columnar and squamous epithelium.
- The TZ must be biopsied to rule out cancer or precancer.

WARD TIP

Cervical dysplasia almost always occurs at the transformation zone or the squamocolumnar junction.

Pap Smear

A 21-year-old G2P2 desires contraception. She has been sexually active for 4 years, with three lifetime partners. Her menses are irregular. Before prescribing oral contraceptive pills, what tests need to be performed?

Answer: A pregnancy test, Pap smear, and STD screening.

A cytologic **screening test** for cervical neoplasia.

TECHNIQUE

- A speculum is placed in the vagina to expose the uterine cervix.
- Cells are circumferentially scraped from the ectocervix with a spatula and from the endocervix using an endocervical brush.
- A conventional Pap smear involved spreading the cells from the spatula and cytobrush on a glass slide, spraying with fixative, and sending to cytopathology for evaluation.
- Liquid-based thin layer cytology (i.e., Thin Prep®) has largely replaced conventional Pap-smear technique. The spatula and cytobrush are placed into a liquid fixative solution and swirled vigorously to collect the cells. This is sent to cytology, where loose cells are trapped onto a filter and then plated in a monolayer on a glass slide to be evaluated.
- If liquid-based cytology is used, the sample may also be tested for presence of gonorrhea, chlamydia, and/or HPV.

SUCCESS RATE

↓ incidence of invasive cervical cancer in the United States by 50% in the last 30 years due to widespread screening.

EXAM TIP

Patients over age 30 should have concurrent HPV testing performed at the time of Pap smear.

SCREENING GUIDELINES

According to the American College of Obstetricians and Gynecologists (ACOG) recommendations as of 2016:

- Women aged 21–29 should be tested with cervical cytology (Pap smear) alone, and screening should be performed every 3 years.
- In women aged 30–65 years, co-testing with cervical cytology (Pap smear with HPV test) should be performed every 5 years. Cytology alone (Pap smear) is also acceptable, and should be performed every 3 years.
- Frequency of Pap smear screening should be individualized, and may need to occur earlier/more often in women who have HIV, are immune compromised, were exposed to DES in utero, or have been previously treated for CIN2, CIN3, or cancer.
- Women under age 21 should not be screened, because the incidence of cervical cancer is very low, and they have an effective immune response that will usually clear the HPV infection in 8–24 months.
- Pap smears may be discontinued after age 65 in healthy women with adequate negative prior screening test (Pap smear) results and no history of CIN2 or higher.
- A pelvic examination should still be performed annually.

CLASSIFICATION OF ABNORMALITIES

- The Bethesda System is used to describe both cytologic (on Pap test) and histologic (on biopsy) findings.
  1. Cytologic (Pap smear) abnormalities are described using the term "squamous intraepithelial lesion" (SIL). (see below).
     - Each cytology report consists of (1) a description of specimen adequacy, (2) a general categorization (i.e., negative, epithelial cell abnormality), and (3) ancillary testing (i.e., HPV test).
     - Management of abnormal Pap smears in women ages 21 to 24 differs from those age ≥25 because of the low incidence of cervical cancer in this age group.
  2. Histologic (biopsy) abnormalities are described using the term "cervical intraepithelial neoplasia" (CIN).
     - CIN1 is a low-grade lesion with mild atypical changes in the lower one-third of the epithelium.
     - CIN2 is considered a high-grade lesion, with atypical changes confined to the lower two-thirds of the epithelium.
     - CIN3 is a high-grade lesion, where atypical cells encompass >2/3 of the epithelium. CIN2 and CIN3 are often classified together and are treated the same.
     - The recommendations for management of CIN differs for women ages 21 to 24 from those age ≥25 because the risk of cervical cancer is very low in this population.

PAP SMEAR RESULTS, WORKUP, AND FOLLOW-UP

- **Negative for intraepithelial lesion or malignancy:** Repeat Pap per age-based protocol described above.
- **Atypical squamous cells of undetermined significance (ASCUS):**
  1. Reflex HPV testing if under age 30, concurrent HPV testing if age 30 and above.
  2. If HPV negative—continue routine screening per protocol.
  3. If HPV positive—colposcopy if age ≥25, repeat cytology (Pap) in 1 year if age 21–24.
- **Atypical squamous cells, cannot exclude high-grade squamous intraepithelial lesion (ASC-H):** Colposcopy with indicated biopsies.
- **Atypical glandular cells (AGC):** Colposcopy with indicated biopsies, endocervical curettage (ECC), and endometrial sampling.

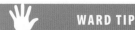

Two things to remember about a Pap smear:
1. It is a screening test.
2. It provides cytologic information, not histologic.

An abnormal screening test (Pap smear) needs a diagnostic test for confirmation (colposcopy with biopsies).

- **Low-grade squamous intraepithelial lesion (LSIL):** Colposcopy with indicated biopsies if age ≥25, repeat cytology (Pap) in 1 year if age 21–24.
- **High-grade squamous intraepithelial lesion (HSIL):** Colposcopy with ECC and indicated biopsies. If there is a discrepancy between the cytology and the biopsy, then an excisional procedure should be performed (loop electrosurgical excision procedure [LEEP] or cold knife conization [CKC]).
- The algorithms are very complex, and vary based on age and history. Protocols are available online at www.asccp.org. (This organization also has a handy app that keeps this information at your fingertips.)

EXAM TIP

Pap-smear screening should not begin until age 21, regardless of sexual activity.

Colposcopy with Cervical Biopsy

A 45-year-old G4P4 presents for a routine annual exam. Her Pap smear returns with a report of ASCUS. Her Pap smears have always been normal in the past. What is the next best step to evaluate her cancer risk?
  Answer: HPV DNA testing. If HPV DNA testing is "positive," indicating the presence of high-risk HPV DNA, then a colposcopy and indicated biopsies should be performed. If the HPV testing is negative, she can be managed as per her age-based protocol.

WARD TIP

Colposcopy and directed biopsies are needed to make a histologic diagnosis.

DEFINITION

- A procedure that utilizes staining and a low-magnification microscope, mounted on a stand, for the viewing of the cervix, vagina, and vulva.
- Provides illuminated, magnified view, which aids in identifying lesions and biopsying suspicious areas to *obtain histologic diagnosis*.

WARD TIP

On biopsy, 5–17% of cases of ASCUS and 24–94% of ASC-H demonstrate CIN2–CIN3.

INDICATIONS FOR A COLPOSCOPY

- Performed to evaluate abnormal Pap smears, as per the guidelines described above.
  - ASCUS with high-risk HPV subtypes (age ≥25).
  - ASC-H. →*immediate*
  - Atypical glandular cells (AGC).
  - LSIL (age ≥25).
  - HSIL.

PROCEDURE

1. Speculum is inserted to expose the cervix.
2. **Acetic acid is applied.** After 30 sec, the acetic acid dehydrates cells and causes precipitation of nucleic proteins in the superficial layers. The neoplastic cells appear whiter because of a higher nucleus/cytoplasm ratio ("acetowhite epithelium").
3. **Colposcopy:** Next, a low-power microscope (colposcope) is used to look for dysplasia. Signs of dysplasia include acetowhite epithelium and abnormal vessels (punctations, mosaicism). The transformation zone must be visualized in its entirety. If the TZ or the entire extent of the lesion is not entirely visualized, then the colposcopy is considered inadequate.
4. **Cervical biopsy:** Neoplastic and dysplastic areas are then biopsied under colposcopic guidance. Contraindications include acute pelvic inflammatory disease (PID) and cervicitis. Pregnancy is **not** a contraindication.
5. **ECC:** A curette is used to scrape the cervical canal to obtain endocervical cells for cytologic examination. An ECC is contraindicated in pregnancy.

WARD TIP

Ninety percent of women with abnormal cytologic findings can be adequately evaluated with colposcopy.

WARD TIP

What must be completely visualized for adequate colposcopic evaluation?
1. TZ.
2. Extent of lesion in its entirety.

WARD TIP

Evaluation of biopsy margins may be difficult with LEEP, because of thermal artifact.

INFORMATION PROVIDED BY COLPOSCOPY AND ECC

If biopsy results or ECC is positive for CIN2 or CIN3, then a cone biopsy or a LEEP should be performed for further diagnosis or treatment.

Cone Biopsy and LEEP

- **Cold knife cone biopsy:** A procedure performed in the operating room in which a cone-shaped biopsy is removed with a scalpel, including part of the endocervical canal. Requires use of general anesthesia.
- **Loop electrosurgical excision procedure (LEEP):** A procedure performed in an office setting or in an operating room. A small wire loop with an electric current is used to excise the TZ and the endocervix. Local anesthesia/analgesia is required.

INDICATIONS FOR CONE BIOPSY/LEEP

- Inadequate view of TZ on colposcopy.
- Positive ECC.
- ≥2 grade discrepancy between colposcopic biopsy and Pap.
- Treatment for CIN2–CIN3.
- Treatment for adenocarcinoma in situ.
- When cancer cannot be excluded after colposcopy, biopsy, and ECC.

LEEP

LEEP can be used to diagnose and treat CIN.

GUIDELINES FOR LEEP TREATMENT

- Never treat during pregnancy.
- Never treat without excluding invasive carcinoma.
- When treating, excise entire TZ.
- Always excise keratinizing lesions.

Cryotherapy

An outpatient procedure that uses a probe cooled with nitrous oxide (N_2O to $-70°F$) to ablate lesions.

INDICATIONS

Treatment of low-grade lesions only if it is a lesion completely visualized on colposcopic exam.

COMPLICATIONS AND SIDE EFFECTS

- Profuse, watery, vaginal discharge.
- Long-term complications include cervical stenosis and a small ↑ in preterm labor.

Laser Therapy

- Light amplification by stimulated emission of radiation (LASER): A high-energy photon beam generates heat at impact and vaporizes tissue.
- Causes less tissue destruction of the TZ compared to other methods.
- Very expensive.

INDICATIONS

Excision or ablation of CIN.

Prevention of Cervical Dysplasia

GARDASIL

- Licensed in 2006 by the FDA as the first quadrivalent HPV vaccine.
- Administered as three doses: 0.5 mL intramuscularly given at intervals of 0, 2, and 6 months.
- Contains virus-like particles from four HPV genotypes: 6, 11, 16, and 18.
- Gardasil-9 is now available, and contains high-risk HPV genotypes 6, 11, 16, 18, 31, 33, 45, 52, 58. The administration intervals are the same.

Gardasil – 4
Gardasil – 9.

CERVARIX

- Licensed in 2010 by the FDA as the first bivalent HPV vaccine.
- Administered in three doses: 0.5 mL intramuscularly given at intervals of 0, 1, and 6 months.
- Contains virus-like particles from two HPV genotypes: 16 and 18.

EXAM TIP

What HPV genotypes are contained in the Gardasil vaccine?
Answer: Types 6, 11, 16, 18.

SUCCESS RATE

Gardasil: Protects against 70% of cervical cancers and 90% of genital warts.

Cervarix: Protects against 75% of cervical cancers caused by types 16 and 18.

INDICATIONS

- Gardasil: Give to males and females age 9–26 years; cervarix: give to females 10–25 years.
- Usually given by pediatrician at age 11–12.
- Pregnancy Class B [not recommended for pregnant women.] → D *!
- Can be given to breast-feeding women.
- Recommended even for previously exposed patients.

SIDE EFFECTS

- Pain.
- Redness.
- Allergic reaction.

FOLLOW-UP

- Routine cervical cancer screening still necessary.
- The need for booster dose has not been established.

NOTES

CHAPTER 25

Cervical Cancer

Cervical cancer is the third most frequent malignancy of the female genital tract. Eighty percent of cervical cancers are squamous cell carcinomas. They are related to human papillomavirus (HPV) infection while adenocarcinomas comprise 20% and can be related to maternal diethylstilbestrol (DES) exposure as well as certain strains of HPV. The lifetime risk in the United States of developing cervical cancer is <1%. Cervical cancer is staged clinically, not surgically. Treatment depends on the stage of disease. Women diagnosed while pregnant face unique considerations, but overall have similar survival rates as nonpregnant patients.

Epidemiology

AGE AFFECTED
- Peak incidence between ages 45 and 55.
- The incidence in the United States in women age ≤20 is 0.1/100,000.
- The incidence in the United states in women age ≥30 is 11–16/100,000.

RACE PREVALENCE
- More prevalent in African-American women and urban Hispanic women than white women.
- African-American mortality rate is two times greater than whites.

WARD TIP

Symptoms of cervical cancer become evident when cervical lesions are of moderate size.

Symptoms

 A 50-year-old G3P3 woman presents with postcoital bleeding and some pain during intercourse. What is the next step?
Answer: Speculum exam with a Pap smear or biopsy if a lesion is visible.

- **Early stages:**
  - None.
  - Irregular/prolonged vaginal bleeding/pink discharge.
  - Postcoital bleeding (brownish discharge).
- **Middle stages:**
  - Postvoid bleeding.
  - Dysuria/hematuria.
- **Advanced stages:**
  - Weight loss, loss of appetite.
  - Bloody, malodorous discharge.
  - Severe pain, due to spread to sacral plexus.
  - Leg swelling (secondary to blockage of lymphatics).

WARD TIP

The incidence of cervical cancer has decreased in countries that have robust screening and vaccination programs.

Differential Diagnosis

- Cervical lesions, i.e., polyps, nabothian cysts.
- Cervicitis or other infections.
- Vaginal malignancies.

Types of Cervical Cancer

SQUAMOUS CELL CANCER

- Accounts for 80% of cervical cancer.
- Associated with HPV infection: Types 16 and 18 are responsible for 80% of cases.

ADENOCARCINOMA

- Accounts for **20%** of all invasive cervical cancers.
- Arises from columnar cells lining the endocervical canal and glands.
- **Early diagnosis is difficult; the false-negative rate with Pap smear is 80%.**
- May be associated with maternal DES exposure and certain strains of high risk HPV, i.e., 16 and 18.

METASTASIS OF CERVICAL CANCER

A. By direct extension:
   - **R**ectal.
   - **I**ntra-abdominal.
   - **B**ladder.
   - **E**ndometrial.
B. By hematogenous spread:
   - Breast.
   - Lung.
   - Bone.
   - Liver.

Clinical Staging of Invasive Cervical Cancer

A 55-year-old G1P1 presents to clinic with a complaint of postcoital bleeding. Her Pap smear and colposcopy with biopsy confirm a diagnosis of squamous-cell cervical carcinoma. Physical exam demonstrates a visible lesion that is 3 cm in size and does not involve the vagina or parametrial tissue. What stage is this patient?
Answer: Based on clinical staging, she is stage IB1.

Clinical staging of cervical cancer is important for prognosis and treatment (see Tables 25-1 and 25-2).

THE INTERNATIONAL FEDERATION OF GYNECOLOGY AND OBSTETRICS (FIGO) STAGING SYSTEM FOR CERVICAL CANCER ALLOWS THE FOLLOWING EXAMINATIONS TO ESTABLISH THE STAGE OF CERVICAL CANCER

- Physical exam (often under anesthesia): Bimanual, speculum, and rectovaginal exams to palpate tumor. Palpation of groin and supraclavicular lymph nodes.
- Colposcopy, ECC, cervical biopsy, cervical conization.
- Endoscopic exams: Hysteroscopy to evaluate the uterine lining, proctoscopy to evaluate rectal involvement, cystoscopy to evaluate bladder involvement.
- Imaging studies: Chest x-ray, intravenous pyelogram (IVP) to evaluate for urinary tract obstruction (CT is used in some centers).

WARD TIP

Cigarette smoking is a risk factor for squamous-cell cervical cancers, but not cervical adenocarcinomas.

lung cer – LABB
– Liver, adrenal, brain, bone.

WARD TIP

Metastasis of cervical cancer to:
RIB Eye steak
Rectal
Intra-abdominal
Bladder
Endometrial

EXAM TIP

Cervical cancer is staged clinically.

WARD TIP

Radical hysterectomy requires removal of:
- Uterus
- Cervix
- Parametrial tissue
- Upper vagina

0—CIS
I— cervix only
II— penetrated uterus, upper vagina
III— pelvic side wall, lower vagina
IV— extend beyond pelvis, bladder or rectal.

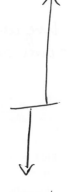

Radical hysterectomy.

chemotherapy + / radiation

TABLE 25-1. FIGO Staging, Revised 2009

STAGE 0—CARCINOMA IN SITU (CIN3)

STAGE I—CANCER CONFINED TO THE CERVIX ONLY

IA—Invasive cancer identified only microscopically. Gross lesions are stage IB.

IA1—Invasion of stroma no greater than 3 mm in depth and no wider than 7 mm.

IA2—Invasion of stroma greater than 3 mm and less than or equal to 5 mm in depth, but no wider than 7 mm.

IB—Clinically visible lesion confined to the cervix or lesions > IA.

IB1—Lesion confined to cervix ≤4 cm.

IB2—Lesion confined to cervix >4 cm.

STAGE II—CANCER EXTENDS BEYOND UTERUS, BUT NOT TO THE PELVIC SIDEWALL; INVOLVES THE UPPER VAGINA, BUT NOT THE LOWER THIRD

IIA—No parametrial involvement.

IIA1—Clinically visible lesion <4 cm with involvement of less than upper 2/3 of vagina.

IIA2—Clinically visible lesion >4 cm with involvement of less than upper 2/3 of vagina.

IIB—Parametrial involvement.

STAGE III—CANCER EXTENDED TO THE PELVIC SIDEWALL; TUMOR INVOLVES THE LOWER THIRD OF THE VAGINA; HYDRONEPHROSIS OR A NONFUNCTIONING KIDNEY

IIIA—No extension to the pelvic sidewall, but involves the lower third of the vagina.

IIIB—Extension to the pelvic sidewall; hydronephrosis or a nonfunctioning kidney.

STAGE IV—CANCER THAT HAS EXTENDED BEYOND THE TRUE PELVIS; INVOLVES EITHER THE MUCOSA OF THE BLADDER OR RECTUM OR BOTH

Stage IVA—Spread of cancer to adjacent pelvic organs (bladder/rectum).

Stage IVB—Spread of cancer to distant organs (outside of pelvis).

TABLE 25-2. Grading of Cervical Carcinoma

GRADE	INVASIVE SQUAMOUS TUMOR	ADENOCARCINOMA
X	Cannot be assessed	
1	Well differentiated	■ Small component of solid growth and nuclear atypia ■ Mild to moderate
2	Moderately differentiated	Intermediate-grade differentiation
3	Poorly differentiated	■ Solid pattern ■ Severe nuclear atypia predominate
4	Undifferentiated	*anaplastic*

Treatment of Invasive Cervical Cancer

- **Non-radical surgery:** Extrafascial (simple) hysterectomy (removal of uterus and cervix, but not parametrial tissue or upper vagina) or cone biopsy may be used to treat women with microinvasive disease (IA1).
- **Radical surgery:** Radical hysterectomy (removal of uterus, cervix, parametrial tissue, upper one-third of vagina) with lymph-node dissection. Performed only in patients with low-stage disease (IB–IIA).
- **Radiation therapy:** High-dose delivery to the cervix and vagina, and minimal dosing to the bladder and rectum:
  - External-beam whole pelvic radiation.
  - Transvaginal intracavitary cesium: Transvaginal applicators allow significantly larger doses of radiation to surface of cervix.

WARD TIP

How does cervical cancer spread? Direct extension and lymphatic spread. Lymph nodes involved are external, internal, common iliac, and para-aortic nodes.

Treatment of Bulky Central Pelvic Disease

- Radical hysterectomy with adjuvant or neoadjuvant radiation therapy.
- Tumor cytoreduction: Use of cytotoxic chemotherapy before definitive treatment with radiation or radical surgery.

Follow-Up of Cervical Carcinoma

- Patients are examined every 3 months for the first 2 years, then every 6 months in years 3–5, and yearly thereafter.
- An exam consists of a history, physical, and Pap.
- A chest x-ray and CT scan of abdomen are performed annually.

Recurrent Cervical Carcinoma

- Thirty percent of patients treated for cervical cancer will have a recurrence.
- Recurrence of cancer can occur anywhere, but occur mainly in the pelvis (vagina, cervix, or lateral pelvic wall).

SCREENING FOR RECURRENCE

Look for:
- Vaginal bleeding.
- Hematuria/dysuria.
- Constipation/melena.
- Pelvic and leg pain.
- Fistulas (in bladder or bowel).
- Sacral backache or pain in sciatic distribution.
- Costovertebral angle and flank pain.

WARD TIP

Leg pain following the distribution of the sciatic nerve or unilateral leg swelling is often an indication of pelvic recurrence.

CAUSE OF DEATH

Uremia is the major cause of death in cervical cancer (found in 50% of patients). **Excretory urogram** can identify periureteral compression by tumor.

Treatment

- Treatment of cervical cancer by stage:
  - **0–1:** If microinvasive disease: Cold-knife cone biopsy (ectocervix); extrafascial (simple) hysterectomy.
  - **1a–2a:** Radical hysterectomy or radiation, pelvic lymphadenectomy, para-aortic lymphadenectomy.
  - **2b–4b:** Chemotherapy (cisplatin) and radiation.
- General principles of treatment:
  - Patients may undergo definitive treatment only if disease is confined to pelvis.
  - Patients with local recurrence after radical hysterectomy are treated with **radiation**.
  - Patients previously treated with radiotherapy are treated only by **radical pelvic surgery**.
- **Chemotherapy:**
  - Response rates are higher with combination therapy.
  - Most combinations include (platinum) *cisplatin*
  - Response rates: 50–70% for 4–6 months of life.

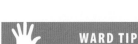

WARD TIP

Causes of death in cervical cancer patients include uremia.

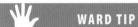

WARD TIP

What is the basic treatment for *invasive* cervical cancer?
- If confined to cervix: Radical hysterectomy, pelvic lymphadenectomy, para-aortic lymphadenectomy.
- If beyond cervix: Chemo and radiation.

WARD TIP

An ECC (endocervical curettage) is contraindicated in pregnancy.

Cervical Cancer in Pregnancy

Three percent of all invasive cervical cancers occur during pregnancy.

Symptoms

- One-third of pregnant patients with cervical cancer are asymptomatic.
- Symptoms in pregnancy include vaginal bleeding and discharge.

Screening

- Cervical cytology should be performed at the initial obstetric visit (if >21 years old).
- Pap results should be managed the same as in a nonpregnant patient.
- Colposcopy and cervical biopsies may be performed during pregnancy, but ECC is contraindicated due to the risk of trauma to the pregnancy, and the risk of heavy bleeding.
- *Therapeutic* conization is contraindicated during pregnancy. *Diagnostic* conization is reserved for patients in whom an invasive lesion is suspected but cannot be confirmed by biopsy *and* the results will alter the timing or mode of delivery. Otherwise, conization is performed postpartum. Cone biopsy, if necessary, should be performed in the second trimester. Complications may include hemorrhage and preterm labor.
- Clinical staging unchanged.

Treatment

- Definitive treatment is incompatible with pregnancy continuation.
- Therapy should be influenced by **gestational age, tumor stage, metastatic evaluation, and patient desires.** If the patient chooses to continue the pregnancy, therapy can be postponed until after delivery. Alternatively, a pregnancy can be terminated in order to begin treatment (subject to local laws). Chemotherapy may be used during pregnancy, but radiation therapy typically is not.
  - In early-stage disease a diagnostic CKC (cold-knife conization) can be done if the patient has a stage IA1 cancer. If the stage is > stage IA2, then after delivery, treatment can be instituted.

- Second-trimester treatments can include platinum-based chemotherapies, which would allow prolongation of pregnancy for fetal maturity. A cold-knife conization during pregnancy can lead to complications such as hemorrhage and loss of pregnancy.
- Third-trimester treatments include radical hysterectomy and pelvic lymphadenectomy after cesarean delivery.
- Delays in treatment have not been reported to ↑ recurrence rates in stage I disease.

DELIVERY

- Consideration of possible tumor hemorrhage and size/shape influence delivery method.
- Patients with small-volume stage IA tumors may be candidates for vaginal delivery.
- Episiotomies should be avoided due to case reports of cancer implantation at such sites.
- Patients with > stage IA1 cancer require a cesarean delivery, followed by appropriate surgical treatment (hysterectomy).

PROGNOSIS

Limited data suggest **no difference** in prognosis of patients with cervical cancer diagnosed in pregnancy compared to nonpregnant patients.

Adenocarcinoma of Cervix

- Makes up 20% of cervical cancers.
- Mean age of diagnosis is early 50s (similar to squamous cell cancers).
- Carcinomas mainly arise from the endocervix.
- Cervical conization with negative margins is required to define microinvasive disease, because noncontiguous or "skip" lesions are common with adenocarcinomas (as opposed to squamous tumors).
- Treatment is largely the same as for squamous cell carcinomas.

SCREENING OF DES-EXPOSED WOMEN

- Annual Pap smear.
- Careful palpation of vaginal walls to rule out adenosis or masses.

TREATMENT

- Similar to treatment of squamous-cell carcinoma of cervix.
- Preferred treatment is radical hysterectomy and pelvic lymph node dissection for stage IB or IIA.
- Vaginectomy if vagina is involved.

DISEASE RECURRENCE

- Most DES-related clear-cell carcinomas recur after ≤3 years of initial treatment.
- Pulmonary and supraclavicular nodal metastasis common; yearly screening chest x-ray recommended.

WARD TIP

Women who took DES during pregnancy have a 1.35% ↑ relative risk of breast cancer.

CHAPTER 26

Endometrial Hyperplasia and Endometrial Cancer

Endometrial Hyperplasia

Hyperplasia is a proliferation of endometrial glands that may progress to or coexist with an endometrial cancer. There are four categories. The terms simple/complex refer to the glandular/stromal architectural pattern. The term atypia refers to nuclear atypia.

- **Simple hyperplasia** *without* **atypia**
  - 1% progress to cancer (most well differentiated).
- **Complex hyperplasia** *without* **atypia**
  - 3% progress to cancer.
- **Simple hyperplasia** *with* **atypia**
  - 10% progress to cancer.
- **Complex hyperplasia** *with* **atypia**
  - 30% progress to cancer.

DIAGNOSIS OF ENDOMETRIAL HYPERPLASIA

- Endometrial **biopsy** (gold standard).
- Pap smear: If endometrial cells are found on a Pap smear in a woman over age 45, suspect endometrial pathology.
- Other procedures might diagnose endometrial hyperplasia:
  - Endocervical curettage (ECC).
  - Thickened endometrial stripe in a postmenopausal woman.
  - Hysteroscopy with uterine curettage if endometrial biopsy is inadequate.

TREATMENT

- Endometrial hyperplasia without atypia may be treated with progestin therapy.
  - Options include oral progestins (cyclic or daily), depo medroxyprogesterone acetate (DMPA, or depo provera), or a levonorgestrel containing IUD (Mirena®).
  - The regression rate is high, and the endometrium should be rebiopsied in 3–6 months to ensure regression.
- Endometrial hyperplasia with atypia is treated with hysterectomy if childbearing is complete.
  - If fertility is desired, may be treated with high-dose progestin therapy and rebiopsied in 3 months. Megestrol acetate is a very potent progesterone that is often used in this setting.

Epidemiology of Endometrial Cancer

- Endometrial carcinoma is a malignancy arising from the lining of the uterus.
- It is the most common gynecologic malignancy in the United States, and is diagnosed in over 35,000 women annually. It is 1.3 times more common than ovarian cancer and twice as common as cervical cancer.
- Because endometrial cancer usually presents with obvious symptoms, it is often diagnosed at an early stage.
- Lifetime risk is 3%.
- The average age at diagnosis is 61 years.
- Two types:
  - **Type I (most common):** An estrogen-dependent neoplasm that begins as proliferation of normal tissue. Over time, chronic proliferation becomes hyperplasia (abnormal tissue) and, eventually, neoplasia. These comprise 80% of endometrial cancers, and histologic types include endometrioid.

WARD TIP

An endometrial thickness of <5 mm in a postmenopausal woman with vaginal bleeding has a negative predictive value of 99% for endometrial cancer.

WARD TIP

Atypical hyperplasia is more likely to progress to cancer in older women compared with younger women.

EXAM TIP

Women with Lynch syndrome (hereditary nonpolyposis colorectal cancer, or HNPCC) have a 40–60% lifetime risk of developing endometrial cancer, which is equal to their risk of developing colorectal cancer.

EXAM TIP

Any factor that lowers the level or time of exposure to estrogen ↓ the risk of endometrial cancer.

- **Type II:** Unrelated to estrogen or hyperplasia. Tends to present with higher-grade or more aggressive tumors. These comprise 10–20% of endometrial cancers, and histologic types include clear cell, serous, mucinous, undifferentiated. These have a poorer prognosis.

Clinical Presentation

👤 A 55-year-old G0P0 presents with a 2-month history of intermittent vaginal bleeding. She completed menopause 3 years ago. She is obese and she has never been pregnant. What is the most likely diagnosis?
Answer: Endometrial cancer.

- **Abnormal bleeding** is present in 90% of cases:
  - Bleeding in postmenopausal women (classic).
  - Meno/metrorrhagia (in premenopausal cases).
- Abnormal Pap smear: 1–5% of cases. Pap smears are *not* diagnostic, but a finding of abnormal glandular cells (AGC) warrants further investigation.

Differential Diagnosis of Postmenopausal Bleeding

👤 A 59-year-old G0 postmenopausal woman comes in with a 2-month history of spotting. She says that the bleeding is minimal, but still requires wearing a panty liner. She has no pain or other symptoms. She weighs 300 pounds. What is the next step?
Answer: Endometrial biopsy. The most likely diagnosis is endometrial cancer. Her risk factors are obesity, and prolonged estrogen exposure.

DIFFERENTIAL DIAGNOSES OF POSTMENOPAUSAL BLEEDING

- Exogenous estrogens (i.e., hormone replacement therapy).
- Atrophic endometritis/vaginitis.
- Endometrial cancer.
- Endometrial/cervical polyps.
- Coagulopathy.
- Endometrial hyperplasia.

RISK FACTORS FOR ENDOMETRIAL CANCER

- Estrogen-producing tumors (i.e., granulosa cell tumors).
- Liver disease (a healthy liver metabolizes estrogen).
- Obesity (2–5 times ↑ risk).
- Early menarche/late menopause.
- Nulliparity (2–3 times ↑ risk; most likely when associated with anovulation).
- PCOS (chronic unopposed estrogen stimulation).
- Diabetes mellitus (2.8 times risk).
- Hypertension.
- Endometrial hyperplasia (highest risk is complex with atypia).
- Tamoxifen treatment for breast cancer (2–3 times ↑ risk).
- Unopposed estrogen stimulation (e.g., menopausal estrogen replacement: 4–8 times ↑ risk).
- Familial predisposition.
- Caucasian race.

WARD TIP

Side effects of progestins:
  Weight gain
  Edema
  Thrombophlebitis
  Headache
  Hypertension

EXAM TIP

Endometrial cancer is the most common gynecologic cancer.

WARD TIP

5–10% of women who present with postmenopausal bleeding will have endometrial cancer.

(handwritten annotations)

Pt factors
obese nulliparus earlymen. latemenop.

Liver dz

Pt Dz
PCOS E secreting tumors DM

drugs: Tamoxifen

EXAM TIP

Any factor that raises the level or time of exposure to estrogen increases the risk for endometrial cancer.

EB ind.:
≥ 45 y/o: AUB or PMB
< 45 y/o: AUB +
– Lynch syndrome
– unopposed Estrogen
– failed medical mgmt
≥ 35 y/o; abnormal glandular cells on PAP.

PROTECTIVE FACTORS

- Regular ovulation.
- Combined oral contraceptives.
- Multiparity.

EVALUATION OF POSTMENOPAUSAL BLEEDING

- Endometrial biopsy.
- Hysteroscopy with D&C if endometrial biopsy is inadequate or suspicious, or if a polyp is diagnosed.
- Transvaginal ultrasound to evaluate endometrial stripe. The stripe should be thin (<5 mm) in a postmenopausal woman. A thickened stripe requires further evaluation.
- If the cause of the postmenopausal bleeding is suspected to be a polyp, office hysteroscopy or saline infusion sonohysterogram (SIS) may be used to visualize. However, tissue sampling (via endometrial biopsy) is still mandatory.

Additional Workup for Endometrial Cancer

After diagnosis of endometrial cancer is made, the following should be performed to evaluate for possible metastasis:

- Physical exam—assess size/mobility of uterus, lymph nodes, ascites.
- Chest x-ray.
- Complete metabolic panel, CBC, type and screen.
- Pelvic or abdominal imaging is not required if surgical staging is planned.
- Take a careful family history to see if the patient is at risk for a hereditary cancer syndrome, i.e., Lynch syndrome.

Staging of Endometrial Cancer

Endometrial cancer is staged surgically.

- The stage of an endometrial cancer is determined by:
  1. The spread of tumor in the uterus.
  2. The degree of myometrial invasion.
  3. The presence of extrauterine tumor spread.
- This assessment is accomplished through a surgical staging operation (similar to ovarian cancer). The staging of a patient's disease directs treatment and predicts outcome (see Table 26-1).

Grading

Grading is determined by the tumor **histology**:

G1	Well differentiated	<5% solid pattern
G2	Moderately differentiated	5–50% solid pattern
G3	Poorly differentiated	>50% solid pattern

Treatment

Basic treatment for all stages (surgical staging is always the first step):

- Hysterectomy (usually abdominal or robotic approach).
- Bilateral salpingo-oophorectomy (BSO).

EXAM TIP

Endometrial hyperplasia with atypia has the highest risk of progressing to cancer (30%).

WARD TIP

Surgical staging of endometrial cancer is both diagnostic and therapeutic.

EXAM TIP

Grade is the most important prognostic indicator in endometrial cancer.

WARD TIP

Grade 3 tumors usually *do not* have steroid hormone receptors, whereas grade 1 tumors usually do.

TABLE 26-1.   Staging of Endometrial Cancer FIGO Revised 2009

STAGE	DESCRIPTION
*I: Tumor confined to the uterus	IA: Limited to endometrium or invades <½ of the myometrium IB: Tumor invades ≥½ of the myometrium
*II: Tumor invades cervical stroma, but does not extend beyond uterus**	
*III: Local and/or regional spread of the tumor	IIIA: Invasion of uterine serosa and/or adnexa IIIB: Invasion of vagina and/or parametrial involvement IIIC: Mets to pelvic/para-aortic lymph nodes
*IV: Tumor invades bladder and/or bowel mucosa, and/or distant mets	IVA: Invasion of bladder and/or bowel mucosa

* Endocervical gland involvement is stage I.

** Positive peritoneal cytology does not change the stage and is reported separately.

- Pelvic and para-aortic lymphadenectomy.
- Peritoneal washings for cytology ("loose or free cancer cells").

ADJUVANT THERAPY

After the above steps in treatment, adjuvant therapy depends on the stage of disease and histology of the tumor, which determines the risk of recurrence.

Low Risk: Grade 1, stage 1A, confined to endometrium.
- No further treatment beyond surgical staging as described above.

Intermediate Risk: Stage 1A or 1B or stage II—involves myometrium or cervical stroma.
- Radiation therapy +/– chemotherapy.

High Risk: Stage III or higher, or any patient with serous or clear-cell histology.
- Chemotherapy (carboplatin and paclitaxel) +/– radiation therapy.

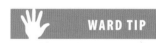

WARD TIP

Side effects:
- Doxorubicin: Cardiotoxicity
- Cisplatin: Nephrotoxicity

Uterine Sarcoma

A 53-year-old G1P1 postmenopausal woman presents with vaginal bleeding and pelvic pain. For the past 3 months, she has noticed that her abdomen has enlarged rapidly. What is the most likely diagnosis?
Answer: Leiomyosarcoma.

- Uterine sarcoma is classified separately from endometrial cancer:
  - <5% of uterine malignancies (a rare cancer).
  - Presents as a rapidly enlarging mass with bleeding.
  - <1% of fibroids progress to cancer.
  - Poor prognosis.

- Risk factors are similar.
- Most cases are diagnosed with exploratory surgery for what was thought to be a uterine myoma (fibroid).

TYPES

A. Homologous (mesenchymal tissue that normally forms in the uterus—most common).

B. Heterologous (foreign tissue to the uterus, i.e., cartilage, bone).

- **Leiomyosarcoma (LMS):**
  - Homologous.
  - One-third of uterine sarcomas.
  - Presents with rapidly growing pelvic mass +/– pain or vaginal bleeding.
- **Endometrial stromal sarcoma (ESS):**
  - Homologous.
  - Ten percent of uterine sarcomas.
  - Low-grade, indolent course.
  - Peak incidence in fifth decade.
  - Tumors contain estrogen and progesterone receptors which are sensitive to hormone therapy.
- **Carcinosarcoma (previously called malignant mixed müllerian tumors):**
  - Heterologous.
  - Rare, comprises <5% of uterine malignancies.
  - Usually found in older patients (>60).
  - Presents with postmenopausal bleeding, pain, and a rapidly enlarging uterus.
- **Undifferentiated sarcomas:** High-grade, aggressive tumors with poor prognosis.

DIAGNOSIS

- >10 mitosis/10 high-powered fields with cytologic atypia.
- Usually diagnosed from specimen sent after hysterectomy.
- Staged just like endometrial cancer.

TREATMENT

- Surgical (TAH/BSO, +/– lymphadenectomy, and peritoneal washings).
- Adjuvant therapy (chemotherapy) may decrease recurrence.
- Radiation may enhance local control after surgery. Unknown survival benefit.
- Multi-agent chemotherapy is prescribed for metastatic sarcomas. Complete responses are rare.

Ovarian Cancer and Fallopian Tube Cancer

Ovarian cancer is a malignancy arising from the cells of the ovary. As such, there are three categories of ovarian cancer: epithelial, germ cell, and sex cord stromal. Ovarian cancer is the most deadly gynecologic malignancy because it is most often diagnosed at an advanced stage.

Epidemiology

- Second most common gynecologic malignancy.
- Fifth most common cancer for women.
- The deadliest gynecologic malignancy.
- Seventy percent of patients are diagnosed as stage III or IV.
- Lifetime risk is 1 in 70.
- Median age at diagnosis is 63 years.
- Epithelial ovarian cancer, fallopian tube cancer, and primary peritoneal cancer all behave in a similar fashion and are treated the same. In addition, there is mounting evidence that they have a common pathogenesis.

Epithelial Cell Ovarian Cancer

 A 65-year-old G0P0 presents with a 4-month history of increasing abdominal girth and bloating. She also reports occasional shortness of breath and nausea. She doesn't understand why her pants are too small when she seems to be eating less. What is the suspected diagnosis?

Answer: Ovarian cancer. Initial steps in diagnosis: Transvaginal ultrasound and CA-125. Definitive diagnosis: Surgery.

 A 61-year-old G2P2 is diagnosed with ovarian cancer after she presented with abdominal bloating. On pelvic ultrasound she is found to have 6-cm bilateral ovarian masses and ascites. What would the next step be in management?

Answer: Total abdominal hysterectomy (TAH) with bilateral salpingo-oophorectomy (BSO), omentectomy, and then chemotherapy with carboplatinum and paclitaxel. The patient will get serial CA-125 levels on follow-up examinations.

The majority of ovarian cancers are epithelial.

HISTOLOGIC SUBTYPES

Six subtypes arising from epithelial tissue:
- Serous: 50%
- Mucinous: 25%
- Endometrioid: 10%
- Clear cell: 6%
- Brenner: 4%
- Undifferentiated: 5%

CLINICAL REMINDER

Initial stages are usually asymptomatic. Signs/symptoms are usually from metastasis to other organs.

SIGNS AND SYMPTOMS

- Pelvic mass/pain.
- Abdominal mass ("omental caking").
- Pleural effusion (dyspnea).
- Ascites.
- Ventral hernia (due to ↑ intra-abdominal pressure).
- Early satiety.
- Nausea/vomiting.
- Change in bowel habits.
- Increasing abdominal girth.

RISK FACTORS

- Early menarche, late menopause.
- Nulliparity.
- Late childbearing.
- Advanced age (50–70).
- Family history of ovarian cancer.
- Personal or family history of breast cancer.
- Caucasian race.
- Talcum powder, high-fat diet, fertility drugs (data inconclusive on these).

WORKUP

- CA-125:
  - A tumor marker that is elevated in 80% of cases of **epithelial** ovarian cancers.
  - It is useful in tracking the progression of the disease and the response to treatment.
  - It may be elevated in many premenopausal medical conditions (i.e., fibroids, endometriosis).
  - It is not effective as a screening tool.

PROTECTIVE FACTORS

- Breast-feeding.
- Oral contraceptives.
- Multiparity.
- Tubal ligation.
- Hysterectomy.

WARD TIP

The serous type of epithelial ovarian cancer is the most common type of ovarian cancer and is bilateral 65% of the time.

EXAM TIP

Ovarian cancer spread is normally through the peritoneal fluid, which carries cancer cells to other abdominal structures.

WARD TIP

Ovarian cancer metastasis to the umbilicus is "Sister Mary Joseph's nodule." This is a palpable umbilical nodule.

WARD TIP

In a postmenopausal woman with a pelvic mass, CA-125 is much more specific for ovarian cancer compared to a premenopausal woman.

Hereditary Ovarian Cancer Syndromes

Ten to fifteen percent of cases occur in association with genetically predisposed syndromes called **hereditary ovarian cancer (HOC) syndromes.** In these patients, ovarian cancer is diagnosed at a median age of 50 years. There are three types:

1. **Breast-ovarian cancer syndrome:** Involves cancer of the breast and ovary and is linked to the mutation of BRCA-1 and BRCA-2 genes in 90% of HOC. BRCA is a tumor suppressor gene that is located on chromosome 17.
2. **Lynch II syndrome—hereditary nonpolyposis colon cancer (HNPCC):** Involves sites that may include breast, ovaries, uterus, and colon.
3. **Site-specific ovarian cancer:** Accounts for <1% and has an extremely strong genetic link. Usually, two or more first-degree relatives have the disease.

Malignant conditions that cause ↑ CA-125:

- Endometrial cancer
- Lung cancer
- Breast cancer
- Pancreatic cancer

Benign conditions that cause ↑ CA-125:

- Endometriosis
- Pelvic inflammatory disease (PID)
- Leiomyoma
- Pregnancy
- Hemorrhagic ovarian cyst
- Liver disease

Large ovarian tumors can cause bowel obstruction and other gastrointestinal symptoms.

Before a staging surgery, a CT scan of the chest/ abdomen/pelvis is helpful to evaluate the extent of the disease, including retroperitoneal lymph-node enlargement and liver metastases.

Krukenberg tumors are ovarian tumors that are metastatic from another primary cancer, usually from the gastrointestinal tract.

Ovarian Cancer Workup

- Unfortunately, ovarian cancer is often diagnosed after the disease has spread beyond the ovary (advanced stage).
- As with any pelvic mass, the first step of evaluation is ultrasound.
- CA-125: Tumor marker for **epithelial** ovarian cancer (not very sensitive or specific).
- Surgical staging procedure if malignancy is suspected (see below).

Screening Recommendations

- Women with **standard risk** (<2 first-degree relatives with ovarian cancer): No routine screening recommended. A first-degree relative is considered a mother, sister, or daughter.
- Women with **high risk** (>2 first-degree relatives with ovarian cancer): Genetic testing and counseling.
- If high risk, perform:
  - Annual CA-125 (poor tool for screening).
  - Annual transvaginal ultrasound.
  - Annual pelvic exam.
  - Consider BRCA screening. Consider prophylactic oophorectomy if positive.

Staging

Ovarian cancer is staged surgically (see Table 27-1). The staging surgery includes:

- Peritoneal washings (for cytology).
- TAH.
- BSO.
- Omentectomy.
- Appendectomy.
- Pelvic and para-aortic lymphadenectomy.

TREATMENT

The purpose of surgery in patients with ovarian cancer is twofold:
1. To accurately stage the patient's disease.
2. To achieve "optimal cytoreduction" of the disease, which means removing all sites of primary or metastatic tumor >1 cm in size. This kind of debulking surgery has been shown to improve survival in patients with *any* stage ovarian cancer.

POSTOP MANAGEMENT

- In selected patients, chemotherapy can improve survival and disease-free intervals.
- First-line chemotherapy: Paclitaxel and cisplatin *or* paclitaxel and carboplatin.

POOR PROGNOSTIC INDICATORS

- Short disease-free interval.
- Mucinous or clear cell tumor.

TABLE 27-1. **Staging of Ovarian Cancer (FIGO)**

STAGE	DESCRIPTION
I: Tumor limited to ovaries	IA: One ovary, capsule intact IB: Both ovaries, capsules intact IC: Tumor on ovary surface, capsule ruptured, ascites with malignant cells, or positive peritoneal washings
II: Pelvic spread	IIA: Involvement of uterus/tubes IIB: Involvement of other pelvic structures IIC: IIA or IIB plus tumor on ovary surface, capsule ruptures, ascites with malignant cells, or positive peritoneal washings
III: Spread to the abdominal cavity	IIIA: Positive abdominal peritoneal washings (indicates microscopic seeding) IIIB: <2 cm implants on abdominal peritoneal surface IIIC: >2 cm implants on abdominal peritoneal surface and/or positive retroperitoneal or inguinal nodes
IV: Distant metastasis	Parenchymal liver/spleen spread Pleural effusion, skin or supraclavicular nodes

- Multiple disease sites.
- High/rising CA-125.

Nonepithelial Ovarian Cancer

Accounts for 15% of ovarian cancers. Histologic types include:
- **Germ cell tumors:** 8% of all ovarian cancers; include teratomas, dysgerminomas, choriocarcinomas.
- **Sex-cord stromal tumors:** 1% of all ovarian cancers; include granulosa-theca cell tumors, Sertoli-Leydig tumors.

OVARIAN GERM CELL TUMORS (GCTS)

Germ cell tumors account for 20–25% of ovarian neoplasms, but only 5% of **malignant** ovarian neoplasms. They are the primary cause of ovarian cancer in women <30 years old. They arise from totipotential germ cells that normally are able to differentiate into the three germ cell tissues. Most are benign.

CLINICAL PRESENTATION
- Abdominal pain with rapidly enlarging palpable pelvic/abdominal mass.
- Acute abdomen.
- Fever.
- Usually found in children or young women.
- Some germ cell tumors produce hormones like hCG and AFP. These patients may present with pregnancy symptoms, abnormal uterine bleeding, or precocious puberty (due to high hCG).

WARD TIP

CA-125 is elevated in 80% of cases of ovarian cancer, but only in 50% of stage I cases. It is most useful as a tool to gauge progression/regression of disease.

WARD TIP

Surgical staging:
Ovarian, endometrial, vulva, and fallopian tube cancers

Clinical staging:
Cervical and vaginal

WARD TIP

While chemotherapy is traditionally administered IV, intraperitoneal (IP) administration has shown promise in treating ovarian cancer.

WARD TIP

Chemotherapy can cause neutropenia. An absolute neutrophil count <500 cells/μL requires prophylactic antibiotic treatment to prevent septic complications.

WARD TIP

Approximately one-third of germ cell tumors found in women <21 years old are malignant.

WARD TIP

A benign (mature) cystic teratoma can undergo malignant degeneration, usually after menopause.

major complication of mature cystic teratoma: ovarian torsion

WARD TIP

Know tumor markers cold for the wards.

Dysgerminoma (most common malignant germ cell tumor)

> A 7-year-old girl complains of abdominal pain, and a workup reveals an adnexal mass. She undergoes an exploratory laparotomy and an excisional biopsy. What is the most likely pathology?
> **Answer:** Dysgerminoma.

- **Most common malignant germ cell tumor** (33% of malignant germ cell tumors); arises from undifferentiated totipotential germ cells.
- Usually affects *young* women (<30 years old).
- Ten percent are bilateral.
- Because these tumors affect young women, they are one of the more common types of malignant neoplasms diagnosed during pregnancy.
- Very chemo and radiation sensitive.
- Lactic dehydrogenase (LDH) is the tumor marker (see Table 27-2).

YOLK SAC Tumor (Endodermal sinus tumor)

- Arises from extraembryonic tissues (resembles a yolk sac).
- 15–20% of malignant GCTs.
- Most aggressive GCT.
- Occurs in young girls and women—median age is 23.
- Characteristic **Schiller-Duval bodies.**
- α-fetoprotein (AFP) is the tumor marker (see Table 27-2).

Teratoma

- Contains tissue from ectoderm, mesoderm, and endoderm.
- Contains hair, teeth, skin, sebum, and bone.
- **Immature** (malignant teratoma): Haphazard tissue from the ectoderm, mesoderm, and endoderm.
- **Mature** solid and/or cystic (also called dermoid):
  - Ninety-five percent of teratomas.
  - Benign: Can lead to torsion >5 cm.
- **Struma ovarii:**
  - Benign teratoma.
  - Mostly thyroid tissue.
  - May cause hyperthyroidism.
- **Carcinoid:** Rare.

TABLE 27-2. Ovarian Tumors and Their Serum Markers

OVARIAN TUMOR	SERUM TUMOR MARKER
Dysgerminoma	LDH
Endodermal sinus tumor (yolk sac tumor)	AFP
Embryonal and choriocarcinoma	β-hCG, AFP
Epithelial ovarian tumor	CA-125
Granulosa cell tumor	Inhibin
Sertoli-Leydig cell tumor	Testosterone

AFP, α-fetoprotein; β-hCG, β-human chorionic gonadotropin, GCT, germ cell tumor; LDH, lactic dehydrogenase.

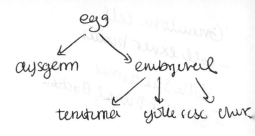

Choriocarcinoma

- Rare nongestational choriocarcinoma; <2% of malignant germ cell tumors.
- Arises from cytotrophoblasts and syncytiotrophoblasts (extraembryonic tissues).
- They are more commonly of placental origin rather than ovarian origin.
- Highly malignant.
- Affects women <20 years old.
- β-human chorionic gonadotropin (β-hCG) is the tumor marker.

Embryonal Carcinoma

- Rare; 4% of malignant germ cell tumors.
- Composed of primitive embryonal cells.
- Affects females aged 4–28, average age is 15.
- Tumors may cause precocious puberty or abnormal uterine bleeding.
- β-hCG and AFP are the tumor markers (see Table 27-2).

Mixed GCTs

- Five percent of malignant GCTs.
- Dysgerminoma and yolk sac tumor is the most common combination.
- LDH, AFP, and β-hCG may be elevated.

TREATMENT OF MALIGNANT GCTS

- Surgery: **Unilateral** salpingo-oophorectomy and complete surgical staging.
- Adjuvant chemotherapy: Recommended for all malignant GCTs except stage IA, grade I immature teratomas. Stage IA, grade 1 immature teratomas have a high cure rate with surgery alone. The BEP regimen is the standard of care:

BEP Regimen	Side Effects
Bleomycin	Pulmonary fibrosis
Etoposide	Blood dyscrasias
Cis**P**latin	Nephrotoxicity (extreme nausea and vomiting)

PROGNOSIS OF OVARIAN GCTS

Prognosis is generally good because most are discovered *early*. Five-year survival is 85% for dysgerminomas, 75% for immature teratomas, and 65% for yolk sac tumors.

OVARIAN SEX-CORD STROMAL TUMORS

- Arise from the sex cords and specialized stroma of the embryonic gonads (before they differentiate into ovaries or testes).
- Some of these tumors are functional tumors and secrete estrogen or testosterone.
- They behave as low-grade malignancies and usually affect older women.
- Rare—comprises only 1% of malignant ovarian neoplasms.

Granulosa Cell Tumor

- Most common type of malignant sex cord stromal tumor. Comprise 2–5% of all ovarian malignancies.
- Secretes **estrogens**.

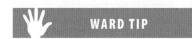

WARD TIP

Up to 80% survival with complete resection.

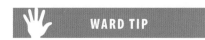

WARD TIP

Granulosa cell tumors are very chemosensitive.

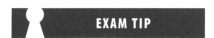

EXAM TIP

The most common solid benign tumor of the ovary is a fibroma.

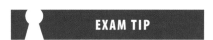

EXAM TIP

Meig syndrome (hydrothorax, ascites) can occur with a fibroma of the ovary.

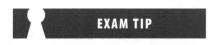

EXAM TIP

A rare type of Sertoli-Leydig tumor is **arrhenoblastoma.** This is found in young women and secretes testosterone. Its treatment is surgery and chemo/radiation therapy.

Granulosa cell
— Call exner bodies
Yolke sac tumor
— Schiller Duval Bodies

early breast develop.

- Can present with **feminization, precocious puberty, menorrhagia**, or **postmenopausal bleeding.**
- Association with endometrial cancer in 5% of cases.
- Characteristic Call-Exner bodies (eosinophilic bodies surrounded by granulosa cells).
- Inhibin is the tumor marker.

Sertoli-Leydig Cell Tumor

- Secretes **testosterone.**
- Frequently presents with **virilization, hirsutism**, and **menstrual disorders.**
- Testosterone is the tumor marker.

TREATMENT OF OVARIAN SEX-CORD STROMAL TUMORS

- **Surgical:**
  - TAH-BSO in women who have completed childbearing.
  - Unilateral salpingo-oophorectomy in young women with low-stage/grade neoplasia.
- **Adjuvant therapy:** Chemotherapy and radiation are not commonly used in patients with stage I disease but is recommended for patients with stage II–IV disease and those with recurrence.

Fallopian tube Carcinoma

- Fallopian tube carcinomas usually are adenocarcinomas.
- The most common histologic subtype is **papillary serous** (90%).
- They spread through the peritoneal fluid in a similar fashion to ovarian cancer.
- Recent data suggest that many serous epithelial ovarian carcinomas have a tubal precursor lesion.
- Fallopian tube cancer behaves like and is treated like epithelial ovarian cancers and primary peritoneal cancers.
- ✳ Removal of fallopian tubes (at the time of hysterectomy or as method of sterilization) has been shown to decrease the lifetime risk of ovarian epithelial cancer.
- It has long been known that tubal ligation decreases the risk of epithelial ovarian cancer.
- **Classic presenting triad:**
  - Pain.
  - Vaginal bleeding.
  - Watery vaginal discharge.
- Many are diagnosed during a laparotomy/laparoscopy for other indications.
- **Hydrops tubae perfluens** is the pathognomonic finding, defined as cramping pain relieved with watery discharge.

— Pain
— PMB
— watery vaginal discharge.

STAGING, TREATMENT, AND PROGNOSIS

Same as ovarian cancer.

CHAPTER 28

Vulvar Dysplasia, Vulvar Cancer, and Vaginal Cancer

Vulvar dysplasia describes precancerous lesions. Dysplasia simply describes cellular changes, characterized by changes in size, shape, hyperchromasia, and presence of mitotic figures.

Vulvar Intraepithelial Neoplasia (VIN)

- Dysplastic lesions of the vulva that have potential to progress to carcinoma.
- VIN refers to squamous lesions.
- VIN is classified into two main categories:
  - **VIN, unusual type.** Associated with HPV. The World Health Organization used to categorize this as VIN 1 (<1/2 epithelium involved), VIN 2 (>1/2 epithelium involved), and VIN 3 (full-thickness involvement). As of 2004, the International Society for the Study of Vulvar Diseases (ISSVD) recommended new nomenclature, whereby:
    - Lesions formerly called VIN 1 are now called condyloma acuminatum.
    - VIN 2: lower two-thirds of epithelium involved.
    - VIN 3: full-thickness involvement of squamous epithelium.
  - **VIN, Differentiated type.**
    - <5% of VIN.
    - Postmenopausal women.
    - **Not** associated with HPV. Possibly a precursor of HPV-negative vulvar cancer.
    - May be associated with lichen sclerosis.

RISK FACTORS

- Like cervical cancer, vulvar cancer risk factors include HPV types 16, 18, 31, and 33, and the precancerous lesions are classified as intraepithelial neoplasia (termed VIN as opposed to CIN).
- HPV types 6 and 11 are commonly found in vulvar warts.
- History of vulvar skin disease.

PRESENTATION

- Pruritus and/or irritation (recent or longstanding).
- Pain, burning, or dysuria.
- Raised white lesions.
- **Often asymptomatic.**

DIAGNOSIS

- **Biopsy** (most important for diagnosis).
- Colposcopic exam (must include vulva, vagina, cervix, and perineum).

TREATMENT

Treatment of VIN is based on symptoms, size, location, and likelihood of invasive disease.
- Surgical excision: This is the treatment of choice, i.e., wide local excision, simple vulvectomy.
- Laser ablation: Must rule out cancer first.
- Topical treatment: Imiquimod, topical 5-fluorouracil.

Vulvar Cancer

> A 64-year-old presents with vulvar itching. On exam, she has a 1-cm white lesion on her labia that bleeds when palpated. What is the first step to make a diagnosis? What other findings in her medical and social history might put her at ↑ risk for cancer?
> **Answer:** The first step in diagnosis is biopsy! Other findings that might put her at ↑ risk for cancer include age, itching, and bleeding on exam.

- Most often found in women age 60–70.
- Vulvar intraepithelial lesions are less likely than cervical intraepithelial lesions to become high-grade lesions or cancers.
- Vulvar cancer is the fourth most common gynecologic cancer (5% of all gynecologic cancers) and can arise as carcinoma of various types:
  - Squamous (90%).
  - Adenocarcinoma (Paget disease, Bartholin's gland).
  - Basal cell carcinoma.
  - Melanoma (4–5%).
  - Metastasis.
  - Sarcoma.
  - Basal cell.

SIGNS AND SYMPTOMS

- Pruritus (most common).
- Ulceration.
- Mass (often exophytic).
- Bleeding.

RISK FACTORS

- Postmenopausal.
- Smoking.
- Immunodeficiency syndromes.
- Other risk factors:
  - Age.
  - HPV.
  - VIN.
  - CIN.
  - HIV.
  - Vulvar skin disease, i.e., lichen sclerosis.
  - Atypical moles.

DIAGNOSIS

Biopsy of the suspicious lesion.

STAGING

See Table 28-1. Vulvar cancer is surgically staged.

TREATMENT

- Surgical excision based on size of lesion.
  - **Radical local excision:** If no extension to adjacent structures.
  - **Modified radical vulvectomy:** If extension to adjacent structures.
  - **Chemoradiation ± surgical excision:** If extension to more distant structures, i.e., bladder mucosa, fixed to pelvic bone.
  - **Inguinofemoral lymphadenectomy:** For stage I–II disease. High morbidity.

WARD TIP

Remember that a dark-pigmented lesion could be a melanoma, even in the vulvar region.

WARD TIP

Most common site of vulvar dysplasia is labia majora.

EXAM TIP

Pruritus is the most common symptom of vulvar cancer. Always biopsy itchy, white lesions on exam.

WARD TIP

Most common vulvar cancer is squamous cell.

WARD TIP

Clear cell adenocarcinoma of the vagina often correlates with in utero diethylstilbestrol exposure (DES); these patients often present young.

TABLE 28-1. Vulvar Cancer Staging, FIGO Revised 2009

STAGE I: TUMOR CONFINED TO THE VULVA OR PERINEUM

IA: Lesions <2 cm in size, stromal invasion <1.0 mm, negative nodes.

IB: Lesions >2 cm in size *or* any size with stromal invasion >1.0 mm, negative nodes.

STAGE II: TUMOR OF ANY SIZE WITH EXTENSION TO ADJACENT PERINEAL STRUCTURES (⅓ LOWER URETHRA, ⅓ LOWER VAGINA, ANUS); NEGATIVE NODES

STAGE III: TUMOR OF ANY SIZE WITH POSITIVE INGUINO-FEMORAL LYMPH NODES

IIIA: (i) With lymph node metastasis (>5 mm), or (ii) 1–2 lymph node metastasis(es) (<5 mm)

IIIB: (i) With 2 or more lymph node metastases (>5 mm), or (ii) 3 or more lymph node metastases (<5 mm)

IIIC: With positive nodes with extracapsular spread

STAGE IV: TUMOR INVADES OTHER REGIONAL (⅔ UPPER URETHRA, ⅔ UPPER VAGINA) OR DISTANT STRUCTURES

IVA : Tumor invades any of the following: (i) upper urethral and/or vaginal mucosa, bladder mucosa, rectal mucosa, or fixed to pelvic bone, or (ii) fixed or ulcerated inguino-femoral lymph nodes

IVB: Any distant metastasis including pelvic lymph nodes

Vaginal Cancer

> 👤 A 72-year-old presents to the office complaining of vaginal spotting. She had a vaginal hysterectomy at age 45. On exam, you notice a 2-cm ulcerated lesion on the posterior wall of the vagina. What is the next step in management?
> **Answer:** Biopsy the lesion.

- Primary cancer arises in vagina.
- A rare gynecologic malignancy (3% of gynecologic cancers).
- Usually presents in **postmenopausal women.**
- Increased risk in premenopausal women exposed to DES in utero.
- Most common type is **squamous cell carcinoma** (other types are the same as vulvar cancer types).
- Having CIN or VIN is a risk factor for development of vaginal cancer.

SIGNS AND SYMPTOMS

- Ulcerated mass.
- Exophytic mass.
- Abnormal or malodorous vaginal discharge.
- Bleeding.
- Asymptomatic.
- Pain in advanced cases.

DIAGNOSIS

Biopsy of suspicious lesion.

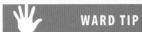

WARD TIP

Vulvar cancer: Surgically staged.
Vaginal cancer: Clinically staged.

cervical + vaginal
= clinical staging
vulvar, endometrial,
ovarian = surgical staging

TABLE 28-2. **Staging of Vaginal Cancer (clinical staging system)**

STAGE
I: Limited to vaginal mucosa
II: Beyond mucosa but not involving pelvic wall
III: Pelvic wall involvement
IV: Involvement of bladder, rectum, or distant mets

STAGING

See Table 28-2. Vaginal cancer is **clinically** staged. The stage of tumor is the most important predictor of prognosis.

TREATMENT

- **Stage I:** Surgical resection ± radiation.
- **Stages II–IV:** Chemoradiation only (platinum-based chemo). → *if extension beyond vaginal wall.*

NOTES

CHAPTER 29

Vulvar Disorders

Vulvar disorders encompass a wide range of conditions, from isolated local findings to systemic illnesses. A good understanding of the vulvar anatomy will help to identify these disorders. Vulvar dystrophies are a group of disorders characterized by various pruritic, white lesions of the vulva. Lesions must be biopsied to rule out malignancy.

Vulvar Dystrophies

A 60-year-old G1P1 presents reporting vulvar itching. She has a history of lichen sclerosis that previously responded well to topical steroids. On exam, she has a raised, white lesion on her vulva. She reports that she can't stop scratching the area. What next step will be most helpful in diagnosing this lesion? Is this patient at ↑ risk for malignancy? What microscopic changes contribute to the white appearance?

Answer: The next step in diagnosis is a punch biopsy. An ↑ risk of vulvar carcinoma is associated with lichen planus and lichen sclerosus. The white appearance is secondary to lichenification.

PAGET DISEASE OF THE VULVA

A 65-year-old who has been menopausal for 10 years presents complaining of an itchy genital lesion that has been present for 2 years. On exam, there is a red eczematous lesion on her vulva. You perform a biopsy, which shows Paget disease. What is the next step in management?

Answer: Solitary lesions need wide local excision down to subcutaneous fat. Paget disease of the vulva may be associated with underlying invasive adenocarcinomas (4–17%). Patients with Paget disease are also more likely to have a noncontiguous cancer (20–30%), and should be evaluated for a synchronous neoplasm.

PRESENTATION

- Pruritic, erythematous, eczematoid lesion. Often multifocal.
- Postmenopausal Caucasian females.
- May be associated with underlying local invasive adenocarcinomas or other synchronous neoplasms, i.e., adenocarcinoma of the gastrointestinal (GI) tract or breast.

DIAGNOSIS

Direct biopsy of lesion. Will visualize Paget cells under the microscope.

TREATMENT

- If solitary lesion without malignancy: Wide excision to subcutaneous fat.
- Assess for underlying malignancy or synchronous neoplasm.
- Recurrences are frequent after treatment.

FOLLOW-UP

Patients with Paget disease of the vulva will need to be followed annually with:
- Breast exams.
- Cytologic evaluation of the cervix and vulva.
- Screening for GI disease.

EXAM TIP

Lichen simplex chronicus carries ↑ risk of malignancy.

LICHEN SIMPLEX CHRONICUS (LSC)

- LSC is a hypertrophic dystrophy caused by chronic irritation resulting in raised, white, thickened lesions.
- It is a skin disorder characterized by chronic itching and scratching.
- Lesions may also appear red and irritated due to scratching.
- Microscopic examination reveals acanthosis and hyperkeratosis.

LICHEN SCLEROSUS

- An atrophic lesion characterized by paper-like appearance on both sides of the vulva, and epidermal contracture leads to loss of vulvar architecture.
- Microscopic examination reveals epithelial thinning with a layer of collagen and inflammatory cells (see Figure 29-1). There is also loss of the rete ridges.

LICHEN PLANUS

- An uncommon condition that may also affect skin, nails, and scalp.
- Usually affects women 50–60 years of age.
- There may be shiny, purple lesions visualized on the vulva.
- Most lesions are found in the inner vulva and the vagina.
- Skin becomes very thickened (hypertrophied) and may cause scarring.
- May present as vulvo-vaginal-gingival syndrome.

DIAGNOSIS OF VULVAR DYSTROPHIES

Keyes 3- to 5-mm punch biopsy of vulva.

EXAM TIP

If an itch-scratch cycle is mentioned, choose LSC!

WARD TIP

Wickham striae are fine, white, lacy lesions, found in lichen planus.

WARD TIP

4 P's of lichen planus:
Pruritic
Planar
Purple
Polygonal

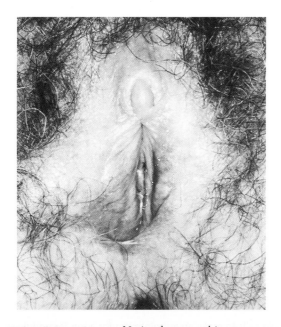

FIGURE 29-1.   Vulvar lichen sclerosus. Notice the paper-thin appearance, bilateral distribution, and pale color, with a loss of architecture. In severe cases, contractures and fissures can occur in the posterior fourchette. (Reproduced, with permission, from DeCherney AH, Nathan L, Goodwin TM, et al. *Current Diagnosis & Treatment: Obstetrics & Gynecology*, 10th ed. New York: McGraw-Hill, 2007: 617.)

TREATMENT OF VULVAR DYSTROPHIES

- Steroid cream (testosterone, clobetasol/temovate); oral steroids in severe cases.
- Diphenhydramine at night to prevent itching during sleep.
- Ultraviolet light for continued scratching.

Psoriasis

- A common dermatologic condition characterized by red plaques covered by silver scales.
- Although it commonly occurs over the knees and/or elbows, lesions can be found on the vulva as well.
- Pruritus is variable.

TREATMENT

- Steroid cream—goal is to decrease scratching and rubbing.
- Topical vitamin D analogs.

Vestibulitis

- Vulvar pain is a common gynecologic problem.
- Inflammation of the vestibular glands → tenderness, erythema, and pain associated with coitus (insertional dyspareunia and/or postcoital pain).
- Etiology is unknown.
- Although the affected area may turn white with acetic acid under colposcopic examination, these lesions are not dysplastic.

DIAGNOSIS

Lightly touch the vulvar vestibule with a cotton-tipped applicator. The diagnosis is made if this touch produces severe pain.

TREATMENT

- Temporary sexual abstinence.
- Tricyclic antidepressants.
- Xylocaine jelly for anesthesia.
- Surgery—if lesions are unresponsive to treatment, vestibulectomy is possible, though with risk of recurrence.

Cysts

BARTHOLIN'S ABSCESS

A 35-year-old calls to make an appointment for a tender nodule she found 3 days ago at the opening of the vagina, on the right. She had some discomfort during intercourse several days ago, but didn't discover the nodule until yesterday morning. Now she says it's uncomfortable to walk. What is the most likely diagnosis?
Answer: Bartholin's abscess.

WARD TIP

Before diagnosing vulvar dystrophy, always rule out more common diagnoses such as a contact dermatitis.

WARD TIP

The vestibular glands (Bartholin's glands) are located at the 5 and 7 o'clock positions of the inferolateral vestibule (area between the labia minora).

- The Bartholin's glands are two pea-sized glands, located at the 4 o'clock and 8 o'clock positions.
- A normal gland cannot be palpated.
- Bartholin's abscesses occur when the main duct draining Bartholin's gland is occluded, forming a Bartholin's cyst. This cyst may become infected due to the occlusion, and cause an abscess.
- Both Bartholin's cysts and abscesses can cause pain and require treatment.
- A Bartholin's cyst may be asymptomatic.

TREATMENT

- If a cyst is asymptomatic, it may be monitored conservatively. However, if the patient is over age 40, it should be excised to exclude malignancy.
- Abscesses require incision and drainage, either with:
  - Marsupialization (suturing the edges of the incised cyst to prevent reocclusion) or
  - Word catheter (a catheter with an inflatable tip left in the gland for 10–14 days to aid healing via an epithelialized tract that allows drainage).
- Inflammatory symptoms generally arise from infection and can be treated with antibiotics.
- Antibiotics and sitz baths may also be prescribed.

SEBACEOUS CYSTS (EPIDERMOID CYST)

- The most common vulvar cyst.
- Usually asymptomatic.
- Occur beneath the labia majora (rarely minora) when pilosebaceous ducts become occluded.
- Exam may show a palpable, nontender, smooth mass. If expressed, a yellow, thick, cheesy material is extruded.
- Most cysts do not require treatment.
- If it becomes infected, it can be treated with incision and drainage.

HIDRADENOMAS

A 30-year-old G3P3 overweight African-American woman presents with painful inflammation of her bikini line. She can't keep her skin dry. On exam, there are draining sinuses and scarring of the skin. What is the diagnosis?
Answer: Hidradenitis suppurativa is most commonly found in intertriginous areas of the body, such as the mons pubis, the genitocrural folds, buttocks, and axillae. Women are four times more likely than men to develop hidradenitis suppurativa.

- This condition is a chronic infection of the apocrine glands, found in reproductive-age women. A foul smelling discharge may be present on exam.
- Hidradenomas (apocrine sweat gland cysts) also occur beneath the labia majora as a result of ductal occlusion.
- As the infection grows over time, scarring and pits can form.
- These cysts tend to be pruritic.
- Diagnosis is made by biopsy.
- Treatment: Topical steroid creams and long-term, oral antibiotics. Severe cases are also treated by excision of the infected skin.

> 40 y/o → excise for malignancy!

OTHER RARE CYSTS

- **Cyst of canal of Nuck:** A hydrocele (persistent processus vaginalis); contains peritoneal fluid.
- **Skene's duct cyst:**
  - Very rare and very small.
  - Ductal occlusion and cystic formation of the Skene's (paraurethral) glands occur, and patients have discomfort.
- Treatment:
  - If asymptomatic, supportive treatment.
  - If symptomatic, excision of cyst.

Gestational Trophoblastic Disease

EXAM TIP

DNA of complete mole is always paternal.

Gestational trophoblastic disease (GTD) is a general term that encompasses a spectrum of interrelated conditions originating from abnormal proliferation of trophoblasts of the placenta. These include complete and partial hydatidiform moles. Gestational trophoblastic neoplasia (GTN) are gestational malignant neoplasms that include invasive moles, gestational choriocarcinomas, and placental site trophoblastic tumors.

Hydatidiform Mole

COMPLETE MOLE

 A 22-year-old G1P0 at 12 weeks by dates presents with vaginal bleeding and an enlarged-for-dates uterus on exam. Her blood pressure is 160/90, there are no fetal heart sounds, and an ultrasound shows a "snowstorm pattern." After dilation and curettage (D&C), what would most likely be the karyotype?
Answer: 46,XX in a complete mole.

EXAM TIP

DNA of a partial mole is both maternal and paternal.

EXAM TIP

The treatment for partial and complete molar pregnancy is prompt removal of intrauterine contents with D&C.

EXAM TIP

Partial mole may contain a fetus or fetal parts.

A placental (trophoblastic) tumor forms when a maternal ova devoid of deoxyribonucleic acid (DNA) "empty egg" is "fertilized" by the paternal sperm (see Figure 30-1).

KARYOTYPE

- Most have karyotype 46,XX, resulting from sperm penetration and subsequent DNA replication.
- Some have 46,XY, believed to be due to two paternal sperms simultaneously penetrating the ova.
- The BHCG value may be higher as compared to a partial mole.

└ BhCG: complete > partial

EPIDEMIOLOGY

Higher incidence in African-Americans, Hispanics, and American-Indians.

PARTIAL MOLE

- A mole with a fetus or fetal parts (see Figure 30-2).
- Women with partial (incomplete) molar pregnancies tend to present later than those with complete moles.

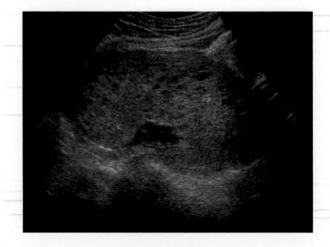

FIGURE 30-1. Complete mole on ultrasonography.

KARYOTYPE

Usually 69,XXY, and contains both maternal and paternal DNA.

EPIDEMIOLOGY

One in 50,000 pregnancies in the United States.

INVASIVE MOLE

- A variant of hydatidiform mole that invades the myometrium or blood vessels.
- It is by definition a malignant gestational trophoblastic neoplasia (GTN), and can spread to extrauterine sites. Twenty percent of patients will develop malignant sequelae after a complete hydatidiform mole, and 1–5% following a partial mole.
- The treatment involves complete metastatic workup and appropriate malignant/metastatic therapy (see below). A D&C is not recommended for treatment, because of the increased risk of uterine perforation. Chemotherapy is the usual treatment.

HISTOLOGY OF HYDATIDIFORM MOLE

- Trophoblastic proliferation.
- Hydropic degeneration (swollen villi).
- Lack/scarcity of blood vessels.

SIGNS AND SYMPTOMS

- The most common symptom is abnormal painless bleeding in the first trimester.
- Passage of villi (vesicles that look like grapes).
- Preeclampsia <20 weeks.
- Uterus large for gestational age.
- High human chorionic gonadotropin (hCG) level for gestational age.

MEDICAL COMPLICATIONS OF MOLAR PREGNANCY

- Preeclampsia.
- Hyperemesis gravidarum. (↑βhCG)
- Hyperthyroidism. (↑βhCG)
- Anemia.
- Pulmonary trophoblastic embolization.

EXAM TIP

A young woman who passes grape-like vesicles from her vagina should be suspected of having a hydatidiform mole.

complete mole
- invades blood vessels / myometrium
- tx w/ chemo.

WARD TIP

The development of preeclampsia before 20 weeks is suspicious for the presence of a molar pregnancy.

↑HCG

WARD TIP

GTD secretes hCG, lactogen, and thyrotropin.

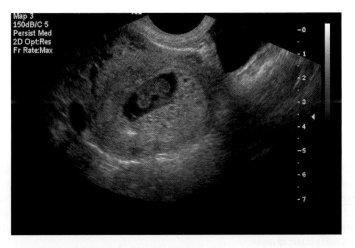

FIGURE 30-2.   Partial mole on ultrasonography.

DIAGNOSIS

- Elevated hCG (usually >100,000 mIU/mL). 15–25% theca lutein cysts visualized (secondary to the high BHCG levels).
- Absence of fetal heartbeat.
- Ultrasound: "Snowstorm" pattern.
- Pathologic specimen: Grapelike vesicles.
- Histologic specimen (see above).

TREATMENT OF COMPLETE OR PARTIAL MOLES

- Dilation and curettage (D&C) to evacuate and terminate pregnancy. Hysterectomy can be considered for women who have completed childbearing.
- Follow up with the workup to rule out invasive mole (malignancy):
    - Chest x-ray (CXR) to look for lung mets.
    - Liver function tests to look for liver mets.
- hCG monitoring: Weekly until negative for 3 weeks, then monthly until negative for 6 months. If the hCG level rises, does not fall, or falls and then rises again, the molar pregnancy is considered malignant gestational trophoblastic neoplasia (GTN).
- Contraception should be used during the follow-up period. A rising hCG should prompt evaluation for a new pregnancy versus GTN.
- Administer RhoGAM for RH negative patients.

METASTATIC WORKUP

- CXR, computed tomography (CT) of brain, lung, liver, kidneys.
- Labs: CBC, comprehensive metabolic panel, clotting studies, and blood type, Rh, and antibody screen.

INVASIVE MOLE

Develops after 15–20% of Complete moles and 1–5% of Partial Moles

TREATMENT OF INVASIVE MOLE

- Chemotherapy with methotrexate or Actinomycin D (as many cycles as needed until hCG levels return to negative).
- These tumors are very sensitive to chemotherapy, and the prognosis is generally excellent.
- If childbearing complete, may treat with hysterectomy ± chemotherapy (fewer cycles needed).

RECURRENCE RISK

One to two percent in subsequent pregnancy.

Choriocarcinoma

May occur after a molar or non-molar pregnancy. Most aggressive type of GTN.

A 31-year-old G2P2 woman, 5 months after a vaginal delivery, reports to the ED complaining of nausea, vomiting, and abnormal vaginal bleeding. Her pregnancy test is positive. A D&C was performed and the histology revealed sheets of trophoblastic cells and no chorionic villi. What is her diagnosis? What is the next step in management?
Answer: Diagnosis is Choriocarcinoma. The workup should be initiated to determine if there is metastatic disease.

[handwritten margin note] po
complete > partial in terms of malignant transformation

EXAM TIP

Twenty percent of complete moles will be malignant. <5% of partial moles will be malignant.

WARD TIP

Any of the following on exam indicates molar pregnancy:
- Passage of grapelike villi
- Preeclampsia early in pregnancy
- Snowstorm pattern on ultrasound

HISTOPATHOLOGY

Choriocarcinoma has characteristic sheets of trophoblasts with extensive hemorrhage and necrosis, and unlike the hydatidiform mole, choriocarcinoma has no villi. These tumors metastasize early. Common sites for metastasis include vagina, lung, liver, and brain.

moles – villi present
choriocarcinoma – villi are absent.

EPIDEMIOLOGY

Incidence is about 1 in 16,000 pregnancies.

DIAGNOSIS

- Increasing or plateauing β-hCG levels.
- Absence of fetal heartbeat.
- Uterine size/date discrepancy.
- Specimen (sheets of trophoblasts, no chorionic villi).
- A full metastatic workup is required when choriocarcinoma is diagnosed.

WARD TIP

Nonmetastatic malignancy has almost a 100% remission rate following chemotherapy.

TREATMENT AND PROGNOSIS OF CHORIOCARCINOMA

- Chemotherapy: Methotrexate or Actinomycin D (as many cycles as needed until hCG levels return to negative).
- If childbearing complete, hysterectomy + chemotherapy (fewer cycles needed).
- Remission rate is near 100%.
- Treatment is determined by the patient's risk (high or low) or prognostic score.
- Low-risk patients (score <7) can be treated with single-agent chemotherapy.
- High-risk patients (score >7) can be treated with multiagent chemotherapy, as they have a higher chance of being resistant to single-agent chemo.
- Chemotherapy is continued until after the hCG levels are negative. hCG levels are monitored for 1 year after normalization. All patients are placed on reliable contraception during this time of monitoring.
- Serial β-hCGs every 2 weeks until negative; then every 3 months, then monthly for 1 year. Give 1–2 additional cycles after first negative β-hCG.
- Risk of recurrence: <1%.

EXAM TIP

Sheets of trophoblasts = choriocarcinoma.

+ hemorrhage / necrosis

PROGNOSTIC GROUP CLINICAL CLASSIFICATION

See Tables 30-1 and 30-2.

Placental Site Trophoblastic Tumor (PSTT)

- A rare form of GTD.
- Characterized by infiltration of the myometrium by intermediate trophoblasts, which stain positive for human placental lactogen. There are no chorionic villi present.
- Unlike other GTDs, hCG is only slightly elevated.

PSTT
– intermediate trophoblasts
– ⊕ hPL staining
– No chorionic villi.
– Hysterectomy + multi-agent chemo!

TREATMENT

- Hysterectomy plus multi-agent chemotherapy.
- Prognosis is poor if there is tumor recurrence or metastasis.

TABLE 30-1. FIGO Prognostic Scoring System (2009)

RISK FACTOR	SCORE			
	0	**1**	**2**	**4**
Age (years)	≤40	>40		
Pregnancy	Hydatidiform mole	Abortion	Term	
Interval from pregnancy event to treatment (in months)	<4	4–6	7–12	>12
hCG (pre-treatment) (IU/mL)	<1000	1000–10,000	10,000–100K	>100K
Largest tumor size uterus (in cm)	<3	3–4	>5	
Site of metastases	Lung	Spleen Kidney	GI	Brain Liver
Number of metastasis	0	1–4	5–8	>8
Prior chemotherapy agent	–	–	Single	≥2 drugs

Scores are added to give the prognostic score.

TABLE 30-2. Treatment According to Score/Prognostic Factors (World Health Organization)

Low risk (score <7)	Single-agent therapy (methotrexate)
High risk (score >7)	Multiple-agent therapy (EMACO therapy—etoposide, MAC, and vincristine)

CHAPTER 31

Sexually Transmitted Infections and Vaginitis

EXAM TIP

Each year approximately 1 million women in the United States experience an episode of symptomatic PID. PID affects 10% of women in reproductive years.

WARD TIP

Rarely is a single organism responsible for PID, but always think of chlamydia and gonorrhea first (these are most common).

WARD TIP

Requirement for a clinical diagnosis of PID:
1. Lower abdominal or pelvic pain
2. Adnexal, uterine, or cervical motion tenderness on exam

WARD TIP

Positive lab tests are not necessary for diagnosis. PID is a *clinical* diagnosis.

Sexually transmitted infections (STIs), also known as venereal diseases or sexually transmitted diseases (STDs), are a major source of morbidity. The group includes bacteria, viruses, parasites, and protozoan infections that are transmitted by close contact. Transmission occurs via mucous membranes of the vulva, vagina, penis, rectum, mouth, throat, respiratory tract, or eyes.

Pelvic Inflammatory Disease (PID)

A sexually active 21-year-old G1P1 presents with a 10-day history of lower abdominal pain and vaginal discharge. She also reports nausea and vomiting. Her temperature is 101.4°F (38.6°C). Examination demonstrates cervical motion tenderness, uterine tenderness, and bilateral adnexal tenderness. You diagnose her with PID. What treatment should be given?

Answer: Inpatient cefoxitin/cefotetan + doxycycline. Criteria for hospital admission include vomiting and fever.

DEFINITION

Inflammation of the female upper genital tract (uterus, tubes, ovaries, ligaments) caused by ascending infection from the vagina and cervix. PID may lead to tubal scarring and an increased risk of ectopic pregnancy and/or infertility.

COMMON CAUSATIVE ORGANISMS

- *Neisseria gonorrhoeae.*
- *Chlamydia trachomatis.*
- *Mycoplasma genitalium.*
- *Gardnerella vaginalis, Peptostreptococcus, Bacteroides, Escherichia coli,* and *Streptococcus.*
- Most PID infections are polymicrobial.

DIAGNOSIS

Physical Exam
- Lower abdominal or pelvic pain.
- Adnexal, uterine, or cervical motion tenderness on exam.
- Other findings may support the diagnosis:
  - Oral temperature >101°F (38.3°C).
  - Purulent cervical or vaginal discharge.

Additional Testing That Supports Diagnosis
- Gram stain of discharge with gram-negative diplococci.
- Presence of abundant white blood cells (WBCs) on microscopy of vaginal secretions.
- Pelvic abscess (i.e., tubo-ovarian abscess).
- Elevated WBC count, erythrocyte sedimentation rate (ESR), C-reactive protein (CRP).
- Culture evidence of N. *gonorrhoeae* or C. *trachomatis.*
- **Laparoscopy**
  - Not often performed to diagnose PID, but may be helpful in patients who do not respond to antibiotic therapy, or in whom the diagnosis is not clear and other diagnoses need to be excluded (i.e., appendicitis).
  - Reveals pus draining from the fallopian tubes, edema, adhesions, purulent drainage in the cul-de-sac.

- Ten percent of women with acute PID will develop perihepatic inflammation, known as Fitz-Hugh–Curtis syndrome. "Violin string" adhesions can be seen at the liver capsule on laparoscopy with this syndrome.

RISK FACTORS

- Age <25 years.
- Multiple sexual partners.
- STI in the partner.
- Unprotected intercourse.
- History of STI or PID.
- Presence of intrauterine device (risk limited to first few weeks after insertion).

CRITERIA FOR HOSPITALIZATION

- Pregnancy.
- Peritonitis or surgical emergency cannot be excluded.
- Gastrointestinal (GI) symptoms, i.e., nausea, vomiting (inability to take oral meds).
- Abscess (tubo-ovarian or pelvic).
- Uncertain diagnosis.
- Outpatient treatment failure.
- Lack of compliance.
- Immunocompromised.
- Severe illness, i.e., high fever >100.9°F (38.3°C), severe pain.

TREATMENT

- Inpatient:
  - Cefoxitin/cefotetan + doxycycline. ✓
  - Clindamycin + gentamicin.
- **Outpatient:**
  - Ceftriaxone + doxycycline ± metronidazole. ✓
  - Cefoxitin + probenecid + doxycycline ± metronidazole.
  - Sexual partners should also be treated empirically.

Gonorrhea

A 19-year-old G2P2 presents with known exposure to gonorrhea 7 days prior. She reports an ↑ in vaginal discharge for the past day, but denies any other symptoms. On physical exam, you notice minimal vaginal discharge. You obtain a nucleic acid amplification test (NAAT) for gonorrhea. What is the next step?
Answer: Treat the patient empirically. Since she admits to a recent exposure to gonorrhea, there is no need to wait for the result to come back. In women, asymptomatic infection is common and symptoms may not begin until 7–21 days after exposure.

- An infection of the urethra, cervix, pharynx, or anal canal, caused by the gram-negative diplococcus, *Neisseria gonorrhoeae*.
- Second most common STI.
- CDC recommends annual screening for gonorrhea in all women age <25 or older with risk factors.

 WARD TIP

Chandelier sign: When you touch the cervix, there is so much pain that the patient jumps to the chandelier.

 WARD TIP

Criteria for hospitalization for PID—
GU PAP
GI symptoms (N/V)
Uncertain diagnosis
Peritonitis
Abscess
Pregnancy

 WARD TIP

Gonorrhea is often asymptomatic in women, and therefore may go untreated, causing complications of adhesions/inflammation such as ectopic pregnancy, chronic pelvic pain, and infertility.

 EXAM TIP

In what media does *Neisseria* gonorrhea grow?
Thayer-Martin in CO_2-enriched environment.

 EXAM TIP

Treat gonorrhea with dual therapy in order to decrease development of antibiotic resistance and treat concurrent chlamydial infections.

if one STI is present, test for the presence of other STIs.

PRESENTATION

■ Asymptomatic (most common, especially in women).
■ Dysuria.
■ Cervicitis.
■ Vaginal discharge.
■ May cause PID, chronic pelvic pain, ectopic pregnancy, infertility.
■ Patients are frequently co-infected with *Chlamydia trachomatis*.

DIAGNOSIS

■ Nucleic acid amplification test (NAAT) is the preferred diagnostic test.
■ Culture in Thayer-Martin agar.
■ Nucleic acid hybridization probes.
■ Patients should be tested for other STIs, i.e., HIV.

TREATMENT

■ Ceftriaxone 125 mg IM single dose plus azithromycin 1 g PO single dose or
■ Cefixime 400 mg PO single dose plus azithromycin 1 g PO single dose.
■ If severe cephalosporin allergy, treat with azithromycin 2 g PO single dose and test of cure in 1 week.
■ Sexual partners should also be treated.

Chlamydia

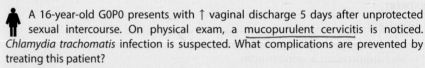

A 16-year-old G0P0 presents with ↑ vaginal discharge 5 days after unprotected sexual intercourse. On physical exam, a mucopurulent cervicitis is noticed. *Chlamydia trachomatis* infection is suspected. What complications are prevented by treating this patient?
Answer: Complications of a *Chlamydia* infection include PID, Fitz-Hugh–Curtis syndrome, ectopic pregnancy, infertility, pelvic adhesions, and chronic pelvic pain.

■ Chlamydia is an infection of the genitourinary (GU) tract, GI tract, conjunctiva, or nasopharynx, caused by *Chlamydia trachomatis*, an obligate intracellular bacteria.
■ Most common STI.
■ CDC recommends annual screening for chlamydia in all women age <25 or older women with risk factors.

PRESENTATION

■ Asymptomatic (most common, especially in women).
■ Mucopurulent discharge.
■ Cervicitis.
■ Urethritis.
■ May cause PID, chronic pelvic pain, ectopic pregnancy, infertility.
■ Fitz-Hugh–Curtis syndrome.
■ Conjunctivitis.

DIAGNOSIS

■ Nucleic acid amplification test (NAAT) of urine or vaginal/cervical swab (preferred method).
■ Antigen testing (requires swab of cervix).

TREATMENT

- Doxycycline 100 mg bid × 7 days or azithromycin 1 g PO single dose.
- Sexual partners should be treated.

LYMPHOGRANULOMA VENEREUM

Serotypes L1–L3 of *C. trachomatis* cause **lymphogranuloma venereum.** Most commonly found in tropical areas. This is a systemic disease that can present in several forms:

- Primary lesion: Painless papule on genitals.
- Secondary stage: Inguinal lymphadenitis with fever, malaise, and loss of appetite.
- Tertiary stage: Rectovaginal fistulas, rectal strictures.

DIAGNOSIS

Nucleated amplification testing of the cervix (NAAT, PCR).

TREATMENT

Lymphogranuloma venereum: Doxycycline 100 mg BID × 21 days.

Syphilis

A 22-year-old G1P1 woman has a positive rapid plasma reagin (RPR) with a titer of 1:4. What is the next step in the workup?

Answer: Order a specific serologic test, such as the fluorescent treponemal antibody absorption test (FTA-ABS) or microhemagglutination test for *Treponema pallidum* (MHA-TP). A false-positive RPR can be seen with certain viral infections (Epstein-Barr, hepatitis, varicella, measles), lymphoma, tuberculosis, malaria, endocarditis, connective tissue disease, and pregnancy.

Syphilis is an infection caused by the spirochete *Treponema pallidum.*

PRESENTATION

Syphilis has various stages of manifestation that present in different ways:

- **Primary syphilis: Painless hard chancre** of the vulva, vagina, or cervix (or even anus, tongue, or fingers), usually appearing 1 month after exposure. Heals spontaneously after 1–2 months.
- **Secondary syphilis: Generalized rash** (often macular or papular on the palms and soles of the feet), condyloma lata, mucous patches with lymphadenopathy, fever, malaise, usually **appearing 1–6 months after primary chancre.** Spontaneous regression after about 1 month.
- **Latent syphilis:** Asymptomatic disease with serologic proof of infection. Further classified as **early latent** if syphilis was acquired within the past year or **late latent** if acquired over a year prior.
- **Tertiary syphilis: Presents years later** with granulomas of the skin and bones (gummas), cardiovascular lesions (e.g., aortic aneurysms), neurosyphilis (e.g., tabes dorsalis, paresis, and meningovascular disease).

DIAGNOSIS

- Syphilis cannot be cultured in vitro, so must be identified by direct visualization or serology.
- **Screening test: Nontreponemal tests** such as Rapid Plasma Reagin (RPR) or Venereal Disease Research Laboratory (VDRL) test. These are

EXAM TIP

Reiter Syndrome (due to chlamydial infection)
Classic triad of conjunctivitis, urethritis, and reactive arthritis: **Can't see, can't pee, can't climb a tree.**

conjunctivitis, urethritis, arthritis

WARD TIP

Use azithromycin rather than doxycycline for pregnant women with chlamydia. Doxycyline causes discoloration of the fetal teeth if used during pregnancy.

WARD TIP

The CDC recommends annual screening for gonorrhea and chlamydia in women age <25 as well as older women with risk factors.

WARD TIP

Syphilis is the most likely diagnosis for a woman with painless genital lesions who then later develops hand, foot, and mouth rashes.

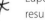

inexpensive and easy to perform, but are nonspecific and can give false-positive results for many conditions.
- **Diagnostic test: Treponemal tests** such as Fluorescent treponemal antibody absorption (FTA-ABS) and microhemagglutination test for antibodies to *T. pallidum* (MHA-TP). These tests are more expensive and complex to perform, and are used to confirm a diagnosis when the RPR/VDRL is positive.
- Direct visualization of spirochetes on darkfield microscopy is an additional test available.

TREATMENT

- **Benzathine penicillin G** for all stages, but dosing regimen differs depending on stage.
- Doxycycline in penicillin allergic nonpregnant patients.
- Treatment during pregnancy is desensitization followed by benzathine penicillin G. It crosses the placenta to prevent **congenital syphilis**.

Genital Herpes

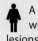
A 17-year-old G1P1 presents with a 5-day history of vulvar pain and discomfort with urination. On physical exam, she has a large number of bilateral ulcerated lesions on the vulva. What lab tests should be obtained?
Answer: Viral culture of ulcerated lesions to diagnose herpes simplex virus.

- Infection caused by herpes simplex virus type 2 (HSV-2) in 85% of cases, and by type 1 (HSV-1) in 15% of cases.
- HSV is a DNA virus.
- Eighty percent of adults have antibodies to HSV-2, most without history of infection.

PRESENTATION

Patients with herpes can be asymptomatic, but may present with the following:
- **Primary infection:** Malaise, myalgias, fever, vulvar burning, or vulvar pruritus, followed by **multiple painful genital vesicles** with an erythematous base that progress to painful ulcers, usually 1–3 weeks after exposure.
- **Recurrent infection:** Recurrence from viral stores in the sacral ganglia, resulting in a *milder version* of primary infection, including vesicles.
- **Nonprimary first episode:** This is defined as **initial infection by HSV-2** in the presence of *preexisting antibodies to HSV-1* or vice versa. The preexisting antibodies to HSV-1 can make the presentation of HSV-2 milder.

COMPLICATIONS

- ↑ risk of meningitis.
- ↑ risk of neonatal infection.

DIAGNOSIS

- Gross examination of vulva for typical lesions.
- Tzanck (cytologic) smear—multinucleated giant cells (low sensitivity/specificity).
- Viral cultures of fluid from an unroofed vesicle/ulcer (first-line method, but sensitivity is only 50%).
- PCR (can also detect asymptomatic viral shedding).
- Western blot assay for antibodies against HSV.

TREATMENT

Treatment for HSV is palliative and not curative.

- **Primary outbreak:** Acyclovir 400 mg TID × 7–10 days; valacyclovir 1 g BID for 7–10 days.
- **Recurrent infection:** Acyclovir 400 mg TID × 5 days; valacyclovir 1 g QD for 5 days.
- **Suppressive therapy for recurrent outbreaks:** Acyclovir 400 mg BID or valacyclovir 1g QD.
- **Pregnancy:** Suppressive therapy should begin at 36 weeks of pregnancy with acyclovir 400 mg TID or valacyclovir 500 mg BID. Primary and episodic treatment same as nonpregnant.
- A vaccine is under development.
- Famciclovir is another antiviral that is dosed less frequently, and can be used in pregnancy.
- Suppressive therapy decreases the frequency of outbreaks AND decreases asymptomatic shedding to prevent transmission to discordant partner.

Human Immunodeficiency Virus (HIV) and Acquired Immune Deficiency Syndrome (AIDS)

 A 30-year-old G3P3 presents requesting STD screening, including HIV. What test should be ordered?
Answer: Fourth-generation HIV 1/2 immunoassay. If positive, HIV-1/HIV-2 antibody differentiation immunoassay should be ordered.

HIV is an RNA retrovirus that causes AIDS. The virus infects CD4 lymphocytes and other cells and causes ↓ cellular immunity.

PRESENTATION

- **Initial infection:** Mononucleosis-like illness occurring weeks to months after exposure—fatigue, weight loss, lymphadenopathy, night sweats. This is followed by a long asymptomatic period lasting months to years.
- **AIDS:** Opportunistic infections, dementia, depression, Kaposi sarcoma, wasting.

RISK FACTORS

- Intravenous drug use.
- Blood transfusions between 1978 and 1985.
- Prostitution.
- Multiple sex partners/unprotected sex.
- Bisexual or homosexual partners.
- Vertical transmission.

DIAGNOSIS

- **Fourth-generation combined antigen/antibody immunoassay.** If positive, a second confirmatory HIV-1/HIV-2 antibody differentiation immunoassay is performed. If the second test is negative or indeterminate, then HIV viral load testing (PCR) is performed.
- **If early or acute HIV is suspected** perform fourth-generation combined antigen/antibody immunoassay PLUS HIV viral load (PCR) testing at the same time in order to pick up early HIV infection.

WARD TIP

Always biopsy an undiagnosed suspicious lesion in order to obtain a definitive diagnosis.

WARD TIP

Cesarean delivery is indicated for active herpes infection or presence of prodromal symptoms.

EXAM TIP

Treatment of AIDS is palliative and not curative.

[handwritten notes:]
fatigue
weight loss
night sweats
LAD.

4th Gen HIV1/2
immunoassay
⊖ / \ ⊕
PCR
(viral load)
HIV 1/2
Ab diff
assay.

If early infection →
4th Gen + PCR viral load.

TREATMENT

- CD4 T-cell counts and plasma HIV-RNA viral load are measured to monitor patient's response to therapy.
- Highly active antiretroviral therapy (HAART) is used. It consists of varying combinations of nucleoside/nucleotide reverse transcriptase inhibitors (NRTIs), non-nucleoside reverse transcriptase inhibitors (NNRTIs), and protease inhibitors (PIs), and integrase strand transfer inhibitors (INSTIs).

Human Papillomavirus (HPV)

A 16-year-old presents complaining of painless growths on her vulva. On exam, numerous irregular, colored, raised lesions are noted. What test can help to make a definitive diagnosis?

Answer: Condylomata acuminata can be diagnosed on physical exam. Biopsy can be done to confirm.

- Subtypes 6 and 11 are associated with genital warts (**condylomata acuminata**).
- Subtypes 16, 18, 31, and 33 are associated with cervical and penile cancer.
- HPV vaccines can help with primary prevention of HPV infection.

PRESENTATION

Warts of various sizes (sometimes described as cauliflower-like papules) on the external genitalia, perineum, anus, vagina, and cervix.

DIAGNOSIS

- Warts are diagnosed on physical exam. Biopsy can be performed for confirmation.
- Cervical dysplasia caused by HPV infection is screened via Pap smear.

TREATMENT

- Treatment is based on either destructive therapy, immune mediated therapy, or surgical therapy.
  - Destructive therapies: Podophyllotoxin, trichloroacetic acid, 5-fluorouracil.
  - Immune-based therapies: Imiquimod cream, interferons.
  - Surgical therapies: Cryosurgery, laser ablation, excision.
- See Chapter 24 for treatment of cervical dysplasia.

Chancroid

A 21-year-old G1P1 presents with a painful genital ulcer on the vulva. On exam, there is an irregular, deep, well-demarcated ulcer with a gray base, along with inguinal lymphadenopathy. The culture and Gram stain returns as chancroid. What is the causative organism?

Answer: *Haemophilus ducreyi*, the diagnosis is confirmed with a culture in a special medium that requires special growth conditions.

PRESENTATION

- Chancroid presents as a soft papule on external genitalia that becomes a painful ulcer (unlike syphilis, which is hard and painless) with a gray, non-indurated, base with ragged edges.
- Inguinal lymphadenopathy, or bubo, also is possible.
- Incubation period is 1 week.

ETIOLOGY

Haemophilus ducreyi, a small gram-negative rod. Uncommon in the United States.

DIAGNOSIS

- Gram stain of ulcer or inguinal node aspirate showing gram-negative rods in chains—"school of fish." The sensitivity of gram stain is low.
- Culture is a more sensitive test, but the culture media required is not widely available.
- Screen for other STIs.

TREATMENT

Ceftriaxone, ciprofloxacin, or azithromycin.

EXAM TIP

Distinguishing painful ulcerating genital lesions with vesicles:

- **Herpes:** Multiple painful ulcers, base red.
- **Chancroid:** 1–3 painful ulcers, base yellow gray.
- **Syphilis:** 1 painless ulcer, indurated.
- **Lymphogranuloma venereum:** 1 painless ulcer, not indurated.
- **Granuloma inguinale:** Ulcer, rolled, elevated, rough.

chancroid
-papule→ulcerates with
yellow grey base;
painful buboes.

Pediculosis Pubis (Crabs)

A 26-year-old presents after unprotected sexual intercourse with intense genital pruritus. You suspect pediculosis pubis. How do you confirm the diagnosis?
Answer: By visualizing the crab louse *Phthirus pubis,* which has a crablike appearance under microscopy.

PRESENTATION

- Pruritus in the genital area from parasitic saliva.
- Ninety percent are commonly seen in the pubic hair, but it can involve any hair-bearing area of the body, i.e., axillae.
- The incubation period is 1 month.

ETIOLOGY

Blood-sucking parasitic crab louse, *Phthirus pubis.* The louse is typically transmitted by close sexual contact, but can less commonly be transmitted by fomites such as clothing or towels.

DIAGNOSIS

- History of pruritus.
- Visualization of crabs or nits.

TREATMENT

- Pyrethrin, permethrin (Nix) cream, or lindane (Kwell) shampoo.
- Proper cleaning of clothing and bedding is also necessary.
- Lindane is contraindicated in pregnancy.
- Reevaluate after 7 days.

Vaginitis

A 25-year-old G2P2 complains of a large amount of foul-smelling vaginal discharge. On physical exam, you notice a frothy, yellow-green discharge and multiple petechiae on the cervix. The wet mount of the discharge shows motile protozoa. What is the treatment of choice?

Answer: Metronidazole is the treatment of choice for trichomoniasis. In addition to the classic frothy, yellow-green malodorous discharge, petechiae are often seen on the cervix during exam (commonly called *strawberry cervix*).

DEFINITION

Inflammation of the vagina and cervix, often resulting in ↑ discharge and/or pruritus, and usually caused by an identifiable microbe (see Table 31-1). The only vaginitis that is sexually transmitted is trichomoniasis.

TABLE 31-1.   Vaginitis

	PHYSIOLOGIC (NORMAL)	BACTERIAL VAGINOSIS	CANDIDIASIS	TRICHOMONIASIS
Clinical complaints	None	**Malodorous discharge**, especially after menses, intercourse	**Pruritus, erythema, edema**, odorless discharge, dyspareunia	**Copious, frothy discharge**, malodorous, pruritus, urethritis
Quality of discharge	**Clear** or **white**, no odor, in vaginal vault	Homogenous **gray** or **white**, thin, sticky, adherent to vaginal walls	**White, "cottage cheese–like,"** adherent to vaginal walls	**Green** to **yellow**, sticky, "bubbly" or "frothy"
pH	3.8–4.2	>**4.5**	4–4.5	>**4.5**
Microscopic findings	Epithelial cells Normal bacteria include mostly *Lactobacillus*, with *Streptococcus, epidermidis, Streptococcus* as well as small amounts of colonic flora	Visualize with saline **Clue cells** (epithelial cells with bacteria attached to their surface) Bacteria include *Gardnerella (Haemophilus)* and/or *Mycoplasma*	In 10% KOH **Budding yeast** and pseudohyphae	In saline **Motile, flagellated, protozoa**
"Whiff" test	Negative (no smell)	**Positive** (fishy smell)	Negative	Positive or negative
Treatment		Oral or topical **metronidazole**; oral or topical **clindamycin**	Oral, topical, or suppository **imidazole** (or other various antifungals)	Oral **metronidazole** (*Note*: Metronidazole has potential disulfiram-like reaction and has a metallic taste)
Treat sexual partners?		Not necessary	Not necessary	Yes

Etiology

- **Antibiotics:** Destabilize the normal balance of flora.
- **Douche:** Raises the pH.
- **Intercourse:** Raises the pH.
- **Foreign body:** Serves as a focus of infection and/or inflammation.
- There are several common organisms that cause vaginitis: *Gardnerella* (bacterial), *Candida*, and *Trichomonas*. The distinguishing features are described with the following characteristics.
  - **Clinical characteristics.**
  - **Quality of discharge.**
  - **pH:** Secretions applied to test strip of pH paper, reveal pH of discharge.
  - **"Whiff" test:** Combining vaginal secretions with 10% KOH: Amines released will give a fishy odor, indicating a positive test.
  - **Diagnosis** is based on microscopic findings.

IUD → actinomyces is the most common infection

EXAM TIP

Clinical diagnosis depends on the examination of the vaginal secretions under the microscope and measurement of the vaginal pH.

WARD TIP

The most common complaint of a patient with candidiasis (yeast infection) is itching.

EXAM TIP

What is the most common infection with an IUD? *Actinomyces:* Sulfa granules, gram positive + rod (like fungi).

NOTES

Painful ulcers

1.) Genital Herpes
- vesicles w/ erythematous base that ulcerate.
- Tzank smear → multinucleated Giant cells.

2.) Chancroid (Haemophilus ducreyi)
- papule → ulcer with grey-yellow base
- severe, suppurative LAD (Bubves)

Not Painful.

1.) Syphilis
- painless chancre: indurated

2.) Lymphogranuloma venirem (Chlamydia L1-L3)
- shallow ulcers
- unilateral painful LAD.

3.) Granuloma inguinale - klebsiella granulomatis
- bleeding ulcer that is rolled and elevated;
  progressively spreads to destroy surrounding
  tissue "beefy red lesions"
- tx: azithromycin or doxycycline

CHAPTER 32

Breast Disease

Benign breast disease and breast lumps may be encountered after a physical exam or noted on imaging studies. The following will provide you with a basic guide in the initial evaluation of breast complaints.

Breast Anatomy

 A 34-year-old G3P3 presents with a 3-month history of right breast pain. She reports that her mother had breast cancer at age 64, and was treated with surgery and chemotherapy. Examination reveals a 2-cm mobile, tender, cystic mass to the right of her areola. Ultrasound (US) demonstrates a simple cystic structure. Aspiration of the mass yields clear fluid and relieves her pain. The cyst resolves with aspiration. What is your next management step?

Answer: Reassure the patient that the mass is benign in nature. Continue annual clinical breast exams (CBE).

The breasts:
- Large sebaceous glands located in the anterior chest wall; weigh 200–300 grams (in premenopausal years).
- Composed of 20% glandular tissue and 80% fat/connective tissue.
- Lymphatic drainage:
  - Drains to regional nodes in axilla and the clavicle.
- Blood supply:
  - Internal thoracic artery.
  - Lateral thoracic artery.
  - Posterior intercostal artery.
  - Thoracoacromial artery.

Approach to Breast Complaints

- Approach to complaints:
  - **B**iopsy, and take a history of complaint.
  - **R**ecord the location of the breast complaint.
  - **E**xamine each breast systematically for at least 3 min.
  - **A**ge: Document age of the patient—biggest risk factor for development of breast cancer.
  - **S**creening mammogram: Every 1–2 years from the age of 40 to 49; after 50, annually.
  - **T**iming of complaints in relation to menstrual cycle.
- Most expert groups do NOT recommend breast self-examination (SBE). Many groups, ACOG included, recommend breast self-awareness be encouraged, which may include SBE. Other groups recommend discussing pros and cons of SBE, and/or viewing SBE as a method of self-empowerment rather than screening.
- A yearly clinical breast examination (CBE) by a health care provider is no longer recommended by the American Cancer Society (as of 2015). However, other groups, such as ACOG and WHO, continue to recommend. ACOG recommends CBE every 1–3 years from age 20 to 39, and annually thereafter. It should take 3–5 minutes for a health care provider to perform a CBE.
- See Chapter 33 for mammogram recommendations.
- **CBE:**
  - Inspect for skin changes and breast asymmetry.
  - Exam in supine and sitting position.

- Use systematic palpation method.
  - Use middle three fingers to palpate the breasts.
  - Apply pressure to the breast with the pads of the fingers.
  - Flatten the breast against the chest wall during palpation.
  - Apply gentle pressure to the nipple to look for a nipple discharge.
- Examine for lymph node enlargement in the axillary and supraclavicular area.

WARD TIP

Examine lymph nodes:
- Supraclavicular
- Infraclavicular
- Medially
- Inferiorly
- Laterally (axillary line)

Common Breast Complaints

BREAST MASS

Breast mass workup.
- **History and physical exam.**
- **Imaging (ultrasound/MMG/MRI).**
- **Aspiration for fluid.**
- **Excisional biopsy (if needed).**
- If a patient palpates a breast mass that the clinician does not palpate, imaging studies should be ordered (see Figure 32-1). Re-examine and/or refer to a breast surgeon in 2–3 months if nothing is appreciated on clinical examination. Always report detection of a breast mass by its quadrant location (see Figure 32-1).
- Palpated masses should be aspirated or biopsied. US may help to localize deep masses and assist in aspiration and/or biopsy.
- Over the age of 40, **diagnostic mammogram** should be the initial imaging modality of choice for a breast lump. If a woman is <40, evaluation of a breast mass should begin with US (ultrasound) because the breast tissue is more dense.
- Ultrasound is the initial imaging modality in women <40 years of age. US helps to differentiate a cystic versus a solid breast mass.

EXAM TIP

Suspicious findings (for a cancer) on exam:
- Fixed, hard, irregular mass
- Mass >2 cm

40/30 ? → uwcrld says 30.

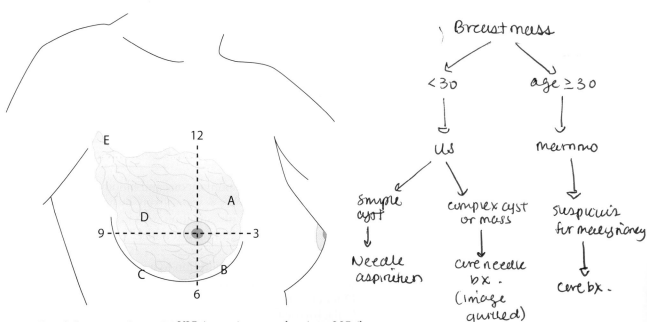

FIGURE 32-1. Female breast quadrants. (A) UIQ (upper inner quadrant); **(B)** LIQ (lower inner quadrant); **(C)** LOQ (lower outer quadrant); **(D)** UUQ (upper outer quadrant), majority of breast cancers are detected in this quadrant; **(E)** Tail of Spence (outer portion of breast toward the axilla).

Suspicious findings (for a cancer) on mammogram:

- Clusters of calcifications.
- ↑ breast density.
- Irregular margins of mass (spiculations).

Risk factors for breast cancer:

- Personal history of breast cancer
- Early menarche
- Nulliparity
- Alcohol intake
- Obesity
- Decreased physical activity
- Use of prolonged HRT (>5 years) during menopausal years.

Risk factors for hereditary breast cancer:

- Ashkenazi Jew
- Personal history of breast/ovarian cancer
- <40 years old
- Two or more relatives with breast cancer (<50 years)

- Aspirate the mass if it is cystic.
- Aspiration:
  - If fluid is cloudy/bloody, → excisional biopsy and imaging.
  - If fluid is clear and the cyst resolves, then monitor.
  - If cyst remains after aspiration, then recommend excisional biopsy.
- A palpable mass not detected on US or mammogram requires surgical referral for biopsy/excision.
- A solid, dominant, persistent mass requires a tissue diagnosis, by aspiration or biopsy.
- A nonpalpable mass, found on an imaging study, requires either following with further imaging or immediate biopsy, depending on how suspicious it appears on the image ("spiculated" masses are very suspicious).
- The **differential diagnoses** of benign breast masses:
  - **Fat necrosis** is usually a result of trauma to the breast with subsequent bleeding into the breast tissue. It is rare but often confused with cancer. The breast may contain a firm, tender, ill-defined mass that requires surgical excision.
  - **Fibroadenoma** is a common lesion seen in patients in the age range of 20–40. They are rubbery, firm, freely mobile, solid, and well circumscribed. Imaging with US can guide biopsy, and if the pathology returns fibroadenoma, it can be followed clinically.
  - **Phylloides tumors** usually occur in older women and are typically larger than fibroadenomas. They should be removed completely.
  - **Fibrocystic breast changes** are a pathologic diagnosis and should not be used to describe clinical findings. The classic symptoms include cyclic bilateral breast pain. The signs include ↑ engorgement, pain, and excessive nodularity. These lesions do not place the patient at ↑ risk for cancer.
  - **Atypical hyperplasia** is usually discovered after mammogram-directed biopsy. Complete excision of this mass is warranted, and these lesions ↑ the risk of future breast cancer *anywhere in the breasts* (not just at the site of the lesion).

NIPPLE DISCHARGE

- This complaint may represent either **benign** or **malignant** breast disease.
- Bilateral milky discharge from multiple ducts is **galactorrhea** and may be normal, although it can be associated with hypothyroidism, prolactin-producing tumor, or medications.
  - Medications that can cause a nipple discharge include antipsychotics, antidepressants, gastrointestinal drugs, and some antihypertensives.
  - If galactorrhea persists more than 6 months from the time of conclusion of breast-feeding, thyroid function tests and prolactin level are warranted.
- Nipple discharge that is spontaneous and bloody, from a single duct, persistent, and stains the clothes is more likely to be an **intraductal carcinoma or papilloma**—requires investigation with imaging and biopsy.
- Imaging begins with mammogram and US. Surgery referral for abnormal findings.
- **Differential diagnoses**, in addition to cancer, include the following:
  - **Intraductal papillomas**
  - **Duct ectasia**
  - **Galactorrhea**

BREAST PAIN

- History and physical exam, noting the cyclicity and duration of the pain. Inquire about menstrual history, hormone use, dietary habits (caffeine, tea, sodas, chocolate), and the presences of breast implants trauma.
  - **Cyclical** pain is bilateral in nature. Pain is ↑ during the luteal phase, dissipating with menses onset. Fibrocystic breast changes and cyclical mastalgia may require more than just reassurance if the exam is negative.
  - **Noncyclical** pain is more likely unilateral, in the following instances: Large breasts, ductal ectasia, inflammatory breast cancer, pregnancy, and some medications.
- If clinical exam is negative and the pain is cyclical, reassurance is reasonable.
- If negative for masses, reassure patient.
- If positive for masses, order imaging studies.
- **Treatment** may consist of reducing intake of caffeine, treatment with nonsteroidal anti-inflammatory drugs (NSAIDs), acetaminophen, and a "support" bra.

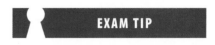

EXAM TIP

Oral contraceptives may cause breast pain.

BREAST SKIN CHANGES

- On exam, the skin is inspected for edema, erythema, or retraction.
- Ulceration, eczema, and redness around the nipple can be Paget disease. Mammogram and surgery referral is warranted.
- Erythema, tenderness, and a mass lead to suspicion for **inflammatory breast cancer.** Mammogram and surgery referral is warranted.
- Warmth, tenderness, induration, and erythema may also be mastitis or a breast abscess, even in the nonlactating woman. If fluctuance is appreciated, a breast US, drainage, and antibiotics are the treatment of choice.

NOTES

Women's Health Maintenance

Obstetricians/gynecologists must be aware of screening tests suggested for their patients. These tools are used for the prevention and/or early detection of serious medical conditions and diseases.

Screening Tests

> A 65-year-old, postmenopausal woman comes to your clinic for a well-woman exam. She has not seen a physician for several years. What screening and health maintenance tests will she need?
>
> **Answer:** This patient will need a Pap smear, annual clinical breast exam, mammogram, colon cancer screening, cholesterol/lipid screening, fasting glucose, complete blood count (CBC), urinalysis, blood urea nitrogen (BUN), creatinine, hemoglobin, influenza vaccine, tetanus-diphtheria (Td) booster, and pneumococcal vaccine.

PAP SMEAR (ACOG, DECEMBER 2012)

- Begin Pap smear screening at age 21. Between ages 21 and 29, Pap test every 3 years. After age 30, Pap test with concurrent HPV testing every 5 years (preferred), or Pap test alone every 3 years.
- This applies to low-risk women. High-risk women require more frequent screening.

BREAST EXAMS

See Chapter 32 for recommendations for breast self-examination (SBE) and clinical breast exam (CBE).

MAMMOGRAPHY

- Women under age 40 are at low risk for breast cancer. Controversy currently exists among professional organizations as to whether to offer mammogram screening to low-risk women under age 50.
- ACOG currently recommends routine annual screening beginning at age 40.
- Most organizations endorse routine mammogram screening annually for women age 50 and older.

BONE DENSITY SCREENING

- Screen with Dual Energy X-Ray Absorptiometry (DEXA) starting at age 65 years.
- Selective women under age 65 should be screened if they are postmenopausal and have one or more risk factors:
  - Personal history of pathologic fracture or parental history of hip fracture.
  - Body weight <127 lb.
  - Current smoker or alcoholic.
  - Rheumatoid arthritis.

COLON CANCER SCREENING

- Begin screening at age 50 in low-risk patients.
  - Preferred options (for prevention and early detection):
    1. Colonoscopy every 10 years.
    2. Flexible sigmoidoscopy every 5 years.

    3. Computed tomographic colonography every 5 years.
    4. Double-contrast barium enema every 5 years.
- Alternative options (for early detection only):
    1. Guaiac fecal occult blood test.
    2. Fecal immunochemical tests.
    3. Stool DNA tests.
- High-risk patients include those with inflammatory bowel disease, colonic polyps, colon cancer, or a family history of familial polyposis coli, colorectal cancer, or cancer predisposition syndrome. These patients should begin screening earlier and more frequently.

LABORATORY TESTING

Thyroid-Stimulating Hormone (TSH)

- Screening begins at age 50, then every 5 years.
- Periodic screening (age 19–64) if strong family history of thyroid disease or if autoimmune disease.

Cholesterol

- One-time screening between ages 17 and 21.
  - If normal and low risk, start screening every 5 years beginning at age 45.
  - If normal and high risk, start screening at age 35.
- Risk factors include:
  - Familial lipid disorder.
  - Family history of premature coronary artery disease (CAD) (<55 years), diabetes mellitus (DM), or multiple coronary heart disease risk factors (smoking, hypertension, obesity).
  - Elevated cholesterol.
  - History of parent or sibling with blood cholesterol ≥240 mg/dL.
  - History of sibling, parent, or grandparent with premature (<55 years) coronary artery disease.

Fasting Glucose (± HbA1c)

- The American Diabetes Association recommends testing every 3 years beginning at age 45 if no risk factors.
- Screening can begin at a younger age and/or more frequently in a patient with risk factors:
  - Family history of DM in a first-degree relative.
  - Obesity.
  - History of gestational DM.
  - Hypertension.
  - High-risk ethnic group (Hispanic/African-American/Native American).
  - History of polycystic ovarian syndrome.
  - History of vascular disease.
  - Age ≥45 years.
  - Sedentary lifestyle.
  - Dyslipidemia.

Tuberculosis (TB) Skin Testing

- Regular testing for teens.
- Human immunodeficiency virus (HIV): HIV-positive patients should be tested regularly.
- Exposure to TB-infected person requires testing.
- Medically underserved/low-income populations.

- Immunocompromised persons.
- Intravenous (IV) drug user.
- Resident of a long-term care facility.
- Recent TB skin test converter.

Sexually Transmitted Infection Testing

- History of multiple sexual partners.
- History of sex with a partner who has multiple sexual contacts.
- Persons whose partner has a sexually transmitted infection (STI).
- History of STI.
- Annual screening for all sexually active females under age 25. 6/6.
- Women with developmental disabilities.
- Women who exchange sex for drugs or money. (prostitutes)
- Women who use IV drugs.
- Women who are in a detention facility.

HIV Testing in Women

Annual testing for those with seeking treatment for any STIs, or with risk factors:

- Who have more than one sexual partner.
- With a history of prostitution/IV drug abuse.
- With a history of sex with an HIV-positive partner.
- Whose partners are men who have sex with men (MSM).
- Who were transfused between 1978 and 1985.
- Who are in an area with high prevalence of HIV infection.
- With recurrent genital tract disease.
- Who have invasive cervical cancer.
- Who are pregnant or planning to become pregnant.
- Who are in a detention facility.

Bacteriuria Testing/Urinalysis

Periodically for women with DM and women who are age 65 or older.

Immunizations

- Td booster once between ages 11 and 18, then every 10 years.
- Measles, mumps, rubella (MMR) for all nonimmune women.
- Hepatitis B vaccine once for those not previously immunized.
- Varicella vaccine, one series, for those not immunized.
- Hepatitis A vaccine if at high risk (such as chronic liver disease, illegal drug user, individuals traveling to endemic countries).
- Influenza vaccine annually for anyone wishing to reduce their chance of becoming ill. Also for high-risk conditions such as:
  - Resident of a chronic care facility.
  - Immunosuppression.
  - Hemoglobinopathy.
  - Diabetes.
  - Asthma.
  - Renal disease.
  - Cardiovascular disease.
  - Health care provider.
  - Pregnancy.
- Meningococcal vaccine before entering high school for those not immunized.
- Pneumococcal vaccine if age 65, or sooner for women with:
  - Sickle cell disease.
  - Asplenia.

WARD TIP

Routine screening for chlamydial and gonorrheal infection is recommended for all sexually active adolescents and high-risk females, even if they are asymptomatic. These tests are done simultaneously as the presence of one of these infections is a high risk for the presence of the other.

- ▪ Alcoholism/cirrhosis.
- ▪ Influenza vaccine risk factors.
- ▪ Revaccination after 5 years in these groups.
- ▪ Human papillomavirus vaccine (HPV): One series for those age 9–26.
- ▪ Herpes zoster vaccine: Single dose in adults age 60 or older.

Health Education

Good diet and exercise are crucial for leading a healthy life. There are many factors that determine each individual's diet and exercise requirements, which all must be considered by the physician.

NUTRITION AND EXERCISE

- ▪ The issues of nutrition and body weight should be emphasized during the three major transitional periods in a woman's life:
  1. Puberty.
  2. Pregnancy.
  3. Menopause.
- ▪ One's body weight is determined by three major factors:
  1. Genetics and heredity, which control:
     - ▪ Resting metabolic rate.
     - ▪ Appetite.
     - ▪ Satiety.
     - ▪ Body fat distribution.
     - ▪ Predisposition to physical activity.
  2. Nutrition.
  3. Physical activity and exercise.

GOALS

- ▪ Maintain a healthy diet consisting of frequent small meals (i.e., 4–6 instead of 2–3).
- ▪ The *2015–2020 Dietary Guidelines for Americans* provides evidence-based recommendations for eating patterns and regular physical activity. The following are recommended:
  - ▪ Follow a healthy eating pattern across the lifespan. This helps to support a healthy body weight and reduce the risk of chronic disease.
  - ▪ Focus on variety, nutrient density, and amount. Choose a variety of nutrient-dense foods from each food group in recommended amounts, including grains, vegetables, fruits, dairy, protein, and oils.
  - ▪ Limit calories from added sugars and saturated fats and reduce sodium intake.
  - ▪ Shift to healthier food and beverage choices.
  - ▪ Support healthy eating patterns for all.
- ▪ Adjust caloric intake for age and physical activity level:
  - ▪ As one ages, there is a ↓ in resting metabolic rate and loss of lean tissue.
  - ▪ Older women who are physically active are less likely to lose lean tissue and can maintain their weight with higher caloric intake.
- ▪ Physical activity is important for all adults. Adults should do at least 150 min/week of moderate-intensity or 75 minutes of vigorous-intensity aerobic physical activity. Adults should also include muscle strengthening activities 2 or more days per week.

EXAM TIP

High-fat diets have adverse effects on lipid metabolism, insulin sensitivity, and body composition.

EXAM TIP

Exercise will ↑ the body's metabolic rate and prevent the storage of fat.

Substance Abuse

A 53-year-old G1P1 presents to your office for a well-woman exam. When asked about alcohol use, she informs you that she drinks several glasses of wine every evening. How should you screen for alcoholism?

Answer: Using the CAGE questionnaire has been shown to be very effective in screening for problem drinking.

- Substance abuse is a serious condition that can affect every aspect of a patient's life. The role of an OB/GYN physician is to provide universal screening for substance abuse. This can be accomplished by direct questioning or via questionnaire.
- An example of screening would be the CAGE questionnaire. Two "yes" answers have a sensitivity of 93% and a specificity of 76% for alcoholism.

ALCOHOL

Women experience more accelerated and profound medical consequences of excessive alcohol than men (a phenomenon called *telescoping*):

- Cirrhosis.
- Peptic ulcers that require surgery.
- Myopathy.
- Cardiomyopathy.
- Stroke.
- Menstrual disorders.
- Early menopause.
- Stroke.
- Malignancies.
- When combined with cigarette smoking, it can cause oral and esophageal cancers.
- Fetal alcohol syndrome:
  - Teratogenic effects are dose related.
  - Includes growth retardation, facial anomalies, and intellectual disability.

TOBACCO

- Cigarette smoking is the most preventable cause of premature death and avoidable illness in the United States. It is important to apply the **5As** to screening women:
  - **A**sk about tobacco.
  - **A**dvise to quit.
  - **A**ssess willingness to quit.
  - **A**ssist in quit attempt.
  - **A**rrange for follow-up.
- Linked to lung cancer, coronary artery disease (CAD), and respiratory diseases.
- Most common factor in chronic obstructive pulmonary disease (COPD).
- **Endocrine effects:** Smokers reach menopause earlier and have ↑ risk of osteoporosis.
- **Obstetric effects:** Reduced fertility, ↑ rates of spontaneous abortion, premature delivery, low-birth-weight infants, fetal growth restriction, and placental abruption.
- Children who grow up exposed to secondhand smoke have higher rates of respiratory and middle-ear illness.

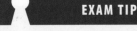

Seat Belt Use

- Deaths due to accidents are leading cause of death in females age 13–18.
- Accidents cause more deaths than infectious diseases, pulmonary diseases, diabetes, and liver and kidney diseases.
- Motor vehicle accidents account for 50,000 deaths/year and 4–5 million injuries/year.
- Seat belts ↓ chance of death and serious injury by >50%.

Safe Sex Practices

Improved and successful prevention of pregnancy and STIs by more adolescents requires counseling that includes:
- Education about *both* abstinence *and also* contraception and condoms.
- Provision of information about contraceptive options, including emergency contraception and side effects of various contraceptive methods.
- Education on safe sex practices, especially condom use, and STIs.

Physical Abuse

INTIMATE PARTNER VIOLENCE (IPV)

- Intimate partner violence (IPV) refers to a relationship in which an individual is victimized (physically, psychologically, or emotionally) by a current or past intimate partner.
- Each year in the United States, 2 million women are abused by someone they know.
- Every woman should be screened for IPV because it can occur with any woman, in any situation.

RECOGNITION OF INTIMATE PARTNER VIOLENCE

- Injuries to the head, eyes, neck, torso, breasts, abdomen, and/or genitals.
- Bilateral or multiple injuries.
- A delay between the time of injury and the time at which treatment is sought.
- Inconsistencies between the patient's explanation of the injuries and the physician's clinical findings.
- A history of repeated trauma.
- The perpetrator may exhibit signs of control over the health care team, refusal to leave the patient's side to allow private conversation, and control of victim.
- The patient calls or visits frequently for general somatic complaints.
- **Pregnant women:**
  - Late entry into prenatal care, missed appointments, and multiple repeated complaints are often seen in abused pregnant women.
  - Pregnant women are at an increased risk to experience IPV during the pregnancy.

DIAGNOSIS (SEE TABLE 33-1)

Use screening questionnaire.

TABLE 33-1. Abuse Assessment Screen

1. Have you ever been emotionally or physically abused by your partner or someone important to you?
2. Within the past year, have you been hit, slapped, kicked, or otherwise physically hurt by someone?
3. Since you've been pregnant, have you been hit, slapped, kicked, or otherwise physically hurt by someone?
4. Within the past year, has anyone forced you to have sexual activities? Has anyone in the past forced you to have sexual activities?
5. Are you afraid of your partner or anyone you listed above?

MEDICAL OBLIGATION TO VICTIMS

- Listen in a nonjudgmental manner, and assure the patient that it is not her fault, nor does she deserve the abuse.
- Assess the safety of the patient and her children.
- If the patient is ready to leave the abusive relationship, connect her with resources such as shelters, police, public agencies, and counselors.
- If the patient is not ready to leave, discuss a safety or exit plan and provide the patient with IPV information.
- Carefully document all subjective and objective findings. The records can be used in a legal case to establish abuse.

If ready to leave → connect w/ resources - shelters, agencies, counselors
not ready to leave → safety or exit plan

SEXUAL ASSAULT

 A 27-year-old G0P0 presents to your office stating that <u>she was raped the night before</u>. What are her options if she desires emergency contraception?
Answer: (1) Plan B: 0.75 mg levonorgestrel q12h × 2 doses; (2) Oral: 2 tabs stat, then 2 tabs 12 hr later; (3) mifepristone (RU486) 600 mg × 1 dose.

- **Sexual assault** occurs when *any sexual act* is performed by one person on another without that person's consent.
- **Rape** is defined as *sexual intercourse* without the consent of one party, whether from force, threat of force, or incapacity to consent due to physical or mental condition.

RAPE-RELATED POSTTRAUMATIC STRESS DISORDER (RR-PTSD)

A "rape-trauma" syndrome resulting from the psychological and emotional stress of being raped.

SIGNS AND SYMPTOMS

- **Acute phase:**
  - Eating and sleep disorders.
  - Vaginal itching, pain, and discharge.
  - Generalized physical complaints and pains (i.e., chest pain, headaches, backaches, and pelvic pain).
  - Anxiety/depression.
- **Reorganization phase:**
  - Phobias.
  - Flashbacks.
  - Nightmares.
  - Gynecologic complaints.

EXAM TIP

Sexual abuse occurs in approximately two-thirds of relationships involving physical abuse.

 WARD TIP

All pregnant women should be questioned about abuse during EACH trimester.

MANAGEMENT

Physician's Medical Responsibilities

- Requirements for forensic evaluations will vary by state. Many institutions have established programs with trained providers to provide this acute assessment and care.
- Obtain complete medical and gynecologic history.
- Assess and treat physical injuries in the presence of a female chaperone (even if the health care provider is female).
- Obtain appropriate cultures; check bloodwork for STIs (HIV, syphilis, hepatitis B/C).
- Counsel patient and provide STI prophylaxis.
- Provide preventive therapy for unwanted pregnancy.
- Assess psychological and emotional status.
- Provide crisis intervention.
- Arrange for follow-up medical care and psychological counseling.

EXAM TIP

Physicians are not obligated to perform procedures if they are morally opposed. There is an obligation to refer patients as necessary.

Physician's Legal Responsibilities

- Obtain informed consent for treatment, collection of evidence, taking of photographs, and reporting of the incident to the authorities.
- Accurately record events.
- Accurately describe injuries.
- Collect appropriate samples and clothing.
- Maintain the chain of command.
- Label photographs, clothing, and specimens with the patient's name; seal and store safely.

EXAM TIP

The greatest danger for spousal abuse to occur involves a threat or an attempt to leave the relationship.

TREATMENT

- **Infection prophylaxis:** Gonorrhea, chlamydia, and trichomonal infections:
  - Ceftriaxone 125 mg IM + azithromycin 1 g PO in a single dose or
  - Doxycycline 100 mg PO BID × 7 days + metronidazole 2 g PO in a single dose.
- Offer the hepatitis B vaccine.
- Offer anti-virals for HIV prophylaxis.
- Administer Td toxoid when indicated.
- **Postcoital regimen:**
  - **Plan B (levonorgestrel):** Consists of two tablets, each 0.75 mg taken 12 hr apart. Failure rate is up to 5% when taken within 24 hr and 11% when taken within 72 hr.
  - **Combined estrogen-progestin pills:** Ovral (50 µg ethinyl estradiol, 0.5 mg norgestrel): 2 tabs PO STAT, then 2 more tabs 12 hr later; 75% effective.

EXAM TIP

The annual incidence of sexual assault is 73 per 100,000 females.

EXAM TIP

Seventy-five percent of rape victims know their perpetrators.

CHAPTER 34

Female Sexuality

Female Sexual Response

It is important to consider every aspect of a woman's health, including her sexuality. Evaluation of sexual function should be a basic part of any well-woman exam.

FEMALE RESPONSE CYCLE

- **Desire:** Begins in the brain with perception of erotogenic stimuli via the special senses or through fantasy.
- **Arousal:**
  - Clitoris becomes erect.
  - Labia minora become engorged.
  - Blood flow in the vaginal vault triples.
  - Upper two-thirds of the vagina dilates.
  - Lubricant is secreted from the vaginal surface.
  - Lower one-third of vagina thickens and dilates.
- **Plateau:**
  - The formation of transudate (lubrication) in the vagina continues in conjunction with genital congestion.
  - Occurs prior to orgasm.
- **Orgasm:** Rhythmic, involuntary, vaginal smooth muscle and pelvic contractions, leads to pleasurable cortical sensory phenomenon ("orgasm").

SEXUALITY: FETUS TO MENOPAUSE

Prenatal and Childhood

- Sexual development begins prenatally when the fetus differentiates into a male or female.
- Sexual behavior, usually in the form of masturbation, is common in childhood.
- As children grow older, they are socialized into cultural emphasis on privacy and sexual inhibition in social situations.
- Between ages 7 and 8, most children engage in childhood sexual games, either same-gender or cross-gender play.

Adolescence

Gender identity and sexual preferences begin to solidify as puberty begins.

Menstrual Cycle

The menstrual cycle can affect sexuality (i.e., in some women, there is a peak in sexual activity in the midfollicular phase).

Pregnancy

- For some women, intercourse is avoided during pregnancy due to fear of harming the baby or a self-perception of unattractiveness.
- Coitus is safe in normal pregnancies.

Postpartum

Women often experience sexual problems within the first 6 weeks of delivery, including:
- Perineal soreness.
- Excessive fatigue.
- Lack of interest in sex.

This is secondary to changing hormone levels.

EXAM TIP

After somatosensory stimulation, orgasm is an adrenergic response.

EXAM TIP

Unlike men, women can experience multiple orgasms without a time lag in between.

WARD TIP

It is normal for children under age 6 to be curious about their own or others' bodies.

EXAM TIP

Sexual intercourse should be avoided in high-risk pregnancies, such as placenta previa, placental abruption, preterm labor, and preterm ruptured membranes.

Menopause

- A ↓ in sexual activity is most frequently observed.
- Advancing age is associated with ↓ in:
  - Intercourse frequency.
  - Orgasmic frequency.
  - Enjoyment of sexual activity: Sexual enjoyment may also be ↓ with the ↑ duration of the relationship and with the partner's increasing age.
- ↓ sexual responsiveness may be reversible if caused by reduction in functioning of genital smooth muscle tissue.
- Psychosocially, middle-aged women often feel less sexually desirable.
- **Hormonal changes:** Low estrogen levels lead to less vaginal lubrication, thinner and less elastic vaginal lining, and depressive symptoms, resulting in ↓ sexual desire and well-being and sometimes dyspareunia due to atrophy.

SEXUAL DYSFUNCTION

It is important to first clarify whether the dysfunction reported is:
- Lifelong or acquired.
- Global (all partners) or situational.

EVALUATION STRATEGIES

- Look for possible etiologies:
  - Medical illnesses.
  - Menopausal status.
  - Medication use (antihypertensives, cardiovascular meds, antidepressants, etc.).
- Rule out other psychiatric/psychological causes:
  - Life discontent (stress, fatigue, relationship issues, traumatic sexual history, guilt).
  - Major depression.
  - Drug abuse.
  - Anxiety.
  - Obsessive-compulsive disorder.

MANAGEMENT STRATEGIES

- Medical illnesses need evaluation and specific treatment.
- Screen for and treat depression with psychotherapy and/or medication.
- Reduce dosages or change medications that may alter sexual interest (i.e., switch to antidepressant formulations that have less of an impact on sexual function).
- Address menopause and hormonal deficiencies.

Female Sexual Dysfunction Disorders

- **Hypoactive sexual desire disorder:** Persistent or recurrent absence or deficit of sexual fantasies and desire for sexual activity.
- **Sexual aversion disorder:** Persistent or recurrent aversion to and avoidance of genital contact with a sexual partner.
- **Sexual arousal disorder:**
  - Partial or total lack of physical response as indicated by lack of lubrication and vasocongestion of genitals.
  - Persistent lack of subjective sense of sexual excitement and pleasure during sex.
- **Female orgasmic disorder:** Persistent or recurrent delay in, or absence of, orgasm following a normal excitement phase.
- **Vaginismus:** Persistent involuntary spasm of the muscles of the outer third of the vagina, which interferes with sexual intercourse.

WARD TIP

Sexual arousal disorders are accompanied by complaints of dyspareunia, lack of lubrication, or orgasmic difficulty.

EXAM TIP

Lack of orgasm during intercourse is a normal variation of female sexual response if the woman is able to experience orgasm with a partner using other noncoital methods.

Flibanserin → female hypoactive sexual desire disorder

EVALUATION FOR A SEXUAL DYSFUNCTION DISORDER

- Take sexual experience into account. Women often become more orgasmic with experience.
- Assess physical factors that may interfere with neurovascular pelvic dysfunction (i.e., surgeries, illnesses, or injuries).
- Psychological and interpersonal factors are very common (i.e., growing up with messages that sex is shameful and for men only).
- Partner's lack of sexual skills.

TREATMENT FOR SEXUAL DYSFUNCTION

Treatment varies and in general involves the couple. Therapy should be instituted for both partners, in addition to the following:
- Treat the ↓ lubrication with the application of lubricants, such as KY Jelly or Astroglide.
- Menopausal symptoms may respond to oral or topical estrogen.
- Pelvic physical therapy can be helpful for women with dyspareunia, pelvic pain, or vaginismus.
- For lifelong, generalized orgasmic disorder, there is rarely a physical cause. Treat with masturbation programs and/or sex therapy.
- Flibanserin (Addyi®) is currently the only FDA-approved drug to treat female sexual dysfunction. It is a serotonin receptor agonist/antagonist that is approved to treat hypoactive sexual desire disorder.

Sexual Pain Disorders

- **Dyspareunia:** Recurrent genital pain before, during, or after intercourse.
  - **Evaluation:** Differentiate between physical disorder, atrophy, vaginismus, lack of lubrication.
  - **Management:**
    - If due to vaginal scarring/stenosis due to history of episiotomy or vaginal surgery, vaginal stretching with dilators and massage.
    - If postmenopausal, vaginal estrogen (cream, vaginal tablet, vaginal ring) to improve vaginal pliability.
    - Low-dose tricyclic antidepressants may be helpful.
    - Pelvic floor physical therapy.
    - Coital position changes.
- **Vaginismus:** Recurrent involuntary spasm of the outer third of the vagina (perineal and levator ani muscles), interfering with or preventing coitus.
- **Evaluation:**
  - Obtain history.
  - Rule out organic causes (i.e., vaginitis, endometriosis, pelvic inflammatory disease, irritable bowel syndrome, urethral syndrome, interstitial cystitis, etc.).
  - Examine the pelvis for involuntary spasm.
  - Rule out physical disorder or other psychiatric disorder.
- **Management:**
  - Treat organic causes.
  - Psychotherapy.
  - Provide reassurance.
  - Physical therapy (i.e., pelvic floor exercises, muscle relaxation massage, and gradual vaginal dilatation). The woman controls the pace and duration.

SSRIs → ↑ serotonin → ↓ sexual response.

CHAPTER 35

Ethics

Physicians in all fields of medicine encounter difficult ethical decisions. Understanding the various aspects of forensic medicine may not make these decisions easier but will likely cause the physician to more closely consider the outcomes of the decision being made.

It is the physician's responsibility to:
- Determine the patient's preferences.
- Honor the patient's wishes when the patient can no longer speak for herself.

End-of-Life Decisions

A 35-year-old G2P2 is scheduled for major surgery. She would like to delineate preferences for her care, in the event that she is unable to speak for herself. What options does she have?

Answer: She can either write a living will (dictates her preferences) or appoint someone as her durable power of attorney to make decisions on her behalf.

- **Advance directives (living will and durable power of attorney for health care)** allow patients to voice their preferences regarding treatment if faced with a potentially terminal illness.
- In a **living will**, a competent adult patient may, in advance, formulate and provide a valid consent to the withholding/withdrawal of life-support systems in the event that injury or illness renders that individual incompetent to make such a decision.
- In a **durable power of attorney for health care**, a patient appoints someone to act as a surrogate decision maker when the patient cannot participate in the consent process.
- The patient's legal spouse is the *de facto* durable power of attorney for health care if no other is appointed; the spouse cannot defy the conditions of a living will or make decisions if another person has been appointed durable power of attorney.

WARD TIP

If a married person has a living will or has appointed another person to be a durable power of attorney, the spouse cannot defy the conditions.

LIFE-SUSTAINING TREATMENT

Any treatment that serves to prolong life without reversing the underlying medical condition.

Reproductive Issues

The ethical responsibility of the physician is:
- To identify his or her own opinions on the issue at hand.
- To be honest and fair to their patients when they seek advice or services in this area.
- To explain his or her personal views to the patient and how those views may influence the service or advice being provided.

Informed Consent

A legal document that requires a physician to obtain consent for treatment rendered, an operation performed, or many diagnostic procedures.

Informed consent requires the following conditions be met:
1. Must be **voluntary.**
2. **Information:**
   - **Risks and benefits** of the procedure are discussed.
   - **Indications** for the procedure are reviewed.
   - **Alternatives** to procedure are discussed.
   - **Consequences** of not undergoing the procedure are discussed.
   - Physician must be willing to **discuss the procedure** and answer any questions the patient has.
3. The patient must be **competent.**

Exceptions

The following are certain cases in which informed consent need not be obtained:
1. Lifesaving medical emergency.
2. Suicide prevention.
3. Normally, minors must have consent obtained from their parents. However, minors may give their own consent for certain treatments, such as alcohol detox and treatment for venereal diseases. *or if emancipated.*

Patient Confidentiality

The information disclosed to a physician during his or her relationship with the patient is confidential. The physician should not reveal information or communications without the express consent of the patient, unless required to do so by law.

EXCEPTIONS

- A patient threatens to inflict serious bodily harm to herself or another person.
- Communicable diseases (i.e., HIV). *→ report to public health dept?*
- Gunshot wounds.
- Knife wounds.

Minors

- When minors request confidential services, physicians should encourage minors to involve their parents.
- Where the law does not require otherwise, the physician should permit a competent minor to consent to medical care and should **not** notify the parents without the patient's consent.
- If the physician feels that without parental involvement and guidance the minor will face a serious health threat, and there is reason to believe that the parents will be helpful, disclosing the problem to the parents is equally justified.
- Documentation of the rationale for these types of decisions is key.

NOTES

Menopause

Menopause signifies the depletion of oocytes and manifests as the absence of menses. The changes in female hormones can have significant morbidity for a woman. A variety of symptoms can occur that may require medical treatment. The treatment options all have pros and cons that must be discussed with patients who are symptomatic.

Definitions

- **Menopause** is the permanent cessation of menstruation diagnosed after 12 months of amenorrhea.
- Menopause signifies ovarian follicular depletion, which results in ↓ estrogen production and ↑ of follicle-stimulating hormone (FSH).
- Menopause is preceded by the **climacteric** or **perimenopausal period**, the multiyear transition from optimal menstrual condition to menopause.
- Most women become menopausal between the ages of 45 and 55 years.
- The **postmenopausal period** is the time after menopause.
- See Figure 36-1.

Factors Affecting Age of Onset

- Genetics.
- Smoking (↓ age by 3 years). ✱✱
- Chemo/radiation therapy.

Physiology During the Perimenopausal Period

OOCYTES DIE

- Women's immature eggs, or **oocytes, begin to die** precipitously (via apoptosis) and become **resistant to follicle-stimulating hormone (FSH)**, the pituitary hormone that causes their maturation.

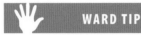

WARD TIP

Average age of menopause in the United States is 61 years.

EXAM TIP

Cigarette smoking is a factor shown to significantly reduce the age of menopause (3 years).

						Final Menstrual Period (FMP) ▽		
Stages:	**-5**	**-4**	**-3**	**-2**	**-1**	**0**	**+1**	**+2**
Terminology:	Reproductive			Menopausal Transition			Postmenopause	
	Early	Peak	Late	Early	Late*		Early*	Late
				Perimenopause				
Duration of Stage:	variable			variable		(a) 1 yr	(b) 4 yrs	until demise
Menstrual Cycles:	variable to regular	regular		variable cycle length (>7 days different from normal)	≥2 skipped cycles and an interval of amenorrhea (≥60 days)	*Amen x 12 mos*	none	
Endocrine:	normal FSH		↑ FSH	↑ FSH			↑ FSH	

*Stages most likely to be characterized by vasomotor symptoms   ↑ = elevated

FIGURE 36-1.   The STRAW staging system. (Reproduced, with permission, from Soules MR, et al. Executive Summary: Stages of Reproductive Aging Workshop [STRAW]. *Fertil Steril* 2001;76[5]: 874–878.)

- Menopause is characterized by an elevated FSH due to:
  1. ↓ inhibin (inhibin inhibits FSH secretion; it is produced in smaller amounts by the fewer oocytes).
  2. Resistant oocytes require more FSH to successfully mature, triggering greater FSH release.

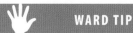

WARD TIP

FSH levels double to 20 mIU/mL in perimenopause and increase to 40 mIU/mL in menopause.

OVULATION BECOMES LESS FREQUENT

Women **ovulate less frequently**: Initially 1–2 fewer times per year, and eventually, just before menopause, only once every 3–4 months. This is due to a **shortened follicular phase**. The length of the luteal phase does not change.

EXAM TIP

Oligo/anovulation leads to abnormal bleeding in perimenopause.

ESTROGEN LEVELS FALL

A 51-year-old G4P4 presents with new-onset pain with intercourse and occasional vaginal itching that started 6 months ago. Workup for sexually transmitted infections (STIs) is negative, and on wet mount you note very few epithelial cells consistent with atrophic vaginitis. What is the major hormonal change implicated in these symptoms?

Answer: There is a decline in estrogen that causes atrophic vaginitis.

- **Estrogen (estradiol-17β) levels begin to decline,** resulting in hot flashes (which may also be due to ↑ luteinizing hormone [LH]).
- There is a major reduction in ovarian estrogen production at 6 months before menopause.
- Hot flashes (also known as hot flushes or vasomotor symptoms) are the most common symptom during the menopause transition.
- Hot flashes can occur for 2 years after the onset of estrogen deficiency begins. Most women will stop having hot flashes within 4–5 years of onset, but a small percentage will report persistent symptoms even after age 70.
- Hot flashes usually occur on the face, neck, and upper chest and last a few minutes, followed by intense diaphoresis. Women often complain of sleep disruption.

EXAM TIP

When menopause occurs after age 55, it is considered late menopause.

Physiology During the Menopausal Period

- ↓ in estradiol level.
- **FSH and LH levels rise** secondary to absence of negative feedback.
- Androstenedione is aromatized peripherally to estrone (less potent than estradiol), which is the major estrogen in postmenopausal women.
- Androstenedione and testosterone levels fall. These two hormones are produced by the ovary.
- The most **important physiologic change** that occurs with menopause is the **decline of estradiol-17β** levels that occurs with the cessation of follicular maturation. Table 36-1 lists the organ systems affected by the ↑ estradiol levels.

estrone is predominant during menopause.

EXAM TIP

Premature ovarian failure is defined as menopause occurring before age 40.

Treatment of Menopausal Adverse Effects

A 50-year-old G1P1 presents with a 3-month history of hot flashes during the day and night sweats so bad she has to change her shirt. On further questioning, she reports that she has ↑ irritability and a lack of libido for that same period of time. What is this patient's diagnosis, and what treatment could you offer her?

Answer: This woman is experiencing menopause. If her symptoms are distressing, she could be offered hormone replacement therapy to alleviate some of her symptoms.

EXAM TIP

Although HRT recommendations changed with the WHI study, there are many flaws in the design. Recommendations will likely change in the near future.

Hormone replacement therapy (HRT) or estrogen replacement therapy (ERT) has been shown to counteract some of the side effects of estrogen loss listed in Table 36-1.

ESTROGEN REPLACEMENT THERAPY (ERT)

ERT—estrogen alone: Indicated in women status post hysterectomy.

TABLE 36-1. **Physiologic Effects of Menopause**

Organ System	Effect of Decreased Estradiol	Available Treatment
Cardiovascular	↑ LDL, ↓ HDL. After two decades of menopause, the risk of myocardial infarction (MI) and coronary artery disease is equal to that in men.	
Bone	Osteoporosis. Estrogen receptors found on many cells mediating trabecular bone maintenance (ie, ↓ osteoblast activity, ↑ osteoclast activity) due to ↓ estrogen levels.	▪ HRT/ERT becoming second line ▪ Calcitonin ▪ Raloxifene ▪ Etidronate (a bisphosphonate osteoclast inhibitor) ▪ Exercise ▪ Calcium supplementation ▪ 50% reduction in death from hip fracture with normal estrogen levels
Vaginal mucous membranes	Dryness and atrophy, with resulting dyspareunia, atrophic vaginitis.	HRT/ERT pill or cream
Genitourinary	Loss of urethral tone, dysuria.	HRT/ERT
Psychiatric	Lability, depression.	+/− HRT/ERT, antidepressants
Neurologic	Preliminary studies indicate there may be a link between low levels of estradiol and Alzheimer disease.	HRT/ERT
Hair and skin	Skin: Less elastic, more wrinkled. Hair: Male growth patterns.	HRT/ERT pill or cream

ERT, estrogen replacement therapy; HDL, high-density lipoprotein; HRT, hormone replacement therapy; LDL, low-density lipoprotein.

HORMONE REPLACEMENT THERAPY (HRT)

- HRT—estrogen + progesterone: The progesterone component is needed to protect the endometrium from constant stimulation and resultant ↑ in endometrial hyperplasia/cancer. It is indicated for women who still have their uterus.
- The Women's Health Initiative (WHI) prompted great changes in the understanding and recommendations for HRT. It specifically demonstrated adverse effects in women over age 60 or women greater than 10 years since menopause. The risk-benefit profile is more favorable in women ages 50–59, which is the age range in which women typically present seeking treatment for menopausal symptoms.
- Cardiovascular: HRT does not seem to protect against cardiovascular disease as previously thought. In fact, combined HRT has been associated with an increased risk of stroke, venous thromboembolism, and coronary heart disease.
- Osteoporosis: Controversial because HRT protects against osteoporosis, but there are other medications, such as bisphosphonates and raloxifene, that can do the same thing with less cardiovascular risk.
- Breast cancer: Combined HRT ↑ the risk of invasive breast cancer, but estrogen alone does not.
- The main indication for HRT is vasomotor symptoms. It may also be helpful for:
  - Vaginal atrophy (but vaginal estrogen is preferred in absence of vasomotor symptoms).
  - Mood lability (alone or in combination with antidepressant).

Recommendations

- Short-term therapy (<5 years) is acceptable for menopausal symptom relief in young, postmenopausal women. Prescribe the lowest dose that relieves the symptoms. Order a mammogram before initiating therapy and yearly thereafter.
- Osteoporosis can be prevented with HRT; however, other medications are as effective and should be used as first-line therapy.
- HRT should not be used to prevent cardiovascular disease.

Risks of HRT/ERT

- ↑ risk of breast cancer.
- ↑ incidence in endometrial cancer (unopposed ERT only).
- Thromboembolism, myocardial infarction (MI), stroke.
- Cholecystitis/cholelithiasis.

Contraindications to HRT/ERT

- Unexplained vaginal bleeding.
- Breast carcinoma. ✱
- Metastatic endometrial carcinoma/ovarian carcinoma. ✱
- Liver disease. ✱ → can't metabolize estrogen.
- History of thromboembolic disease.
- History of MI or stroke.
- May worsen hypertension or migraines.

[Handwritten margin notes:]

- Hot flushes
- sleep disturbances
- night sweats
- atrophic vaginitis
- osteoporosis
- CAD.

vasomotor sx = HRT.

✋ **WARD TIP**

Menopause wreaks HAVOC:
Hot flashes
Atrophy of the
Vagina
Osteoporosis
Coronary artery disease

EXAM TIP

Estrogen creates a hypercoagulable state due to ↑ production of hepatic coagulation factors.

} ✱ -

NOTES

Menopause sx

1.) neuro
- Hot flushes
- sleep disturbance
- night sweats
- mood Δ's

2.) genital
- atrophic vaginitis - dryness, pruritis
- vulvar pruritis

3.) GU
- dysuria, frequency, urgency
- stress incontinence
- pelvic floor prolapse.

4.) CV
- CAD

5.) Bone
- osteoporosis

Hot Flashes, night sweats
Atrophic ⎰ — dryness , dysuria, incontinence/
Vaginitis ⎱ pruritis   freq, urg. prolapse
Osteoporosis
CAD. (↑LDL, ↓HDL)

CHAPTER 37

Pelvic Relaxation

age
↑ abdominal pressure

With aging and ↑ pelvic pressure, there is a risk that the pelvic musculature will no longer be able to keep pelvic organs in their proper position. Prolapse can occur in various organs and is usually associated with a sensation of ↑ pressure. Diagnosis must be made by examining the patient when supine and standing. When prolapse becomes symptomatic, treatment is warranted with surgery or a pessary device.

Anatomy of Pelvic Floor Support

Several crucial structures make up the support of the female pelvic floor. Disturbance of any of the following can result in prolapse:
- Bony structure.
- Cardinal, broad, and round ligaments.
- Endopelvic fascia.
- Pelvic diaphragm.
- Urogenital diaphragm.
- Perineum.

> **EXAM TIP**
>
> The pelvic diaphragm is made up of the levator ani and coccygeal muscles.

Pelvic Organ Prolapse (POP)

 A 57-year-old G3P3 overweight woman (250 lb) who has had three vaginal deliveries comes to your office complaining of pressure and a bulge in her vagina that is worse at the end of the day. What is your next step in management?
Answer: Perform a complete pelvic exam to assess for prolapse. Examine the patient in both the supine and standing position to help determine the severity of the prolapse.

> **EXAM TIP**
>
> In general, think of prolapse as either limited to the upper vagina, to the introitus, or protruding through the vagina.

Pelvic organ prolapse (POP) is the failure of pelvic musculature to maintain the pelvic organs in their normal position. There are several types.

TYPES

POP can be classified according to the location of the herniated pelvic organ:
- **Anterior compartment:**
  - Cystocele (bladder).
  - Anterior vaginal wall herniation.
- **Posterior compartment:**
  - Rectocele (rectum): See Figure 37-1.
  - Posterior vaginal wall herniation. *(middle ⅓)*
- **Enterocele:** *(posterior vaginal wall, upper ⅓)*
  - Herniation of intestines to or through vaginal wall. See Figure 37-1.
- **Apical:**
  - Uterine prolapse.
  - Vaginal vault prolapse.
- **Uterine procidentia:** Herniation of all three compartments, including uterus, through the vaginal introitus.

GRADING (BADEN-WALKER CLASSIFICATION)

Organ displacement:

To the level of the ischial spines:	Grade I ↑ *above introitus*
Between ischial spines and introitus:	Grade II ↑
Up to introitus:	Grade III @ *introitus*
Past introitus:	Grade IV *below introitus.*

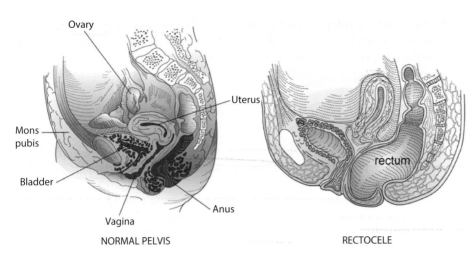

FIGURE 37-1. **Types of prolapse.** (Reproduced, with permission, from Pernoll ML. *Benson & Pernoll's Handbook of Obstetrics and Gynecology*, 10th ed. New York: McGraw-Hill, 2001: 807–808.)

RISK FACTORS

Many conditions can cause prolapse: Disturbing the anatomical supports (childbirth), disrupting the innervations, or increasing abdominal pressure. Examples include:

- ↑ abdominal pressure: Obesity, cough (e.g., chronic obstructive pulmonary disease), heavy lifting, chronic constipation.
- Loss of levator ani function: Postpartum.
- Transection of supporting tissue: Postsurgical, i.e., hysterectomy.
- Loss of innervation: Amyotrophic lateral sclerosis (ALS), paralysis, multiple sclerosis.
- Loss of connective tissue: Spina bifida, myelomeningocele.
- Atrophy of supporting tissues: Aging, especially after menopause.
- Race: Hispanic and Caucasian > African-American.

SIGNS AND SYMPTOMS

- Feeling of "pressure" or "bulge."
- Organ protrusion, especially upon exertion.
- Incontinence.
- Groin pain.
- Dyspareunia.
- Spotting.
- Splinting to defecate.

Symptom alleviation/exacerbation is often related to gravity (i.e., better when prone, better in the morning, worse with standing, worse in evening).

DIAGNOSIS

- Diagnosis is made by direct visualization of prolapsed organ during complete pelvic examination.
- Patient should be **examined in the supine and standing position**.

TREATMENT

Nonsurgical

- **Asymptomatic prolapse:**
  - Usually requires **follow-up,** but no immediate intervention needed.
  - Pelvic-strengthening exercises (i.e., **Kegel** maneuvers) and/or hormone/estrogen replacement therapy may be beneficial.

EXAM TIP

Risk factors for developing prolapse:
- Advancing age
- Chronic obstruction
- Constipation
- Genetic predisposition
- Menopause *aging*
- Parity
- Prior surgery
- Pulmonary disease
- Tumor/mass

WARD TIP

Remember to examine the patient in **both** the supine and standing positions.

↑age (atrophy)
childbirth (perineal tear)
↑abd pressure
- obesity

consider lifestyle mods
e.g. if pt is obese →
lose weight!

- **Symptomatic prolapse:** Can be treated with a pessary or surgically. A **pessary** is an object (prosthetic) placed in the upper vagina designed to help maintain support of the pelvic organs. Types include:
  - Smith-Hodge (oval ring).
  - Doughnut (ring).
  - Inflatable.
  - Gehrung (U-shaped).

Surgical

- Indications for surgery: Childbearing is completed and/or symptoms are interfering with patient's functioning and do not respond to nonsurgical treatment.
- There are several types of surgical repairs for each type of prolapse. New, minimally invasive techniques are being developed.
  - **Cystocele: Anterior colporrhaphy (anterior repair):** Bladder buttress base sutures proximal to the bladder neck.
  - **Rectocele: Posterior colporrhaphy (posterior repair)**—posterior vaginal wall reinforcement with levator ani muscles via vaginal approach.
  - **Enterocele: Moschcowitz repair**—approximation of endopelvic fascia and uterosacral ligaments via abdominal approach to prevent an enterocele. Similar transvaginal repair exists.
  - **Apical prolapse:** Vaginal approach: Sacrospinous ligament fixation (SSLF), uterosacral ligament suspension (USLS). Abdominal approach: Sacrocolpopexy.
  - **Uterine prolapse: Hysterectomy**—a uterine prolapse often occurs in conjunction with another prolapse, so combined repairs are usually performed.
  - **LeFort procedure/colpoclesis:** Surgical obliteration of the vaginal canal in a female who is NOT sexually active. This procedure can be performed with any type of prolapse.

WARD TIP

Pessaries are especially useful in the elderly population or when surgery is contraindicated.

WARD TIP

Complications of pelvic organ prolapse:
- Urinary retention
- Constipation
- Urinary tract infections
- Ulcerations
- Vaginal bleeding

asx
observation vs. Kegel Exercises/ERT

sx
pessary vs. surgery
non responders to surgical tx
un-
child bearing complete + fx impairment.

Urinary Incontinence

Urinary incontinence is an involuntary loss of urine that can be due to a variety of conditions. It can cause social embarrassment, sexual dysfunction, and hygiene issues. It is important to differentiate between the different types of urinary incontinence, because the management of each type is different.

Definition

Involuntary loss of urine that is a symptom of a pathological condition. Incontinence can be due to reversible or irreversible (but treatable) causes. A careful history will help to determine the underlying cause(s).

Causes

REVERSIBLE

- Delirium, infection, atrophic vaginitis, drug side effects, psychiatric illness, excessive urine production, restricted patient mobility, and stool impaction are *reversible* causes of urinary incontinence.
- It is helpful to explore these easily correctable causes before moving on to the more expensive and invasive workup for the irreversible causes.

IRREVERSIBLE (THREE MAIN TYPES ARE STRESS, URGE, AND OVERFLOW)

Stress Incontinence

- Loss of urine (usually **small amount**) with ↑ **intra-abdominal pressure** (i.e., with coughing, laughing, exercise).
- Caused by **urethral hypermotility** and/or **intrinsic sphincter deficiency (ISD)** that maintains enough closing pressure at rest (sphincter tone), but not with exertion.

Urge Incontinence

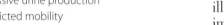 A 52-year-old G4P4 active female complains of sudden urgency to go to the bathroom followed by loss of urine before she makes it to the bathroom. The urge is not precipitated by laughing or coughing, and she does not leak constantly throughout the day. What is the underlying cause of her incontinence?
Answer: This woman has urge incontinence that is caused by unopposed detrusor muscle contraction.

- Sudden feeling of **urgency** followed by involuntary leakage of urine (can be small or large volume loss).
- Caused by unopposed detrusor contraction. Also called "overactive bladder."

Overflow Incontinence

- Constant dribbling +/– urgency with inability to completely empty the bladder.
- Caused by detrusor underactivity (due to a neuropathy) or urethral obstruction.

WARD TIP

Reversible causes of urinary incontinence—
DIAPPERS
Delirium
Infection
Atrophic vaginitis
Pharmacologic causes
Psychiatric causes
Excessive urine production
Restricted mobility
Stool impaction

WARD TIP

Causes of urinary incontinence—
This **U**rine **F**low is **S**o **O**utrageous

Total
Urge
Functional
Stress
Overflow

WARD TIP

Incontinence that presents as continuous urinary and/or fecal leakage ("total incontinence") is often due to a fistulous tract. This occurs as a result of:
- Prior pelvic surgery
- Obstetric trauma
- Radiation

Mixed Incontinence

Combinations of above (usually stress and urge).

Evaluation

HISTORY

Ask about aforementioned symptoms, medications, medical history (diabetes mellitus, neuropathies), and impact on quality of life. It is also helpful to have the patient keep a **voiding diary** (i.e., volume, frequency, fluid intake).

PHYSICAL

- Pelvic exam: Check for POP, masses, atrophic changes, and Q-tip test.
- Rectal exam: Check for impaction and rectocele; assess sphincter tone.
- Neurological exam: Assess for neuropathy.
- Cough stress test: In clinic, place patient in standing (or supine) position with full bladder. Visualize urethra and ask patient to cough to see if direct visualization of leaking from urethra is possible.
- Postvoid residual (PVR) (normal is <50–100 mL).

LABS

Urinalysis and culture to rule out urinary tract infection.

Q-TIP TEST

- A cotton swab is placed in the urethra. The change in angle between the Q-tip and the woman's body is measured upon straining.
- Normal upward change is <30 degrees, and a **positive test** is one with **>30-degree change.**
- **A positive test indicates** (urethral hypermobility.) → stress incontinence

CYSTOMETRY

- Cystometry provides measurements of the relationship of pressure and volume in the bladder.
- Catheters that measure pressures are placed in the bladder and rectum, while a second catheter in the bladder supplies water to cause bladder filling.
- Measurements include post **residual volume, volumes at which an urge to void occurs, bladder compliance, flow rates,** and **capacity.**
- **Diagnoses:** Stress, urge, and overflow incontinence.

URODYNAMIC STUDIES

- A set of studies that evaluate lower urinary tract function.
- Studies may include **cystometry** (see above), **bladder filling tests, cystoscopy, uroflowmetry,** and **leak-point pressure tests.**
- Can help diagnose and differentiate between types of incontinence.

Treatment

Lifestyle modification is recommended for all patients with incontinence of any type. This may include weight loss, dietary changes (i.e., reduction of caffeine, alcohol), correction of constipation, and smoking cessation.

WARD TIP

Functional incontinence: A person can recognize the need to urinate, but cannot make it to the bathroom in time because of immobility.

WARD TIP

Q-tip test: ↑ upward motion of the Q-tip is caused by loss of support from the urethrovesicular junction, indicating urethral hypermobility.

EXAM TIP

Stress incontinence is treated with α-adrenergic agonists and surgical repair.

1.) Lifestyle Mods
- weight loss
- diet: ↓ coffee, caffeine
- tobacco ↓
- ↓ constipation

1.) lifestyle mod
2.) kegel excersises
3.) Pessery
4.) Midurethral sling vs. Burch colposuspensin for urethral hypermobility; Bulking procedures for intrinsic sphincter deficiency.

1.) lifestyle mods
2.) Bladder training aka timed voiding
3.) antimuscarinics or mirabegron.

can also use cholinergic agonist.

STRESS INCONTINENCE

- **Kegel exercises** strengthen pelvic floor muscles. Referral to a physical therapist who specializes in pelvic floor health can be beneficial.
- **Topical estrogen therapy.**
- Incontinence **pessary**.
- Surgical repair.
  - Burch retropubic colposuspension is the gold standard in the literature, but is not often performed as primary treatment anymore due to similar outcomes with less invasive procedures.
  - Midurethral slings are more popular due to ease of placement and excellent outcomes.

URGE INCONTINENCE

- **Medications:**
  - Antimuscarinic agents ($\uparrow$ bladder capacity, $\downarrow$ urge by blocking release of acetylcholine during bladder filling). Most common side effects are dry mouth and constipation.
    - Mirabegron (beta-3-adrenoreceptor agonist).
- **Timed voiding:** Patient is advised to urinate in prescribed hourly intervals before the bladder fills. (Bladder training)
- Surgery is rarely used to treat urge incontinence.
- Avoid stimulants and diuretics (i.e., alcohol, coffee, carbonated beverages).

OVERFLOW INCONTINENCE

- **Due to obstruction:** Relieve obstruction.
- Due to detrusor underactivity: Treat possible neurological causes—diabetes mellitus, B_{12} deficiency.
- intermittent self catheterization

TOTAL INCONTINENCE

Surgical repair for fistulas.

Medical Student Information of Interest

Opportunities

AMA-MSS COUNCILS

The Medical Student Section of the AMA (AMA-MSS) has several councils for which it seeks medical students. Please see the website ama-assn.org for further details.

Application involves a current curriculum vitae, an essay on why you want to be a member of an AMA Council, which Council(s) you prefer, what you consider to be your major strengths and qualifications for the position, and what benefits you feel are likely to result from your participation.

- AMA-MSS Governing Counsel (GC)—eight-member council that directs MSS agenda and strategies.
- AMA Government Relations Advocacy Fellowship (GRAF)—experience organized medicine and federal government as it relates to advocacy and policy making.
- The AMA-MSS GC appoints medical student members to serve on its Standing Committees. Application deadline is usually July 1 (check website).
- Council on Constitution and Bylaws
  - Committee on Bioethics and Humanities
  - Committee on Legislation and Advocacy
  - Committee on Long-Range Planning
  - Committee on Medical Education
  - Minority Issues Committee
  - Committee on Scientific Issues
  - Committee on Economics and Quality in Medicine
  - Committee on Global and Public Health
  - Membership and Recruitment Committee
  - Communication and Engagement Committee
  - Committee on Health Information Technology
  - HOD Coordination Committee
  - Community Service Committee

AMA POLITICAL ACTION COMMITTEE (AMPAC)

AMPAC is a bipartisan group that serves to advance the interest of medicine within Congress, specifically by supporting candidates for office that are friendly to medicine. They also provide numerous programs to educate physicians, medical students, and their families on political activism. The Board directs the programs and activities of this extremely important political action committee. Adding medical students to the leadership of this group will provide for better medical student representation within the group as well as greater student involvement in this important process. Terms are for 2 years.

Websites of Interest

ACOG.ORG

ACOG.org is the official website for the American College of Obstetricians and Gynecologists. The website has several items of interest to medical students, including a career guide for medical students interested in the specialty.

MEDICAL STUDENT MEMBERSHIP IN ACOG

- ACOG publications.
- Reduced meeting fees.
- Entry into their member-only website.
- Updates in the specialty.
- Scholarships available to national or regional meetings.

APGO.ORG

APGO is the Association of Professors of Obstetricians and Gynecologists. It is the organization for OB/GYN Educators. They have a section of medical student resources, which includes:

- Residency directory.
- Medical student guide for interaction with industry.
- *The OBGYN Clerkship: Your Guide to Success.*
- *Comprehensive Women's Health Care: A Career in Obstetrics and Gynecology.*
- **uWISE** (Web-Based Interactive Self-Evaluation)—a 542-question interactive self-exam designed to help medical students acquire the necessary basic knowledge in OB/GYN.

JOIN AMWA (AMERICAN MEDICAL WOMEN'S ASSOCIATION)

Become a medical student life member of AMWA. Membership benefits include:

- Networking opportunities at the national and local levels—60 physician branches and 120 student branches.
- Continuing Medical Education (CME) programs.
- Leadership and mentoring opportunities.
- Professional and personal development programs.
- AMWA's legislative network.
- AMWA's Annual, Interim, and Regional Meetings offering career and personal development curricula.
- Gender Equity Information Line to assist you with concerns on sexual harassment, gender bias, racial discrimination, and other matters.
- Women's Health Advocacy.
- Subscription to the *Journal of the American Medical Women's Association* (JAMWA), a quarterly peer-reviewed scientific publication.
- AMWA Connections, a bimonthly newsletter keeping you connected to your colleagues.
- Women's health projects and innovative "Train-the-Trainer" programs.
- Discounts for AMWA publications such as *The Women's Complete Healthbook*, *The Women's Complete Wellness Book*, and *Developing a Child Care Program.*
- Advanced access and reduced fees to AMWA's Career Development Institute.
- Members-Only sections on the AMWA website.

AMA-ASSN.ORG

- FREIDA Online—computer access to graduate training program data (members receive up to 30 free mailing labels).
- Airline discounts for travel to residency interviews (graduating seniors only).
- USP Drug Information for the Health Care Professional.
- Discounts up to 35% in AMA's Medical Student Catalog.

- PaperChase—discounted online subscription to MEDLINE searches (free access after 5 pm).
- Policy Promotion Grants for chapter and community projects.
- Educational loans consolidation.

MEDSCAPE.COM

This website's medical student section includes features such as "today's headlines," a medical student discussion forum to vent and exchange study tips, a weekly "focus" story from a med student's perspective, free apps for your smart phone, test-taking skills, study tips, and a "clerkship clues" section that summarizes the latest advances relevant to OB/GYN, medicine, surgery, and other clerkships.

NOTES

Index